Caring for Patients from Different Cultures

Fifth Edition

Caring for Patients from Different Cultures

Fifth Edition

Geri-Ann Galanti

PENN

UNIVERSITY OF PENNSYLVANIA PRESS

PHILADELPHIA

Published by
University of Pennsylvania Press
Philadelphia, Pennsylvania 19104-4112

Printed in the United States of America on acid-free paper
10 9 8 7 6 5 4 3 2 1

Library of Congress Cataloging-in-Publication Data

ISBN 978-0-8122-2311-8

To the many students and clinicians
who generously shared the case studies within this book.
Thank you!
And to my family . . . always

Contents

Preface to the Fifth Edition

People are endlessly fascinating. I wrote this book because I think it is important that clinicians see that. When I wrote the first edition back in 1990, I had never heard the term "cultural competence." Today, it is a very popular term and one I use frequently in this book. However, in all honesty, I'm not very concerned about definitions. Many other people are, and that's fine. But I think the real key to attaining cultural competence is developing honest curiosity about other people.

I'm a medical anthropologist. What first drew me to anthropology was the realization that all the different aspects of a culture were interconnected. For example, people who live in traditional agricultural societies tend to value large families (more workers), live in permanent (they're tied to the land) multigenerational houses (grandparents can help raise the grandchildren), practice warfare (they can support an army because efficiently growing crops means many people are freed from the task of food production), exhibit social stratification (due to varying degrees of wealth related to land ownership) and have strict sexual mores (since they own property, men don't want to pass on their wealth to another man's child). I found the interconnectedness comforting. It meant that things were (almost) predictable.

The other thing that appealed to me about anthropology was that it shows us how we are all simultaneously similar (we love, we hurt, we get angry, we need relationships, we like material goods, etc.) and yet so different. The difference is where culture comes in. We all want to feel self-esteem, for example, but what gives us self-esteem and what causes us to lose it varies from culture to culture. I find that interesting.

My goal is to help you, the reader, to see what I see. I do this by using case studies. I spend little time on theoretical issues. Over the years, I have found that the most effective way to make a point is to tell a story. People remember anecdotes much better than they do dry facts and theories. Theories that grow out of stories are much easier to grasp and retain than ones presented in a vacuum because they create a sense of empathy and resonate with our emotions. Thus, the emphasis is on case studies and the lessons we can draw from them. For that I must thank the thousands of health care professionals who over the years have shared with me the frustrations and joys of dealing with the huge variety of ethnic populations in the United States.

I should also point out that the writing style in this book may not be what one expects from an academic book published by an Ivy League press. I use contractions and write in the first person. I do this because I want to communicate to a nonacademic audience—to clinicians—and I want my writing to be as clear and understandable as possible. I trust this won't be a problem for the academics who read it.

When I first began teaching nursing classes, I was incredibly idealistic. I thought I could give my students the knowledge they would need to provide culturally appropriate care. I found, however, that most nurses are overworked and have little time to make adjustments for ethnic differences. They work in the "real world," not an academically idealized version of it. Were my classes of no value, then, beyond mere curiosity?

Fortunately, no. I found I could significantly reduce the nurses' stress by explaining *why* their patients acted as they did. The ethnic populations were not deliberately trying to irritate the staff; they were simply behaving according to what was appropriate within their culture. Now, when people ask me what I do, I explain that I teach health care providers why their patients are *interesting* rather than *annoying*. It makes a difference.

Throughout the book I make references to "a nurse who was taking a class in cultural diversity"; the class was mine, taught in the School of Nursing at California State University, Dominguez Hills. The class is called Cultural Diversity and Health Care. At the end of each class, I asked students to write an essay on how they've applied what they've learned in class to their clinical practice. (Confession: one reason I gave this assignment was so that throughout the term they would make a point of applying what they were learning.) I was delighted when one student wrote about an orthodox Jewish family who kept going to the nurse's station to ask someone to change the channel for them on Saturday. She said, "If I were not in this class, I would have thought that this family was demanding and annoying. Taking this class has helped me to be more open and aware of different cultures around me." Another student wrote that what she learned in class, "has helped me not be so irritated with patients or co-workers. My shifts flow much easier now and I have seemed to enjoy what I do even more." I have accomplished what I had hoped.

Although many of the case studies emphasize the clash of cultures, I have also included many examples that illustrate how potential problems can be *avoided* when health care providers practice culturally competent health care. Those cases are marked by having their case number in *italics*.

The biggest danger of cultural competence training is that, no matter how often you remind people *not* to stereotype, there is a strong tendency to misuse cultural information. Culturally competent health care is at its core *patient-centered care*. The most important aspect of that is learning to ask the right questions. Cultural competence will never be achieved by memorizing lists of information which may or may not apply to the individual. Therefore, the section on the 4 Cs of Culture (a mnemonic for asking key questions) has been expanded with numerous case studies.

I've added a new chapter, "Improving Adherence." Lack of adherence is one of the most frequent complaints of physicians and a source of both poor health outcomes and rising health care costs. Some of the causes of lack of adherence stem from cultural factors, while others are due to communication issues. Common causes—and solutions—are discussed.

The final chapter, "Making a Difference," has been expanded, and presents some of the changes various hospitals have made in order to provide more culturally sensitive care. It is certainly not an exhaustive list, but my hope is that it will inspire other health care institutions to make additional changes. I've also added examples of how individual clinicians—in this case, nurses—can bring about changes within hospitals to better serve the community. One person *can* make a difference.

Working with patients from a variety of ethnic groups can be challenging, but when health care practitioners make an effort to be sensitive to the cultural needs of their patients it can add an interesting and pleasurable dimension to the work, and often reduce their own stress while increasing patient satisfaction. This in turn can lead to greater adherence and, ultimately, better patient outcomes. Although many clinicians fear that "cultural competence" will just add one more thing to their already overburdened workload, in reality, it overwhelmingly makes for win-win situations.

I have expanded the appendix containing profiles of various cultures and religions. Keep in mind that the profiles are merely meant to be a quick guide to broad culture areas; it must always be remembered that the descriptions will never fit individuals perfectly. They are simply intended to give practitioners a place to *start* to understand the behavior of others. I have not covered all aspects of all cultures; that would be impossible. I also believe it's unnecessary. My hope is to help clinicians shift their thinking to be more open to cultural variation in general. For that reason I also include a few rare cases that most clinicians will probably never run across. Rather than serving as a guide to what to do or avoid, these cases are meant to exemplify the range of human experience. The examples are all based on actual cases, although sometimes I have taken minor liberties in order to make a point.

Some of the case studies that appeared in earlier editions were deleted from the current one, not because they weren't good, but in the interest of space. I have added over 60 new cases. Most of what is missing is covered in a new case or in one of the remaining original cases. Those who have earlier editions of my book will now have a larger pool of cases studies.

I should mention that there is some repetition throughout the book. This is because some ideas are relevant to a number of topics. Because a reader may choose to read a chapter appropriate to his or her specialty rather than the entire book, when I thought it important, I included the same material in more than one chapter. Some material did not fit well into any chapter but did not warrant a separate one. Life does not always fit into neat categories.

Unlike most books, this one can be read in almost any order, a few pages at a time, although the first chapter should be read first. Each case is self-contained and can be understood on its own.

The general organization of the book is identical to that of the previous edition. The first chapter covers basic theoretical concepts. The rest of the book contains the best of the thousands of incidents of conflict and misunderstanding—or cases where conflict has been avoided through the application of cultural competence—that my students and colleagues experienced. I have tried to give solutions or ways to avoid problems whenever possible, although it is not always possible. In every case, however, I've attempted to explain why people acted the way they did. I hope that the book will help readers to see things through the eyes of people from cultures that are different from theirs. For me, the most important contribution of anthropology is that it can provide us with new perspectives.

My only fear is that people reading this book will feel their ethnic group has been presented in a bad light or that the individual in the case described is a poor representative of his or her ethnic group. Such accusations would not be entirely unjustified. I have chosen cases that created the greatest trouble for the hospital staff, and the individuals involved may not be the best representatives of their ethnic groups. I have tried to choose examples of behavior that reflect cultural values or customs, even if the behavior is an extreme version. It is my intention to promote understanding, not prejudice. (Troublesome members of my own ethnic group are also well represented here.) I will make a blanket apology at the outset, lest I offend anyone. Truly, no offense is meant. I should also add that I intend no disrespect to any members of the health care profession. Some of the nurses and doctors depicted do not come across as very admirable. Individuals should *not* be taken to represent all members of that group. Hopefully, the examples of things clinicians have done *right* will counterbalance the negative examples.

I decided to use names for all the patients and hospital staff in the various case studies; it makes the stories more accessible. I have tried to use ethnically appropriate names whenever possible. All names are fictitious. If I inadvertently use someone's real name, it is accidental. I use first names for the nurses and last names for the doctors to reflect their common usage. For the patients, I generally use first names for individuals under eighteen and last names for those older, consistent with recommended usage.

I should also note that the terms "Hispanic" and "Latino" are both used throughout the book. Both are in common usage at the time of writing, and each reflects the preferences of different individuals. Over time, however, preferred terminology may change. In the first edition, Black was the accepted term; in this edition, it is African American.

The major goal of the book is to help health care professionals recognize the cultural dimensions of problems that occur in hospitals between and among patients, their families, and staff. Obviously, not every possible problem can be documented. There is no easy "recipe" for solving problems; each individual and situation is different. My hope is that this book will give the reader some idea of the range of cultural behaviors and the need to understand others' actions from the perspective of the other person's culture, as well as offer clinicians some alternatives for providing culturally competent care.

The bibliography is intended as a resource guide for those who want to do more research, either out of general interest or to deal with specific problems. It also contains the references I used in writing this edition. In earlier editions, I divided it into sections by topic and by ethnic group, for those wanting to do further research on specific areas. However, since most research can now be easily done via the Internet, I didn't feel that was necessary. For recommended Internet sites, check the "Resources" section of my website at www.ggalanti.org.

Acknowledgments

First, second, and third, I want to thank the hundreds of health care practitioners who generously shared with me the cross-cultural misunderstandings they encountered in their work. Without them, there would be no book. Ideally, each case study would include a note stating the name of the individual who shared it with me. However, because I didn't keep such records when I first began collecting cases, I'm unable to do that for all of them. And it doesn't seem right to give credit for some and not others. As a result, no one gets credit. But you know who you are . . . and I hope you know that you have my gratitude. This book is dedicated to you.

Next, I am indebted to the School of Nursing at California State University, Dominguez Hills, and the Department of Anthropology at California State University, Los Angeles, where I have taught the courses that gave me access to the many nurses who shared their experiences. I would particularly like to acknowledge Carole Shea, who believed in my approach, and Laura Inouye, for always supporting me. Next, I want to thank all those who hired me to conduct workshops on cultural diversity. Lecturing is a two-way street; I always learn from those I teach.

I would also like to thank Jerry Hoffman, Michael Wilkes, Susan Stangl, Lacey Wyatt, Art Gomez, and Margi Stuber for helping me see the world through the eyes of physicians, and who have been instrumental in training a new generation of caring physicians. Jerry Hoffman has been a great friend and mentor, working behind the scenes to make things happen for me and helping me better understand the world of medicine. Michael Wilkes has been particularly generous in including me on numerous grants to develop training materials for medical students and residents. It has given me an additional entrée into the culture of medicine, as well as the opportunity to organize my thoughts. Jean Gilbert, Robert Like, and Noel Chrisman have earned my eternal gratitude by generously sharing their comprehensive knowledge with me and answering all my many questions. Angela Jo, my first longterm Doctoring partner and dear friend, gave me important insights into Korean culture and taught me so much about what it means to be a caring physician. Stephanie Han also shared her insider's knowledge of Korean culture with me. Micky Obradovic, my Doctoring partner and good friend, has become my "go to" physician for all questions pediatric. I'd also like to thank Martin Gerretsen and Harvey Strydhorst who run Sea Courses for making it possible for me to live my dream of teaching about cultural diversity on cruise ships as part of their wonderful CME programs. I also want to thank my editors at University of Pennsylvania Press, Alison Anderson and Eric Halpern for making this book a reality.

I'd like to recognize Michael Woods for helping me get my work out into the public arena. Through our collaboration I've written a cultural sensitivity booklet, now being published by Joint Commission Resources, and an e-learning course on cultural competence, being used at numerous hospitals and offered through PerforMax.[3] Hopefully, through our joint efforts, my work will reach more clinicians than ever before.

In researching the material for the last chapter ("Making a Difference"), I was aided by many individuals. In particular, I would like to acknowledge the many members of the CLAS-talk listserv who responded to my request about what hospitals are doing to provide more culturally competent care: Doug Green, Min Lui, Susanne Salimbene, Riikka Salonen, Lynn Stoller, and Matthew Wynia. Special thanks to Julia Puebla Fortier for running the listserv.

Without my husband, Donald Sutherland (not the actor), there would be no book. I am eternally grateful. Thank you, Don, for everything.

I also want to thank my huge Sephardic family. I never realized how different my upbringing was from that of most Americans until I was in college and read the classic article "The Folk Society" by Robert Redfield. My first reaction was: *The folk society? This sounds just like* my *family.* Being raised in my family gave me insight into more traditional cultures as well as surrounding me with the love and security that gave me the courage to make my way in the world.

Finally, I want to thank my friends who, to me, are like family. As always, you make the world a much better place.

Chapter 1

Basic Concepts

If the United States is a melting pot, the cultural stew still has a lot of lumps.

Introduction

What happens when an Iranian doctor and a Filipino nurse treat a Mexican patient? When a Navajo patient calls a medicine man to the hospital? Or when an Anglo nurse refuses to take orders from a Japanese doctor? Generally, the result is confusion and conflict, unless they all have some understanding of cultural differences.

The goal of the medical system is to provide optimal care for all patients. In a multiethnic society, this goal can be accomplished only if the health care providers understand such things as why Asian patients rarely ask for pain medication whereas patients from Mediterranean countries seem to need it for the slightest discomfort; why Middle Easterners will not allow a male physician to examine their women; and that coin rubbing is an Asian form of medical treatment, not a form of child abuse.

Disparities in Health Care

The health care system in the United States has been in a state of crisis for some time. An obvious problem is the cost and apportionment of medical care. Over the last decade or so, much attention has been paid to the health care disparities that exist in this country. According to the National Conference of State Legislatures (2013), infants born to African American women are 1.5 to 3 times more likely to die than those born to women of other races/ethnicities; American Indian and Alaska Native infants die from SIDS at nearly 2.5 times the rate of white infants; African American men are more than twice as likely to die from prostate cancer than whites; Hispanic women are more than 1.5 times as likely to be diagnosed with cervical cancer; African Americans, American Indians, and Alaska Natives are twice as likely to have diabetes as white individuals; and diabetes rates among Hispanics are 1.5 times higher than those for whites.

Such disparities result from multiple factors including poverty, inadequate access to care, and poor quality of care. A study by Hasnain-Wynia and colleagues (2007) found that minority patients tend to receive care from lower-quality hospitals. The gap was particularly large in terms of patient counseling. This finding underscores the need for better communication.

One way to improve health outcomes is to improve patient adherence to health care provider recommendations. Essential to adherence is trust; if the patient trusts the provider, he or she is more likely to follow recommendations; if not, then not. Good communication is a key to developing trust. And understanding the patients' perspective—often influenced by their culture—can go a long way toward achieving a positive outcome. Thus, this book looks at ways in which health care providers can improve communication and enhance trust through more culturally sensitive care.

Cultural Competence

This book addresses the cultural differences that can create conflicts and misunderstandings and that may result in inferior medical care. The goal is to help the reader achieve *cultural competence.* It begins with understanding your own culture and biases, becoming sensitive to the cultures of others, and appreciating the differences. The next step involves acquiring knowledge and understanding of other cultures, especially their values and beliefs. The final step is to apply that knowledge. Culturally competent health care will lead to greater patient satisfaction, improved clinical outcomes, and greater cost efficiency. Note that throughout the book, I use the terms "cultural competence" and "cultural sensitivity" somewhat interchangeably. It should also be acknowledge that cultural competence is a journey, not an end point.

1   Sometimes, however, even the best of intentions can go awry. Carolyn, an American physician, was part of a medical team that flew to an Islamic Arab nation to operate on a member of the royal family. Interestingly, one of the reasons the patient wanted American doctors to perform the surgery was that he wanted doctors who could be impartial and do what was medically indicated regardless of the loyalty they might feel toward him. For example, if he wanted something to drink while intubated—a medically unwise action—his own personal doctors would

find it difficult to refuse his requests; American physicians would have no trouble doing so. In addition, his doctors did not want him to experience even the slightest discomfort, and would overmedicate and sedate him for even the most minor procedure, such as changing bed sheets. In any case, Carolyn was concerned that she show respect for Islamic traditions, and had one of the flight attendants on the plane show her how to properly cover her head. On her second day in the country, she went to the mall to buy an *abaya*, a traditional, loose, robe-like garment worn over the clothing by many Arab women. After receiving a dirty look from the guard at the mall, she quickly took it out of her shopping bag and put it on. From there, she went to the hospital to see the patient in the ICU, joining the male physicians on their rounds. When she walked in wearing her *abaya* and headscarf, she was stopped by a royal advisor. He didn't want her wearing that kind of dress: "In here, dress like a professional." The patient was paying millions of dollars to bring in a western team to do his surgery; he wanted *western* doctors, not women in traditional dress. She quickly changed into a white coat, to the approval of the royal advisor. The lesson here is clear; rules may exist, but they are often specific to a situation. You may have every intention of following the rules, only to find that they don't apply to that situation. Always expect to be surprised.

As indicated earlier, cultural competence is something we continually strive for, rather than attain. I was reminded of this when I was a speaker at a conference in the South. The setting was lunch in the grand ballroom. There were over 100 people in the room. Salads sat waiting at every plate. My presentation was over; I was hungry. I waited several minutes for people to begin eating. No one did. Finally, I asked one of my hosts if there was some reason no one was eating. He was rather nonresponsive, and I was starving, so I began to eat. No one else followed suit. A few minutes later, a member of the clergy came to the podium and said grace. Then, everyone picked up their fork and began to eat. What I hadn't considered was that people in the South tend to be more religious than those in the West Coast urban center where I live. Apparently, my host hadn't wanted to embarrass me by pointing out my ignorance when I asked about eating. I wish he had. Sometimes we forget that there can be cultural differences even within our own culture. And no matter how much we think we know, we can still make mistakes.

Asking the Right Questions: The 4 C's of Culture

Culturally competent care is essentially patient-centered care. Effective communication is vital. Although the case studies used in this book focus on a variety of ethnic groups, the principles of cultural competence should be applied to *all* patients. The key factor in achieving cultural competence is learning to ask the right questions to elicit an understanding of the patient's point of view. A number of mnemonics have been developed to help practitioners remember what questions to ask. A simple one, which I developed with physicians Stuart Slavin and Alice Kuo, is called "The 4 C's of Culture." It was inspired by "The 8 Questions" proposed by Arthur Kleinman and his colleagues (1978).

The first C is for "Call," as in *What do you* call *your problem?* This is to remind the clinician to ask, "What do *you* think is wrong?" (You wouldn't want to *literally* ask someone "What do you call your problem?") It's a way to get at the patient's perception of the problem. This is an important question because the same symptoms may have very different meanings in different cultures and may result in barriers to adherence. For example, among the Hmong, epilepsy is referred to as "the spirit catches you, and you fall down." Seeing epilepsy as spirit possession (which has some positive connotations for the possessed; after all, a powerful spirit is within you) is very different from seeing it as a disruption of the electrical signals in the brain. This should lead to a very different doctor-patient conversation and might help explain why a Hmong patient may be less anxious than the physician to stop the seizures. For an excellent example of what can happen when caring, competent physicians do not understand the patient's perspective, see Anne Fadiman's 1997 book *The Spirit Catches You and You Fall Down.* Understanding the patient's point of view can help the health care provider deal with potential barriers to adherence and improve the patient-practitioner relationship.

3   Another medical anthropologist and I were shadowing a pediatric attending on rounds. A young Mexican boy named Pablo Medina presented with cyclic vomiting. His mother reported that the episodes had occurred in conjunction with specific events. The first was when Pablo saw his dog run over in the street and he watched his father carry the dog's bloody body into the house. The second was when a friend of the family was shot while he was standing next to him. Just before his most recent admission, his father informed the family that he (dad) was moving back to Mexico. On the day of admission, Pablo's teacher yelled at him for something he did wrong. His mother was called to pick him up from school for vomiting. My colleague and I both immediately shared a single thought: *susto.* This is a Hispanic folk disease in which a shock— such as the ones the boy experienced—causes the soul to leave the body. (For more on *susto,* see Chapter 12.) No one mentioned *susto*—not the mother, nor the attending, nor the interpreter. My colleague and I wanted to, but as observers, we didn't feel it was our place to do so. But

we left wondering, what if the attending had said something like, "What do you think is wrong with your son?" What if she had answered, "I think he might have *susto*." Perhaps the mother didn't see it that way. But what if she did? Would it have changed the clinical management of the boy's condition? Probably not. His symptoms were treated successfully. But what might it have done for the relationship between the patient and the physician if the physician had nodded and acknowledged her belief?

We tend to think that everyone respects the knowledge of doctors, but that's not always the case. What if you had just moved to a foreign country and were diagnosed with soul loss by the traditional healer who was held in high esteem by all the villagers? Would you be impressed with his diagnostic skill, or would you think he's not very smart and doesn't really understand what's going on? Might some of your patients feel the same way?

A fifty-year-old Mexican woman named Sandra Ramirez came to the ER with epigastric pain. She told the nurse that she had been experiencing the pain constantly for the past week, but denied any nausea, vomiting, diarrhea, or constipation. There had been no changes in her diet or bladder or bowel function. She revealed that when she had experienced similar pain in the past, she was treated with an unknown medication that helped her greatly. The nurse who was interviewing her had just been introduced in class to the concept of the 4 C's, so she also asked the patient what *she* thought the problem was. The patient called her condition "stressful pain," and elaborated that it wasn't the pain that caused stress, but that stress caused the pain. It turned out that the medication that had helped her in the past was Xanax. She had stopped taking it eight days earlier; the pain began seven days ago. Had the nurse not gotten the patient's perspective on her condition—that it was related to stress—they would have done just a standard abdominal workup and perhaps not discovered that it was due to anxiety.

No one is expecting physicians or nurses to work within the health model of their patients, but by showing some respect and understanding for it, they can greatly increase patients' trust. Finding out and acknowledging patients' interpretation of what is wrong can aid in that. *However, it's crucial that providers not fall into the trap of focusing only on what the patient thinks the problem is and ignoring other possibilities. Fixating on one possibility can defeat the purpose of making a differential diagnosis.*

The second C is for "Cause." *What do you think caused your problem?* This gets at the patient's beliefs regarding the source of the problem. Not everyone believes that disease is caused by germs. In some cultures, it is thought to be caused by upset in body balance, breach of taboo (similar to what is seen in the United States as diseases due to "sin" and punished by God), or spirit possession. Treatment must be appropriate to the cause, or people will not perceive themselves as cured. Doctors thus need to find out what the patient believes caused the problem, and treat that as well. For example, it may sometimes be appropriate to bring in clergy to pray with them if they believe God is punishing them for some transgression.

5   Emma Chapman, a sixty-two-year-old African American woman, was admitted to the coronary care unit because she had continued episodes of acute chest pain after two heart attacks. Her physician recommended an angiogram with a possible cardiac bypass or angioplasty to follow. Mrs. Chapman refused, saying, "If my faith is strong enough and if it is meant to be, God will cure me." When her nurse asked what she thought caused her heart problems, Mrs. Chapman said she had sinned and her illness was a punishment. Her nurse finally got her to agree to the surgery by suggesting she speak with her minister. If she hadn't learned about Mrs. Chapman's religious beliefs while asking what she that was the *cause* of her heart problems, she might not have thought to contact her clergyman. This case will be discussed again in Chapter 12, with an additional possible solution suggested. [See case #287]

6   Roberto Cruz, a sixty-three-year-old Hispanic male, developed pneumonia two days after surgery to remove a thoracic tumor. Emma, his nurse, asked him was he thought *caused* him to get the pneumonia. His wife answered for him, saying that he wasn't wearing socks during the surgery, and that he always gets a cough when exposed to the cold in that way. The patient nodded in agreement. Learning this led Emma to change the way she educated her patients prior to surgery. In the past, she had always told them what to expect—things such as catheter placement for collecting urine and compression devices on the legs to increase circulation. After her experience with Mr. Cruz, she also talked to her patients about temperature management and assessed their need for warming blankets and made sure that every part of the body not being operated on would stay warm and unexposed to the cold. Until this time, she hadn't realized that temperature could make such a difference to patients. (See Chapter 12 for more information on similar beliefs.) She stated that she hopes that by doing this, she can help relieve some of the anxiety of patients who believe they will become ill due to exposure to cold in the operating room.

The third C is for "Cope." *How do you* cope *with your condition?* This is to remind the practitioner to ask, "What have you done to try to make it better? Whom else have you been to for treatment?" This will give the health care provider important information on the use of alternative healers and treatments. As is discussed in Chapter 12, most people will try home remedies before coming in to the physician; however, few will share such information due to fear of ridicule or chastisement. It's important that health care providers learn to ask about such remedies in a nonjudgmental way, because the occasional traditional remedy may be dangerous or could lead to a drug interaction with prescribed medications.

Olga Salcedo was a seventy-three-year-old Mexican woman who had just had a femoral-popliteal bypass. Anabel, her nurse, observed that Mrs. Salcedo's leg was extremely red and swollen. She often moaned in pain and was too uncomfortable to begin physical therapy. Yet during her shift report, her previous nurse told Anabel that Mrs. Salcedo denied needing pain medication. Later that day, Anabel spoke with the patient through an interpreter and asked what she had done for the pain in her leg prior to surgery. Mrs. Salcedo said that she had sipped herbal teas given to her by a *curandero* (a traditional healer; see Chapter 12); she didn't want to take the medications prescribed by her physician. Anabel, using cultural competence, asked Mrs. Salcedo's daughter to bring in the tea. Anabel paged the physician about the remedy and brought it to the pharmacist, who researched the ingredients. Because there was nothing contraindicated, the pharmacist contacted Mrs. Salcedo's physician, who told her she could take the tea for her pain. The next day, Mrs. Salcedo was able to go to physical therapy and was much more motivated and positive in demeanor. Although it took some time to coordinate the effort, in the end, it resulted in a better patient outcome. Had Anabel not asked what she had been using to cope with her pain, it is likely Mrs. Salcedo would have delayed physical therapy and thus her recovery.

Celine was caring for Roberto Gomez, a young Hispanic patient admitted for possible Kawasaki Syndrome. His mother explained that Roberto was suffering from high fevers, irritability, redness, and swelling in both hands and feet. Although these are typical symptoms of Kawasaki Syndrome, Roberto's skin was not peeling from his hands and feet, one of the major markers a doctor uses for Kawasaki Syndrome, and thus throwing the possible diagnosis into question. When Celine asked Mrs. Gomez what she had done to treat Roberto at home (*cope*), Mrs. Gomez hesitated. Celine encouraged her, saying that most people use home remedies, and Mrs. Gomez finally admitted that she had been applying a cream made of snake oil to Roberto's genital area, hands, feet, and face at least three times a day. Celine then understood that the snake oil had prevented the skin peeling patients with Kawasaki syndrome normally experience. Roberto's mother was afraid to share this information with the doctor; she did not want him to think she was ignorant and she was afraid she would get into trouble with him. Celine explained that it was very important to tell the doctor everything she had done at home to treat Roberto. She reassured Mrs. Gomez that the doctors know that many people use traditional home remedies. After Celine shared the information with the doctor, she also asked the doctor to talk to the mother and explain to her that he understood that home remedies were used before seeing medical services. Not knowing what the patient had used to cope with the condition might have hindered making the correct diagnosis.

The fourth and final C is for "Concerns." *What concerns do you have regarding the condition?* This should address questions such as "How serious do you think this is?" "What potential complications do you fear?" "How does it interfere with your life, or your ability to function?" It is important to understand the patient's perception of the course of the illness and the fears they may have about it so you can address their concerns and correct any misconceptions. You also want to know what aspects of the condition pose a problem for the patient; this may help you uncover something very different from what you might have expected and lead to different solutions. For example, one patient with a back injury may be concerned about the pain, while another may be more concerned with the ability to work and support a family. The first patient would benefit from a referral to a pain management specialist, while the second would gain more from consulting a social worker. This C also includes *What are your concerns regarding the recommended treatment?* It is also important to know a patient's concerns in order to avoid problems of nonadherence, because some patients may have misplaced concerns based on their own or others' past experience.

Jorge Valdez, a middle-aged Latino patient, presented with poorly managed diabetes. When Dr. Alegra, his physician, told him that he might have to start taking insulin, he became upset and kept repeating, "No insulin, no insulin." Not until Dr. Alegra asked Mr. Valdez what concerns he had about insulin did he tell her that both his mother and uncle had gone blind after they started taking insulin. He made the logical—though incorrect—assumption that insulin caused blindness. In this case, the patient expressed his fears, and because the physician was competent enough to pick up on them and explore them, she was able to allay them. In many cases, however, unless the physician specifically asks about concerns, patients will say nothing and simply not adhere to treatment. By asking, the health care provider can correct any misconceptions that can interfere with treatment.

The 4 C's, though designed to be used with patients, can also be of value in other areas of the hospital, as one of my nursing students who works in Infection Control and Employee Health suggested. Using employee needle stick monitoring as an example, she would ask an employee who came to her with a needle stick what *they* thought was wrong. In other words, did the needle stick occur due to the technique that was used, or a specific product? She'd also ask what they believed *caused* it—for example, poor technique, a combative patient, or product failure. She would then discuss *coping* with them—the need to take prophylactic medication or get counseling. She'd also discuss their willingness to test new products. Finally, she would ask them about their *concerns* such as potential complications, their disease risk, or a repeat of the event. By getting the employee's perspective on what happened, she can make any necessary changes to equipment, policy, and procedures. Since the basic approach of the 4 C's is to ascertain another person's perspective, it can be applicable in many different areas.

It should be noted that although the 4 C's can be an excellent tool for practicing more culturally competent healthcare, such questions can also backfire.

Mrs. Phan, a Vietnamese patient, had been urinating far more than usual for several weeks. After taking a medical history, Dr. Madison, a physician and medical educator, asked the two questions she had taught thousands of medical students to ask: "What do you think is wrong, and how would you treat the illness?" She worried that Mrs. Phan had diabetes so she ordered some blood tests and asked that she return in a few days for the results. Mrs. Phan didn't return, so over the next two weeks Dr. Madison's office called and left several messages for her. Still, she did not return. Dr. Madison finally asked a Vietnamese medical student to leave a message in Vietnamese on Mrs. Phan's telephone machine. To Dr. Madison's surprise, Mrs. Phan answered the phone and spoke to the student for some time. Mrs. Phan explained that she wasn't coming back to see the doctor. She explained that she couldn't trust a doctor who asked *her* what was wrong and then asked *her* how she would treat the illness. "That is doctor's job," she explained. The medical student tried to explain why Dr. Madison asked those questions and that it was an attempt to respect her culture. Mrs. Phan wasn't convinced.

The remainder of this chapter is devoted to several anthropological concepts that may help the reader understand the source of many of the conflicts and misunderstandings contained within the book. Many will be reviewed in the chapters that follow as well, when additional incidents that illustrate the principles are described.

Culture

A basic working definition of culture is that it encompasses beliefs and behaviors that are learned and shared by members of a group.

The example I have always used is that of a man who removes his shoes when he enters the house. He has indoor shoes and outdoor shoes and will not wear one for the other. I would then ask, "Is this a cultural trait or a personal idiosyncrasy?" From the information given, it is impossible to tell. One must know his ethnic background. If he were Japanese, I point out, it would be a cultural trait. He is not. He is a white Anglo-Saxon Protestant from New York. Thus, I would argue, this trait is a personal idiosyncrasy. For behavior to be cultural, it must be learned and shared by members of a group. New York WASPs do not make a practice of removing their shoes when entering a house. The Japanese do. It turns out, however, that the man's mother is from Germany, where it is common to remove your shoes in a home. And, today, many Anglo Americans trying to be "green" will also remove their shoes. Deciding what is cultural can be tricky.

Subcultures

Within most cultures, smaller groups of people share certain characteristics not shared by the culture at large. Anthropologists call such groups subcultures. Subcultures may be based upon a variety of things, including ethnicity (Hispanic Americans, Asian Americans), occupation (nurses, physicians), activity (gangs), or sexual orientation (lesbians). When one subculture has more power than another, it is referred to as the "dominant" culture. Those subcultures with less power—even when they are in the numerical majority—are called "minority" cultures and are often discriminated against.

Every culture and subculture has its own values, worldview, language ("jargon"), and norms (rules of acceptable behavior). For example, Anglo American culture values independence, a value not shared by many of the other ethnic groups found in the United States. Part of the American worldview is to believe that humans control nature. American social norms include the following rule of behavior: if someone offers you something you want, you may accept it with thanks the first time it is offered. Iranian cultural rules, in contrast, dictate that you wait until it is offered a second time; the first is to be polite; the second is sincere. Chinese cultural rules would have you wait until it is offered a third time. Another American cultural rule is that the needs of your children come before those of your parents, directly opposite to the norm in most Asian cultures. A third American rule of behavior is that you firmly shake hands in greeting someone. This may violate the norms of many Middle Eastern cultures, which prohibit touching between members of the opposite sex, or Navajo norms that view a firm handshake as too aggressive.

Nursing and medicine are two examples of subcultures. If you are a health care practitioner, consider what values, worldview, language, and norms describe your subculture. When I was teaching a nursing class several years ago, several of us were in the restroom during a break. I noticed one of the nurses following an elaborate ritual. After using the toilet, she went to the sink, turned on the water, and scrubbed her hands and arms with much more vigor than I thought necessary for the occasion. She then left the water running while she went to get a paper towel to dry her hands, and finally turned off the faucets using her elbows. I stood there staring. When I brought this up in class, the students—all nurses—thought her behavior sounded quite normal. From the perspective of an outsider, it was actually quite bizarre. The handwashing ritual is one of the norms of the nursing subculture; it is based on the worldview belief that germs cause disease.

Stereotype Versus Generalization

I will be making many generalizations in this book. They should not be mistaken for stereotypes. The difference between a stereotype and a generalization lies not in the *content*, but in the *usage* of the information. An example is the assumption that Mexicans have large families. If I meet Rosa, a Mexican woman, and I say to myself, "Rosa is Mexican; she must have a large family," I am stereotyping her. But if I think, "Mexicans often have large families," and then ask Rosa how many people are in her family, I am making a generalization.

A generalization is a beginning point. It indicates common trends, but further information is needed to ascertain whether the statement is appropriate to a particular individual. Generalizations may be inaccurate when applied to specific individuals, but anthropologists do apply generalizations broadly, looking for common patterns, for beliefs and behaviors that are shared by the group. It is important to remember, however, that there are always differences between individuals; each case must be considered by itself. So why even bother with a generalization? Because it can help us understand and anticipate behavior. Rather than becoming annoyed because my Mexican patient is moaning and groaning in the absence of any serious problems, I might note, "Ah, Mexican culture encourages emotional expressiveness." Or, knowing that Asians value stoicism might help me remember to pay more attention to an Asian patient's pain needs rather than draw (incorrect) conclusions

based on the fact that the patient isn't moaning or requesting pain medication. Of course, this should be done with *all* patients. A *stereotype* is an
ending point. No attempt is made to learn whether the individual in
question fits the statement. Given the tremendous variation within each
culture, stereotypes are often incorrect and can have negative results.

11   Courtney recounted the case of Lamar Johnson, a thirty-three-year-
old African American patient who had been deemed a "frequent flyer"
(a term used to describe those who keep coming to the hospital for the
same reason, often assumed to be drug seekers) by the nurses and doctors in the emergency department. Each time he came in complaining
of extreme headaches he was given pain medication and sent home. On
this last admission, he was admitted to the ICU, where Courtney had just
begun working. When she heard him described as a frequent flyer, she
asked another nurse why he was thought to be a drug seeker. She was
told, "He has nothing else better to do; I'm not sure why he thinks we
can supply his drug habits." Although Courtney says her instincts told
her that something else was going on, she saw his tattoos, observed his
rough demeanor, and went along with what everyone else was saying.
While she was wheeling him to get a CT scan, Mr. Johnson herniated
and died. It turned out that he had a rare form of meningitis and truly
was suffering from severe headaches. If some of the staff had not stereotyped him as a drug seeker on one of his earlier visits, perhaps his life
could have been saved. This incident left a lasting impression on Courtney, who vowed not ever to judge a patient on his looks, and to trust her
instincts, rather than let others influence her nursing care.

12   Casey worked as a nurse in a busy Pediatric Unit in the middle of a
low-income town. Many of the patients were Hispanic, and some did not
speak any English at all. Most of the staff in the unit automatically assumed that any Hispanic patient that came in did not speak English.
One day Casey admitted a very sick Hispanic infant with fever, dehydration, and respiratory signs and symptoms from an outside hospital. He
gathered all vital signs and measurements and did an intake interview
with Mrs. Sanchez, the child's mother. He started explaining to Mrs.
Sanchez the procedures he was about to perform on her child. She
asked appropriate questions. At that point, the doctor walked into the
room, and immediately asked, "Is there a translator around here?" and
then walked out of the room. Mrs. Sanchez was really offended by this,
as she spoke English. One of the other nurses on the team explained
to the doctor that the mother spoke English. He later apologized for
stereotyping her. The lesson Casey learned that it is very important to
first speak to patients in English, and then if they say that they don't
understand, to ask if they would like an interpreter. If they do want an

interpreter, it's important to follow up and make sure that an interpreter has arrived, as having a child in the hospital can be very frightening. Stereotyping is always a mistake.

Lily Khalid was a forty-eight-year-old woman from the Middle East. She was in the county hospital to have surgery for gallstones. Sandy, a Mexican American nurse, was caring for her prior to surgery. Sandy cared for Mrs. Khalid for three nights and describes them as a nightmare. Mrs. Khalid did nothing but moan and groan and demand pain medication. She pushed the call light continually. Sandy did her job but resented Mrs. Khalid's behavior. She chalked it up to her ethnic background—Middle Easterners are often demanding and express their pain freely and loudly. She looked forward to Mrs. Khalid's surgery; at last, her gallstones would be removed and she could go home.

When Sandy returned to work a week later, she learned that Mrs. Khalid had not had gallstones after all. When the surgeons opened her up, they discovered that cancer had invaded her entire gastrointestinal system. She died on the operating table. Sandy's heart sank. She had stereotyped Mrs. Khalid as just another loud, complaining Middle Easterner. It turned out that she had been moaning and groaning and requesting pain medication not because she was Middle Eastern, but because she was riddled with cancer and in excruciating pain. It was an important lesson for Sandy about the dangers of stereotyping.

While taking a course on cultural diversity, Anike Oghogho, a nurse from Nigeria, recognized his tendency to stereotype. He related an example of an African American male patient who presented with a swollen left foot. The patient, Jefferson Bell, kept ringing the call light and asking for more pain medication. Anike said that in the past, he would have assumed Mr. Bell was merely seeking pain meds. This time, however, he reassessed the patient. He discovered that Mr. Bell's fourth and fifth toes were more red and swollen and had pus. Anike summoned the physician and Mr. Bell was eventually taken to the operating room for incision and drainage of his left foot. Stereotyping could have severely harmed the patient; fortunately, Anike had learned the lesson of *not* stereotyping in his class.

One of the reasons stereotyping is so inappropriate is that no one ever belongs to just one culture. We belong to numerous cultures, including those of ethnicity, religion, region of the country, generation, sex, occupation, education, and socioeconomic status. All of them have some varying degree of influence on us. Add to that the degree of assimilation, which includes such factors as the length of time spent in the United States, age at immigration, desire to assimilate, and residence in an ethnic community or an "American" one. When you also consider the influence of personality factors and individual life experiences, it

13

14

should be obvious why stereotyping is not just dangerous, but more likely to be incorrect than anything else. Often, people from similar economic strata, but different ethnic backgrounds have more in common than those from similar ethnic backgrounds and different economic strata.

I have purposely chosen examples of individuals who have not assimilated to a great degree and whose beliefs and behaviors deviate from those expressed in the American health care system. It should not be inferred that all or even most members of these groups would act in the manner described. The ones who are most Westernized do not generally present problems. It is those who adhere to traditional ways that are most likely to do so, hence their inclusion in this book. It should be remembered, however, that assimilation occurs in unpredictable stages. Individuals may be quite Westernized in some areas but traditional in others. I remember teaching a university anthropology class many years ago in which most of the Asian students claimed to be 100 percent American. And yet when we discussed the notion of premarital loss of virginity, most of the young women claimed that they intended to be virgins when they got married. I had to laugh; that was certainly *not* an *American* cultural trait. They may have been Americanized in other areas, but not in terms of sexual mores.

I will be making many generalizations throughout this book. I will also be lumping together groups that are actually quite distinct from each other. The term "Hispanic" or "Latino" includes people from such diverse cultures as Mexican, Puerto Rican, Argentinean, and Peruvian. "Asian" refers to people from a variety of countries, including China, Japan, Korea, Vietnam, Cambodia, and the Philippines. It is dangerous and inaccurate to think they are all alike. When I do make such generalizations, it is because there are some traits that are fairly consistent across cultures within the designated group. But never forget individual differences.

Also remember when you come into contact with people from different cultures that it is often highly offensive to them to be labeled by the wrong country. Many are historical enemies. There is also a tremendous amount of prejudice and stereotyping within each larger culture area. A Chinese student shared that many Chinese think that Vietnamese have prominent cheekbones, Koreans have small eyes, and Japanese are short. These are all seen as characteristics that are inferior to those of the more "beautiful" Chinese. A Chinese person would probably be insulted if mistaken for a Korean, and vice versa. Ethnocentrism is universal, and stereotyping occurs even within ethnic groups.

Generalizations made in this book about large cultural groups such as Asians or Hispanics may be seen as a way of distinguishing broad geographical groupings from each other while recognizing that there are differences within them. Also, on occasion, the only ethnic identity given for a patient is Asian or Hispanic because more detailed information was not known, but the case illustrated a general point common to many cultures within that group.

It is important to recognize that the cases chosen for this book were selected specifically because the misunderstandings were due to cultural differences. Many interactions between individuals of the same two cultures will occur without conflict or misunderstanding, because not every member of an ethnic group adheres to all the traditional beliefs and practices of that group. Alternately, conflicts and misunderstandings will occur between members of different ethnic groups that have nothing to do with culture, but result from individual differences and personality clashes. That is why it is extremely important *not* to stereotype individuals. The generalizations provided in this book are meant to be suggested guideposts, not precise, detailed maps. Ideally, they will help health care providers anticipate possibilities that should be considered, and make sense of behavior that has already occurred.

Prejudice and Discrimination

An important related issue in today's world, given strained inter-ethnic relations, is that of prejudice and discrimination. The long history of slavery in this country, followed by Reconstruction and its aftermath, along with less institutionalized racism, has led many African Americans to distrust the health care system. This was compounded by the infamous Tuskegee experiment. In 1932, the U.S. Public Health Service began the Tuskegee Study of Untreated Syphilis. They were looking at 399 Black men. It was not the only organization conducting such a study. Stanford University was also doing a similar study, but primarily with Caucasian men. At the time, the only treatment for syphilis was heavy metals, which, needless to say, was ineffective. In the 1940s, after it was discovered that penicillin was an effective treatment, the Stanford study was ended, and the patients treated with penicillin. However, at Tuskegee it was decided to continue the experiment, to see what would happen if the disease were left untreated. The experiment was finally ended in 1972, after it came to public attention.

If you were African American and knew that the government had purposely withheld treatment from you, just to "see what would happen," how much trust would you have for white medical institutions? Furthermore, prejudice and discrimination are real. Not surprisingly, if you have been a frequent victim of discrimination, you are likely to come to expect it, even, as in the next two cases, when it is not there.

15   During a prenatal exam, an obstetrics resident asked the patient whether she had considered having her tubes tied at the time of delivery. The patient, Lotty Parker, was a forty-three-year-old African American woman, pregnant with her twelfth child. Mrs. Parker immediately became angry, saying, "I ain't gonna have no white doctor messin' with my insides!" The resident may have felt that it was his responsibility to explain increased pregnancy risks after forty, but the African American woman apparently viewed his suggestion as a form of racial genocide. Health care personnel must be especially sensitive to this issue when dealing with patients from minority ethnic groups. Rather than directly asking if she wanted her tubes tied, a culturally competent physician might have begun by asking Mrs. Parker if she enjoys having such a large family. If she said she loves it, the doctor wouldn't need to pursue the issue and would avoid asking a racist-sounding question. If, however, she said that it's difficult raising so many children, the physician could then ask if she would like to limit her family size to twelve. If she said yes, the physician could suggest having her tubes tied. In general, health care providers should try to ascertain the *patient*'s attitude, rather than imposing their own.

16   Another case, which could have ended as badly as the previous one, was rescued by the cultural sensitivity of the clinician. Mrs. Washington, a fifty-year-old African American woman, had had a surgical release for carpal tunnel syndrome, which was a work-related injury. Linne was assigned to her case. Five months after the surgery, Linne called to see how she was doing. Mrs. Washington replied that she was still having some discomfort when driving and doing household chores. Linne commented that as per their clinical guidelines, she should have been showing improvement after six to eight weeks post op. Linne was concerned that five months later, Mrs. Washington was still having problems. Mrs. Washington, however, immediately became defensive and hotly replied, "I'm not in it for the money. I don't want to be in pain."

Linne felt terrible. She didn't mean to imply that Mrs. Washington was trying to scam the system. She then remembered learning that years of discrimination have led many African Americans to be acutely attuned to signs of prejudice. She realized that Mrs. Washington thought she was implying that rather than return to work, she preferred to stay home and receive worker's compensation. She perceived Linne as prejudiced and thinking of African Americans as lazy and shiftless.

The situation could have gone very badly from here. Linne could have become defensive as she tried to defend her comment. Mrs. Washington might have responded argumentatively, justifying why she was still off work and receiving worker's compensation benefits. In fact, several times in the past, that is exactly what had happened to Linne, which resulted in the patients hiring an attorney, which further delayed their release to work and increased the cost of care. This time, however, Linne used cultural competence skills to restore the situation. She immediately apologized for her comment and explained that she only meant to educate her regarding what she could expect following a carpal tunnel release. She wanted to let her know that if she was still having pain, she needed to talk with her physician to see if there were other treatments to help her. Linne told her that as her case manager, she would also speak with Mrs. Washington's physician about her ongoing pain. As a result, Mrs. Washington calmed down and became more receptive. A combination of understanding the impact of prejudice and discrimination, followed by a sincere apology, changed a potentially negative outcome to a positive one.

An Anglo American nurse shared that when she is accused of being a racist by an African American patient because she hasn't yet given a patient pain medication or a food tray, rather than becoming defensive, she'll apologize and calmly explain why she hasn't gotten to it yet and assures them that she will do it as soon as possible. When she does get them what they need, she'll ask them what else they need to feel more comfortable and what she can do to help them. She finds that to be a much more effective and productive approach.

There is good reason for African Americans to be wary of the predominantly white health care institution. Unless one has had the experience of being stopped by the police simply for driving a nice car in a good neighborhood, or been asked by a white salesperson, "Are you sure you can afford it?" when buying a high-ticket item, it is difficult to understand what it is like to be the recipient of racial prejudice. We are all individuals and want to be treated as such, but, unfortunately, minorities are often judged simply by the color of their skin.

At the same time, however, years of discrimination may have led some individuals to be acutely sensitive and to perceive prejudice when it does not exist. Health care providers should be aware of this and do what they can to ensure that their words and actions do not unintentionally hurt their patients. An African American student in one of my classes interviewed twelve elderly African Americans. They all said they preferred African American physicians because they thought they were the only ones who would treat them fairly, without discrimination. Because their "radar" was always up for discriminatory treatment, if something could be interpreted in two ways, they would usually interpret it as a sign of racism—for example, if the physician was running late, or didn't spend much time with them. Culturally competent physicians will take the time to apologize and explain such situations—to *all* patients.

Values

Values are the things we hold important. Just as each individual holds certain values, so does each culture. U.S. culture (I use this term loosely because there are literally hundreds of subcultures within the United States) currently values such things as money, freedom, independence, privacy, health and fitness, and physical appearance.

One way to assess a culture's values is to observe how it punishes people. In the United States wrongdoers are punished by being fined (taking away their *money*) or incarcerated (taking away their *freedom*). The Mbuti pygmies of Africa value social support, and they punish people by ignoring them (Turnbull 1962). The kind of health care provided by the American medical system is often influenced by financial considerations, whereas concern for family, lower on the list of "American" values, influences much behavior in patients from other ethnic groups. Hence conflict may develop between health care providers and patients.

In the United States, *independence* is manifested by the desire to move away from home as soon as one is financially able. In many cultures that value family more than independence, adult children rarely move out before marriage and often not thereafter. The health care culture also supports the values of *independence* and *autonomy* in its efforts to teach self-care.

Privacy is also very important to most people from the United States, who build fences to separate their houses from each other. The U.S. health care culture tries to provide privacy for patients by often giving information only to the patient, excluding other family members, by limiting visiting hours, and by offering no sleeping accommodations for visitors. Many non-Anglo patients, however, prefer just the opposite.

Health and fitness are popular movements. There are hundreds of food products labeled "low fat" and "low cholesterol." People can be seen jogging on most city streets, and attendance at gyms is high. This obsession with health leads the medical profession to expect patients to comply with suggestions regarding changes in diet and exercise, assuming that health and fitness is a value shared by all. It is not. Furthermore, what is considered "healthy" varies across cultures.

Concern for *physical appearance* is manifested at every magazine stand. There are few women's magazines that do not have articles on the latest diet, makeup, hairdo, and clothing. The incidence of cosmetic surgery for both men and women is at a record high. Surgical techniques are developed to minimize scarring and maintain youth and beauty. What is considered "beautiful," however, is not the same for every culture.

Understanding people's values is the key to understanding their behavior, for our behavior generally reflects our values. A dramatic example occurred in the early 1980s, when a Japanese ship captain was bringing a boatload of cars to the United States. There was a disaster at sea, and the cargo was ruined. The captain had done nothing to cause the disaster, and he could not have prevented it. If an American ship captain had had a similar experience, the first thing he probably would have done when he reached land was call his insurance agent to see who would pay for the damages. The Japanese captain killed himself.

There is obviously a big difference between calling one's insurance agent and killing oneself. The different reactions are dictated by different values. The hypothetical American captain would probably value *money*; his concern would be for the financial loss. The Japanese captain was concerned about his *honor*. As the captain of the ship, he considered himself responsible for the accident. The loss of the cargo meant the loss of his honor. Without honor, he felt he could not live. Committing ritual suicide was the only way for him to regain his honor.

Values influence our everyday behavior as well. Why are you reading this book? Is it because you value knowledge and hope to learn something? Is it because you are required to read it for a course and you value good grades? If so, are you motivated because good grades will get you a better job, and with a better job you will earn more money, and you value money? Nearly everything we do reflects our values on some level.

Values and the American Health Care Culture

One reason for so many conflicts and misunderstandings in hospitals is the great disjunction between the values of the health care culture and that of the patient population.

As mentioned earlier, the health care culture values autonomy and independence. Patients, in contrast, often value the family over the individual. The family may prefer to make decisions as a group and to assist the patient in "self-care" functions the staff thinks the patient should do on his or her own. Furthermore, many patients prefer to have family members with them at all times, leading to chaos and loss of control from the perspective of the nurses.

The health care culture's value of *efficiency* often conflicts with patients' value of *modesty*. Many doctors and nurses find concern about keeping patients covered difficult when their primary focus is performing an appropriate procedure. The health care culture also values *self-control*. Many patients, however, come from cultures in which emotional expressiveness is the norm. This can lead to resentment toward such patients on the part of the staff.

Privacy is another dominant health care value, institutionalized in the Health Insurance Portability and Accountability Act known as HIPAA. One of the important aspects of HIPAA is the requirement that protected health information be kept confidential. Many health care providers interpret this to mean that information about a patient cannot be shared even with family members unless the patient has given permission for information to be shared with that specific person. In fact, this is not the case. HIPAA regulations stipulate that health care providers may share information with others *unless* the patient objects. Confusion over the laws and fear of lawsuits has led many health care providers to be overzealous in the protection of patient privacy (see Gross 2007). For patients that come from cultures where the family (including aunts, uncles and cousins), rather than the individual, is the primary unit, this can be problematical.

Worldview

The second most important concept for understanding people's behavior is to understand their worldview. Problems can result from a disparity between the worldview of the health care culture and that of the patient population. People's worldviews consist of their basic assumptions about the nature of reality. These become the foundation for all actions and interpretations. For example, people whose worldview includes the notion that everything happens for a reason will tend to find meaning in all events. A childless thirty-five-year-old woman who goes through the emotional agony of finding a breast lump, only to have the biopsy turn out to be negative, may interpret the experience as a message from the universe reminding her that now is the time to decide whether or not she wants to have children (breasts metaphorically representing nurturing). As another example, someone who believes that the world is a hostile place and "out to get them" may perceive a health care provider who is late for an appointment due to a sudden emergency as deliberately displaying prejudice.

An individual's worldview can have an important influence on his or her health care behavior. For example, someone with a scientific worldview might perceive birth defects as a mistake in the transcription of DNA during the process of meiosis, while someone whose worldview encompasses the notion of reincarnation might see it as resulting from improper behavior in a past life, and someone who believes that God rewards good behavior and punishes bad behavior might interpret it as punishment for one's sins. Thus, one's worldview might affect one's interest in genetic counseling during pregnancy. Again, if part of an individual's worldview is that the physical body is all there is, that person might want everything possible done to extend their life. A person who believes that this life is but a precursor to the next, however, might be more willing to "let go." If one's worldview holds that life begins at conception, abortion might be viewed as murder; if, however, life is thought to begin at the point that the fetus becomes viable, a first-trimester abortion is more likely to be seen as a medical procedure.

While we all have our own individual worldview, our culture can influence the way we perceive things. Religion often defines the world-view of people who are devoutly religious. Belief in the existence of God, for example, might be part of their worldview. If people believe God confers both health and illness, it may be very difficult to get them to take certain medications or change their health behavior. They might not share the health care culture's belief that germs cause disease and that diet and exercise contribute to one's health. They may see no need to quit smoking and no point in worrying about high blood pressure or bacteria when moral behavior is the key to good health.

Mona had the opportunity to use her understanding of worldview *17* when caring for Ramón Diaz, a Hispanic male who had been admitted to the hospital three times in a single year for uncontrolled diabetes. Despite being given a strict diet and insulin orders to follow, he contin- ued to eat whatever he wanted and refused to monitor his blood sugar. When Mona questioned him about this, he replied, "Okay, I'll start my diabetic diet tomorrow, but it's not going to make any difference. It's in God's hands now." Mona's initial reaction was to become frustrated with him, but instead, noted his fatalistic worldview. She realized that her usual "lecture" and instructions were not going to be enough. So she took the time to explain to him and his wife that if not managed daily, diabetes can have fatal complications. She also went over with them ways to gradually change his diet, which made adherence more likely than would a demand for a complete and sudden change. Mona also used cultural competence skills by including his wife in the teaching, since the family is the primary unit in traditional Hispanic cultures. Since she was also the family cook, it was important to get her on board with the plan. Mona took a further step by talking to her coworkers about a fatal- istic worldview, hoping this knowledge would keep them from getting frustrated and "giving up" on their patients as they often did. Cultural competence can be contagious; health care practitioners should be encouraged to share their knowledge and experiences with co-workers.

Since people's worldviews consist of their *assumptions* about the nature of reality, they rarely question the veracity of their beliefs. For example, a devout Christian might not be likely to conclude that God does not exist on the basis of the accidental slaughter of innocent children. Rather, the Christian might simply remark, "God works in mysterious ways." No matter how much "evidence" is presented to the contrary, people rarely change or even question their worldview. Instead, they reinterpret events in a manner consistent with their beliefs.

People's Relationship to Nature

Another aspect of worldview involves people's relationship to nature. The culture of the United States, for example, believes people can control nature. If the land is dry, they irrigate. If bacteria cause disease, they destroy them. If the heart does not work, they replace it. This also relates to the health care culture's view of the body as a machine; if it becomes broken, one should simply turn it over to the mechanics (doctors and nurses) to be fixed. To the consternation of many health care professionals, not all cultures share that belief.

Other cultures, such as Asian and Native American, see people as a part of nature. They strive to maintain harmony with the earth and look to the land to provide treatment for disease. Herbal remedies are important in their cultures. Still other cultures, such as Hispanic and Middle Eastern, believe people have little or no control over natural forces. *Que será, será.* What will be, will be. *Insha'Allah.* If God wills it. Preventive health care measures are likely to be ignored; they would do no good anyway. Thus worldview can have important implications for health-related behavior.

Emic and Etic

The terms "emic" and "etic," derived from linguistics and rarely used in ordinary life, are extremely important in anthropology. They refer to perspectives. Emic perspectives are the insiders' perspectives, natives' views of their own behavior. Etic perspectives are those of outsiders. The two simply represent different vantage points, and knowing both helps provide a more complete picture, a fact caregivers would do well to remember when treating patients from different cultures. Try to understand *their* perspective on their condition, as well as your own.

An Etic Perspective on American Medicine

Anne Fadiman, in the now classic book *The Spirit Catches You and You Fall Down* (1998), contrasts biomedicine with traditional Hmong medicine. In doing so, she helps us to see biomedicine from an *etic* perspective, while looking at traditional Hmong medicine from an *emic* perspective. American medicine doesn't come off as well as Hmong medicine.

- A traditional Hmong healer might spend as much as eight hours in a sick person's home, whereas American doctors forced their patients, no matter how weak they were, to come to the hospital, and then might spend only twenty minutes at their bedsides.
- Traditional Hmong healers were polite and never needed to ask questions; American doctors asked many rude and intimate questions about patients' lives, right down to their sexual and excretory habits.
- Traditional Hmong healers could render an immediate diagnosis; American doctors often demanded samples of blood (or even urine or feces, which they liked to keep in little bottles), took x-rays, and waited for days for the results to come back from the laboratory. And then, after all that, sometimes they were unable to identify the cause of the problem.
- Traditional Hmong healers never undressed their patients; American doctors asked patients to take off all their clothes, and sometimes dared to put their fingers inside women's vaginas.
- Traditional Hmong healers knew that to treat the body without treating the soul was an act of patent folly; American doctors never even mentioned the soul.
- Traditional Hmong healers could preserve unblemished reputations even if their patients didn't get well, since the blame was laid on the intransigence of the spirits rather than the competence of the negotiators, whose stock might even rise if they had had to do battle with particularly dangerous opponents; when American doctors failed to heal, it was their own fault.

Ethnocentrism and Cultural Relativism

Two key anthropological concepts are ethnocentrism and cultural relativism. They refer to attitudes. *Ethnocentrism* is the view that one's own culture's way of doing things is the right and natural way. All other ways are inferior, unnatural, and perhaps even barbaric. *Cultural relativism* is the attitude that other ways of doing things are different but equally valid. It tries to understand the behavior in its cultural context. Most humans are ethnocentric. It is natural to think one's own culture's way is best. Anthropologists, however, strive to be culturally relativistic.

If I were to tell most Americans about a group of people in Africa who sometimes kill healthy newborn infants, they would probably take the ethnocentric attitude that these people were barbarians. If I were to explain that they were hunters and gatherers living on the edge of starvation and that if a second child is born too close to the first, chances are close to 100 percent that both will die because the mother does not have enough milk to support both, their attitude might change. They still might not condone infanticide, but they might understand it as the only viable choice in a desperate situation. Rather than seeing the Africans as barbarians, they might realize that the people were forced to extreme measures by difficult circumstances. Their attitude would thus change from ethnocentric to culturally relativistic.

The Western health care system tends to be ethnocentric because practitioners believe that their approaches to healing are superior to all others. There is a lot we can learn, however, from other cultures. Many modern drugs, including quinine, were derived from plants used by native peoples. Westerners are beginning to acknowledge the effectiveness of acupuncture for certain conditions. The goal of all systems of healing is the same; to help people get well. If all cultures could study each other's techniques with a culturally relativistic perspective, the cause of modern medicine would be greatly advanced.

It should be noted, however, that cultural relativism does not extend to all behavior. Many anthropologists draw a line where cultural practices cross over into human rights issues. But one hopes that we would all learn to be more culturally relativistic.

Time Orientation

Time orientation, one's focus regarding time, varies in different cultures. No individual or culture will look exclusively to the past, present, or future, but most will tend to emphasize one over the others. Chinese, British, and Austrian cultures have a past orientation. They are traditional and believe in doing things the way they have always been done. Interestingly, in many cases countries that emphasize the past are ones that were once more powerful than they are now. This may be their way of recognizing and valuing that time in their history. Time orientation can have an important impact on health-related behavior. People from past-oriented cultures, for example, usually prefer traditional approaches to healing rather than accepting each new procedure or medication that comes out.

People with a predominantly present time orientation may be less likely to use preventive health measures. They reason that there is no point in taking a pill for hypertension when they feel fine, especially if the pill is expensive and causes unpleasant side effects. They do not look ahead in hope of preventing a stroke or heart attack, or they may feel they will deal with it when it happens. Poverty often forces people into a present time orientation. They are not likely to make plans for the future when they are concerned with surviving today. A sudden unpredictable change in life circumstances, such as a car accident that leaves one paraplegic, can also lead one to be present-oriented. A present time orientation, while generally negative from a preventive health care perspective, can also be positive. For example, the ability to focus on the present, rather than the future, can be beneficial for someone living with a cancer diagnosis.

Middle-class Anglo American culture, along with health care culture, tends to be future-oriented. That is reflected in the medical system's stress on preventive medicine and enthusiasm for each new medical technique or drug. In contrast to past-oriented cultures, progress and change are highly valued. China is also shifting to a future orientation, as evidenced, for example, by the long-term plan to reduce the country's population by limiting family size. Patients with a future time orientation are often more amenable to preventive medicine. They may also be eager for the newest drugs on the market, assuming "newer" is "better."

Hispanics and African Americans tend to have a present time orientation. This does not mean that they do not recognize the past or the future, but that living in the present is more important to them. Their concept of the future may also be different from the Anglo concept. For example, African Americans are more likely to say "I'll see you" than "I'll see you tomorrow." The former implies the future but is not specific. The future arrives in its own time. From this point of view, one cannot be late. Conflict may occur, however, in interactions with white middle-class people, for whom time is very specific.

As the last statement implies, time orientation can also refer to degree of adherence to clock time versus activity time. From the perspective of one oriented to the clock, someone who arrives at 3:15 for a 2:30 appointment is late. For someone who does not focus on clock time, both represent midafternoon. The time to arrive at the afternoon appointment is after the morning activities are completed.

This type of time orientation appears to be related to subsistence economy. In countries with economies based on agriculture, people tend to be more relaxed about time; as I like to say, "The crops don't care what time they get picked." Many people in traditional agricultural villages do not own clocks; the pace is slower and more attuned to nature's rhythms. They tend to focus more on activities, rather than on the clock. In contrast, industrialized nations must pay attention to clock time. There are large numbers of people to organize, and each must complete his or her task according to schedule in order for the next person to begin. Without clocks, chaos would reign.

Hierarchical Versus Egalitarian Cultures

Just as cultures differ in time orientation, they also vary in social structure. American culture is organized according to an egalitarian model. Theoretically, everyone is equal. Status and power are dependent on an individual's personal qualities rather than characteristics such as age, sex, family, or occupation. In reality, things may operate differently, but we hold equality as our ideal. Many Asian cultures are based on a hierarchical model. Everyone is not equal. Status is based on such characteristics as age, sex, and occupation. Status differences are seen as important, and people of higher status command respect. Hospitals are based on a hierarchical model. Social structure, then, can have an important influence on the way people interact, as will be seen in many of the examples given later in this book.

Family of Orientation Versus Family of Procreation

During the course of their lives, many people are members of two different family groups; the family they are born into and the one they create through marriage and children. Anthropologists distinguish the two as "family of orientation" and "family of procreation." The family of orientation is the one a person is born into, the one to which one first orients oneself. It includes the individual, parents, brothers and sisters, and any other household members. The family of procreation is the one formed through marrying and procreating. It includes the individual, spouse, and children. Some cultures, particularly those in which the married couple continues to reside with the parents of the bride or groom, emphasize the family of orientation. Other cultures emphasize the family of procreation. Americans tend to set up their own nuclear family households, and that family takes precedence over all others. The result is a differing set of loyalties.

Models of Disease

Medical anthropologists have identified three primary health belief models. They are the following:

Magico-religious model: The world is an arena in which supernatural forces dominate. One's health depends upon the action of gods or other supernatural forces, which can act on their own or be manipulated by other humans. In some cases, illness is seen as punishment for transgression.

Biomedical model: Life is seen as being controlled by a series of physical and biochemical processes, which can be studied and manipulated.

Holistic model: The forces of nature must be kept in balance or harmony, both within the body and between the individual and the physical and metaphysical universe. Health is a positive state of well-being, and encompasses broader environmental, sociocultural, and behavioral determinants. Healing is aimed at restoring balance.

Note that within any given cultural healing system, elements of more than one paradigm or model may apply. As you read the next section, notice which "causes" of disease belong to which paradigm. Also keep in mind that a common reason for lack of adherence is a conflict between the patient's model of disease and that of the biomedical practitioner. Why adhere to a treatment regime that makes no sense to you?

Disease Etiology

Most Americans believe that germs cause disease. Not all cultures share that belief, however. Other causes of disease include upset in body balance; soul loss, soul theft, and spirit possession; breach of taboo; and object intrusion. Treatment for diseases resulting from such etiologies must vary to be appropriate to the cause.

Upset in body balance is a notion that appears to have originated in China and spread from there to influence beliefs in Asia, India, Spain, and Latin America. It refers to the belief that a healthy body is in a state of balance. When it gets out of balance, illness results. In Asia, the balance is between *yin* and *yang*. All things in the universe are primarily either yin or yang, including diseases, which may result from excess yin, excess yang, deficient yin, or deficient yang. Yin and yang are generally translated as hot (yang) and cold (yin), although these refer to qualities, not temperatures.

The balance between hot and cold can be upset by a number of factors, including an improper balance of foods and strong emotional states. The goal of treatment is to restore balance to the system. This is generally accomplished through the use of foods (for example, cold foods should be eaten to cure a hot illness), herbs, or other treatments. To prevent disease, one should avoid extremes, such as ice water. Diet is exceedingly important. (Dietary staples such as rice are generally thought to be neutral, a fortunate and practical designation.)

Foods that are hot in one culture may be cold in another, so it is difficult to make a comprehensive list. Patients' beliefs in hot and cold qualities can generally be ascertained only by observing their behavior. If they refuse certain foods or medications, it may be that an illness they perceive as hot is being treated with a hot food or medication. Offering other foods or liquids to take with the pill to "neutralize" it may solve the problem. If they will not take a pill with ice water, they might take it with hot tea, orange juice, or hot chocolate.

Although the importance of maintaining a balance between hot and cold is not recognized in Western medicine, it is recognized that stress plays an important role in affecting the immune system's ability to fight disease. Stress represents a kind of imbalance. Recent studies indicate that a person's emotional state may also have a significant influence on the immune system. Thus, though the words we use are different, body balance is a notion to which we should be able to relate.

Paradoxically, China is moving away from traditional medicine in favor of Western medicine, while there is increasing interest in the United States in traditional Chinese healing practices. When I asked several Chinese nurses how they integrate the concept of yin and yang with germ theory, they explained that when yin and yang are out of balance, germs can cause disease. This is nearly identical to the Western notion of the relationship between stress and disease.

Soul loss, along with *soul theft,* is another category of disease etiology. The concept is self-explanatory. The soul has either left the body on its own or been stolen, leaving the body in a weakened and ill state. The goal of treatment is to return the soul to the body. It usually requires a specialist, such as a shaman, who can "leave" his or her own body to search for and return the missing soul. Although Western medicine lacks a similar etiological category, catatonic schizophrenics can be described metaphorically as bodies with "no one home."

Spirit possession involves the taking over of the victim's body by a spirit being. The victim usually acts in ways that are inappropriate for him or her. In some cultures, this may give the victim a form of power. It is generally the poor, the oppressed, and minorities who become "possessed." For example, in Ethiopia, powerful Zar spirits may possess women. When this occurs, their husbands must treat them with unaccustomed kindness and respect, for they are no longer dealing with their wives but with powerful Zars. The negative side of possession by a Zar is that the woman is thought to be crazy and must seek help through a Zar cult (Kennedy 1967). Exorcism is the treatment for spirit possession.

The next etiological category is *breach of taboo*, which means doing something forbidden—for example, eating food cooked by a menstruating woman, speaking directly to one's mother-in-law, or, among some Christian sects, having extramarital or homosexual relations. Disease is the punishment meted out by a supernatural force such as God. Treatment involves penance and atonement.

The final major category is *object intrusion*. It refers to the condition in which a magical foreign object enters the body and causes the individual to become ill. Treatment involves removing the object. In most cases, a shaman will suck it out from the afflicted part of the patient's body. The shaman then produces the offending object. On analysis, the object often turns out to be bits of hair, animal parts, teeth, or plant material, mixed with blood from the shaman's mouth. One shaman, accused by an anthropologist of practicing legerdemain, freely admitted to secreting the object in his mouth prior to sucking it out of the patient's body. He explained that the real object he removed was invisible, but that it was important for the patient to see something tangible, so he practiced a bit of sleight of hand (or mouth) for the patient's psychological benefit.

Two important points should be made regarding disease etiology. *First, the treatment must be appropriate to the cause.* If germs cause disease, kill the germs. If the body is out of balance, restore balance. If the soul is gone, retrieve it. If a spirit has taken over the body, exorcise it. If a rule has been violated, do penance. If an object has entered the body, remove it. All these remedies are perfectly logical. Whether these etiologies are the true causes of the disease is irrelevant. A patient who believes he or she is ill because of soul loss will not be completely cured by any amount of antibiotics. The mind is very powerful, as the placebo effect demonstrates. The patient's beliefs, as well as body, must be treated. Many Americans feel they have not been treated properly if they do not receive an antibiotic for a virus, even though antibiotics are effective only against bacteria. Psychologically, they need the pill to get well. This has unfortunately led to a selection for ever more powerful and antibiotic-resistant bacteria.

Second, we must not let our ethnocentrism blind us to the merits in the beliefs of other cultures. They may be right. It is easy to look down on other systems, citing science to support Western medical beliefs. But all medical systems are based on observed cause-and-effect relationships. The major difference with the scientific approach is that science is falsifiable. A scientific hypothesis can be proven wrong. The beliefs of other systems cannot.

At the level of the individual, however, Americans demand no more proof than do people of any other culture. Most believe germs cause disease because their mothers told them so. Few have ever actually seen a germ, and fewer demand to see proof of viruses or bacteria at work. The experts have done that, and their word, along with our mothers', is enough. The same is true in other cultures. People believe disease is caused by spirit possession or object intrusion because their mothers and cultural experts told them so. They have seen people become ill when that happens and get well when treated. What further proof is necessary?

Even within biomedicine, treatments once thought to be the best medicine had to offer were later discredited. Siddhartha Mukherjee in *The Emperor of All Maladies* (2010) describes how the radical mastectomy, at one time the gold standard treatment for breast cancer, was based on the experience and reputation of its proponents rather than actual data. When at long last it was subjected to clinical trials, the survival, recurrence, and mortality rates were statistically identical with lumpectomy followed by radiation. Today the radical mastectomy is rarely, if ever, performed.

Theoretical Perspective: Adaptation Theory

As can be inferred from the preceding sections, the underlying theoretical perspective of this book is based on adaptation theory. I believe that, in most cases, people have developed traditions designed to achieve success in the broader environment in which they live. These include adaptations to both the physical and social environments. Obviously, there are exceptions, and there are other theoretical approaches that are equally fruitful in explaining people's behavior. However, this is the theory that will inform the interpretations given in this book. When cultural conflicts occur, it is often because what is successful under one set of environmental circumstances may be less so under others.

We can better understand the relationship between environment and culture by looking at some examples. These generalizations are very broad, but they should serve to illuminate the underlying principles.

Arabs, for example, developed their culture in a harsh desert environment. Humans can have a limited effect on such an environment without the benefit of advanced technology. It makes sense, then, to have a fatalistic worldview, and to see a supernatural entity (God, or Allah) in control. Many Arabs were traditionally herders. Because men tend to be in charge of the herds, this leads to male authority. Because males are often away from home, tending the herds, female purity becomes important. Otherwise, men would often be raising other men's children. Because it is difficult to keep watch over the herds at all times, they are vulnerable to theft. Without an external policing force, the best way to protect one's animals is through one's reputation. Everyone must know that if your animals are stolen, the consequences will be swift and great. Honor and reputation thus become highly valued. In this way, we can see that the environmental factors of the desert environment and a pastoral (herding) subsistence base led to a fatalistic worldview, a social structure that emphasizes male authority, and the values of female purity and family honor.

These cultural characteristics have important implications with regard to health care. For example, preventive care may be underutilized. Since Allah is in control, what's the point? Wives may defer to husbands when it comes to decision making due to male authority. Women may refuse to be examined by a male physician due to concerns about female purity.

Another example is the Japanese. Japan is old and densely populated. Thus the Japanese have had both the time and the need to develop rules that will help avoid chaos. These include a hierarchical social system and the value of emotional control. The Japanese were traditionally agricultural, thus leading to an emphasis on the group over the individual. The combination of an agricultural subsistence base and a hierarchical social structure combined to place great value on the elderly (something which is changing in light of the industrialization of Japan) because they are the ones with the most experience and thus the most useful knowledge.

How do these characteristics influence Japanese health care behavior? Because the Japanese see themselves as a members of a family group, rather than as individuals, family members may want to decide what information is to be given to the patient, and choose to withhold a negative prognosis. Respect for the hierarchy may lead patients to agree verbally to what the physician requests, even if they have no intention of following through; to disagree would be seen as disrespectful. The emphasis on emotional control may lead them to exhibit little sign of pain, no matter how much discomfort they may be feeling.

Adaptation theory can also help us understand the U.S. health care system. The United States was founded by immigrants who came to avoid religious persecution and a kind of class system where who you were depended on the status of your family, so freedom and individualism became highly valued and success was measured by your individual worth. One "objective measure" of worth is money, and thus wealth became highly valued. Those who prospered in the early days of this open land were often those who were independent, worked hard, and developed the land, in other words, those who controlled nature. Once the country became industrialized, people had to go where there jobs were available or could be created, and thus family became less important than mobility.

As discussed earlier, these characteristics are closely related to the U.S. health care culture. The view that humans control nature leads to extensive use of life support, fetal monitoring, organ transplants, and so forth. The emphasis on money not only influences the level of health care one receives, but also leads to the notion that with enough money, we can cure any disease. The values of individualism and freedom lead us to give information directly to the patient, rather than the family, and to expect that the patient will make all the decisions concerning his health. The value of independence leads to an emphasis on self-care.

Adaptation theory can help explain many of the similarities between cultures. For example, most agriculturalists, whether from Asia, Latin America, or Africa, will value the family over the individual, because successful small farming requires the combined efforts of all members of the family. Large families will also be desired, because more family members mean more workers, which often translates to greater success.

Cultural Customs

Utilizing adaptation theory, it can be argued that most cultural practices originate for very practical reasons. People, however, do not always act in a practical manner if the benefit to them is not obvious and immediate. They may need a "higher" purpose. Ideological injunctions are much more likely to be followed, as anthropologist Marvin Harris (1974), a leading proponent of the cultural materialism approach, points out.

For example, the Hindu prohibition against killing cows may seem bizarre in a country where many people are starving, but it has a practical basis. Most cows are malnourished and if slaughtered would provide very little food. Living, however, cows are good substitutes for tractors. Their milk provides food. Their dung provides fertilizer, fuel for cooking, and, mixed with water, an excellent household flooring material. Far more use is made of living cows than could ever be gained from dead ones. Hungry individuals might look at a cow and see dinner. Forgetting the animal's other practical uses, they might kill and eat it. But if the animal is made sacred, religious ideology will prevent such killing.

Circumstances sometimes change, obliterating the practical need for a custom. Ideology, however, is enduring and soon becomes tradition. Although many cultural and religious traditions no longer have any practical value, they have an important psychological one—they provide a sense of identity and belonging. They serve as a strong reminder that the individual is not like everyone else; he or she belongs to a special group. Abstaining from meat when everyone else is having hamburgers reminds the Hindu that he is Hindu. Walking to temple instead of driving on the Sabbath reminds the Jew that she is Jewish. In fact, the more difficult or impractical the custom, the stronger the reminder of ethnic or religious identity. Thus the benefits of adhering to seemingly outmoded customs can be enormous in a country like the United States, where feelings of isolation and anomie may be strong.

Key Points

- Culturally competent care is patient-centered care.
- Learn your patient's point of view by asking the right questions.
- One model of the questions to ask is "The 4 C's of Culture":
  - What do you *call* your problem? (What do *you* think is wrong?)
  - What do you think *caused* your problem?
  - What have you done to *cope* with your problem?
  - What *concerns* do you have about your problem? About my recommended treatment?

Chapter 2

Communication and Time Orientation

Miscommunication is a frequent problem in hospitals. The most obvious case is when the patient and the hospital personnel do not speak the same language. Although interpreters should always be available, either in person or by telephone, they are not always used. Bilingual family members may not possess the necessary vocabulary, or have their own agendas. There are also more subtle problems that result from cultural differences in verbal and nonverbal communication styles and patterns. This chapter explores these problems in communication as well as another subtle but provocative source of difficulty—cultural differences in time orientation. Patients and staff members may operate on different "time clocks," causing confusion and resentment for all parties.

Language Issues

Idioms

18 Idioms or other nonliteral expressions can often create misunderstanding. A Chinese-born physician called the night nurse one evening to check on a patient scheduled for surgery the next day. The nurse advised the physician that she noticed a new hesitancy in the patient's attitude. "To tell you the truth, doctor, I think Mrs. Colby is getting cold feet." The physician, not familiar with this idiom, suspected circulation problems and ordered vascular tests.

19 A nervous patient jokingly asked his surgeon if he were going to "kick the bucket." The Korean physician, wanting to reassure the patient that his upcoming surgery would be successful, responded affably, "Oh, yes, you are definitely going to kick the bucket!" The patient was not reassured.

In general, it is best to avoid using idioms with people who speak English as a second language, since they may often be misunderstood.

Another English

Language problems can also occur among native English speakers. In England, South Africa, and Australia, the word "fanny" is a derogatory term referring to a woman's vagina. Imagine the shock and horror of a British woman—or the confusion of a British man—when told to prepare for a shot in the fanny. (A South African nurse was appalled when an American aerobics instructor called out to her class, "Tighten your fanny, shake your fanny!")

Lynette was educating a patient and her husband on the pain-free method of moving up in bed. Part of her instructions was to "slide your fanny up to the middle of the bed." Both started giggling. They were from England. Fortunately, rather than be offended, the patient called Lynette "a fun nurse." 20

Similarly, birth control instruction to speakers of the "Queen's English" could be confusing if the instructor referred to a condom as a "rubber." Erasers are not a very effective means of preventing pregnancy.

Same Language, Different Meaning

Words can have different meanings in the same language. In Mexico, the word *horita* means right now. In Puerto Rico, it means in an hour or so. This could cause confusion between two Spanish speakers. Similarly, "just now" in South Africa means "later" in the United States. A South African immigrant reported frequent problems with her boss when she first moved to the United States. At times, when he asked her to do something, she would reply, "I'll get to it just now." He'd come back an hour later, asking for the work, which hadn't been done. He would be angry; she had said she would do it right away, but hadn't. She, on the other hand, would be upset because she told him she would get to it later, and now he was expecting her to have it done immediately.

Same Word, Different Language

Sometimes the same word can have different meanings in different languages. Consuela, a Filipina nurse, had for several days been caring for Ramon Ibañez, a Mexican premature baby in intensive care. Everything seemed fine, until the Ibañezes suddenly requested that another nurse be assigned to their baby. Consuela was shocked, particularly since they had not given the social worker any explanation. 21

Consuela had Graciela, a Spanish-speaking coworker, ask them to explain the problem. They were a bit hesitant, but finally told her that they had overheard Consuela talking to a coworker and mentioning that she had a *puto*. In Spanish, *puto* refers to a male prostitute. Their baby's health had gotten worse; they assumed it was because Consuela had picked up a disease from her male prostitute and passed it on to their child. They were in fact a bit surprised that the hospital would employ such a woman to care for the infants.

Was Consuela really seeing a male prostitute? No. In the Philippines, a *puto* is a rice cake. Consuela had been telling her coworker that she was having a rice cake for lunch. Graciela explained this to the Ibañezes and clarified that babies born severely premature often got worse before getting better; Ramon's condition had nothing to do with Consuela. Fortunately, they understood their misunderstanding. The next week, Consuela brought the Ibañezes some *puto* to eat. Mrs. Ibañez hugged her and again expressed their apologies.

22   Sometimes words sound the same, but mean something different. Gail Price-Wise, author of "An Intoxicating Error: Language, Culture, and Medical Tragedy," writes about the famous case of Willie Ramirez, who became quadriplegic in large part due to confusion over the word "intoxicado." Willie lost consciousness several hours after eating a hamburger. His Cuban family believed that a bad hamburger had caused him to get sick. In Spanish, this reaction can be described as "intoxicado." Among Cubans, according to Price-Wise, "*intoxicado* is kind of an all encompassing word that means there's something wrong with you because of something you ate or drank. *I ate something and now I have hives or an allergic reaction to the food or I'm nauseous*" (Price-Wise 2008). Willie was erroneously treated for drug intoxication because a bilingual family friend used the English word "intoxicated," believing the words meant the same thing. She was a native Spanish speaker who spoke fairly good English. Unfortunately, this was a case where a little bit of knowledge is a dangerous thing. Had she not been bilingual, the medical staff might have used a professional interpreter and might not have been led to the misdiagnosis. They may have looked for the real reason Willie became unconscious—a brain aneurysm. The aneurysm was finally discovered and surgically repaired 36 hours after Mr. Ramirez was admitted. Unfortunately, by that time extensive bleeding had left him quadriplegic.

23   Jerry treated a Hispanic male patient who was hospitalized with a suspected drug overdose. It wasn't, at least, not intentionally. As it turned out, the instructions on the medication stated, "Take once a day." The patient, who spoke limited English, thought it said to take *eleven* a day; in Spanish, *once* means eleven. Now the instructions read "one time daily" instead of "once a day."

Different Connotations in Different Countries

Most Anglo Americans realize that the term "boy" is offensive to African Americans due to its use among white slave owners. Many non-Americans, however, are not familiar with the history of slavery in this country and the significance of that word. Colleen, an Anglo nurse from Canada, learned the meaning of "boy" the hard way. Her first job when she moved to the United States was at an inner city hospital. The cafeteria was crowded the first day she was there, but she found an empty place across from two African American men. She went over to them and asked very sweetly, "Do you boys mind if I sit down here?" One answered her by picking up his plate of food and throwing it at her.

Most people would agree that he overreacted, but his response is understandable in the context of race relations in this country. The misunderstanding occurred because Canada has not had the same racial problems as the United States, and in the part of the country Colleen was from, adult men and women commonly refer to each other as boys and girls. No insult is meant or taken. Once someone explained the reason for the man's reaction to Colleen, she did not make that mistake again.

Most people in the United States know that "boy" is highly insulting to an African American man, but fewer are aware that the term "gal" has similar connotations for many African American women in the South. Black slave women were called "gals," which explains why several Anglo nurses reported receiving cold and hostile glares from African American nurses whom they innocently referred to as "gals."

Two other words that can cause problems due to different connotations in different languages are "mama" and "papa." In Filipino culture, these terms convey a sense of respect, and Filipino health care workers will sometimes refer to elderly patients in this way. In other cultures, however, it can be interpreted as a *lack* of respect. Health care professionals from the Philippines should be informed of this cultural difference.

When "Yes" May Mean "No"

Cultural values can also create communication problems. Jackie, an Anglo American nurse, was explaining the harmful side effects of the medication that Adela Samillan, a Filipina patient, was to take at home after her discharge. Although Mrs. Samillan spoke some English, her husband, who was more fluent, served as interpreter. Throughout Jackie's explanation, the Samillans nodded in agreement and understanding and laughed nervously. When Jackie verbally tested them on the information, however, it was apparent that they understood very little. What had happened?

Dignity and self-esteem are important for all individuals, but particularly so for most Asians. Because the family, rather than the individual, is the primary unit, if you look bad, everyone looks bad. In a sense, it multiplies the humiliation. Had the Samillans indicated that they did not understand Jackie's instructions, they would have lost their self-esteem for not understanding or they would have caused Jackie to lose hers for not explaining the material well enough. By pretending to understand, Mr. and Mrs. Samillan felt they were preserving everyone's dignity.

Jackie's first clue should have been their nervous laughter. Giggling is often a sign of discomfort and embarrassment. Once Jackie realized they had not understood the material, she went over it until they were able to explain it back to her. It is important not to take smiles and nods of agreement for understanding when dealing with Asian patients—or *any* patients. Elderly patients who are hard of hearing commonly nod in agreement, even when they can't hear what is being said. Patients should always be asked to demonstrate their understanding. This will be discussed in more detail in Chapter 13 on Improving Adherence.

26   A second incident involved Linh Lee, a sixty-four-year-old Chinese woman hospitalized for an acute evolving heart attack. At discharge, her physician suggested that she come back in two weeks for a follow-up examination. She agreed to do so, but never returned. It is likely that she never intended to do so but agreed because he was an authority figure. Chinese people are taught to value accommodation. Rather than refuse to the physician's face and cause him dishonor, Mrs. Lee agreed. She simply did not follow through, sparing everyone embarrassment.

27   In a similar incident, when Dr. Jacks told Cha Xeng, a Hmong patient, that she needed to have gallbladder surgery, she agreed. Several days later, however, she told the interpreter that she did not plan to have the surgery. The interpreter asked her why she had changed her mind. She hadn't changed her mind, she said; she never intended to have the surgery. But she didn't want to show disrespect to the surgeon by disagreeing with his recommendation. It is not clear that the surgeon could have done anything different in this case, other than present the options to her more objectively, and ask about her concerns rather than simply giving his recommendation.

Grammar

The cases described above involved the use of the word "yes" to avoid the embarrassment of saying "no." "Yes" may also be used inappropriately (from the American perspective) for reasons of grammar. According to common English usage, if someone were asked, "Haven't you taken your medication yet today?" and they had *not* taken it, they would answer, "No." According to the rules of grammar found in most Asian languages, the accurate response would be "Yes," as in "Yes, it is a true statement that I have not yet taken my medication today." The English speaker would be misled by the Asian patient's affirmative response, thinking that person had already taken the medication when he or she had not. To reduce possible confusion, it is generally best to avoid sentences with negatives.

A related source of misunderstanding involves the phrase, "Do you mind . . . ?" If you ask an Asian, "Do you mind . . . ?" you will probably receive the answer "yes." Americans would generally interpret that to mean the other individual *does* mind, but they would be wrong. It is the Asian way of showing agreement or willingness.

Pronouns

Different languages have characteristics that are not directly translatable, as any English speaker who has struggled with remembering the gender of inanimate objects in French or Spanish knows well. English poses a similar problem for many Asians. Mieko, a Japanese nurse, was assigned to care for six patients, two male and four female. During reports, she consistently referred to the female patients as "he." Her supervisor interrupted to point out that there were no male patients in the bed numbers she mentioned. Mieko acknowledged that fact and continued in the same manner. The supervisor became confused. Had four transsexuals slipped in?

The explanation is simple. Many Asian languages do not have pronouns that reflect gender; "he" and "she" do not exist. Thus Asians have no model for using the pronouns "he" or "she" and often mix them up, confusing everyone else in the process. This may seem surprising, given the importance of gender in Asian hierarchical cultures. It might help to think of it in this way—gender is of *such* importance that it is not diminished by the use of a mere pronoun. An individual would be referred to as "that man" or "that woman." Knowledge of this characteristic of the language can lessen the confusion.

Common Misunderstandings

Even American English can have different meanings for hearing and deaf people. While Kelly, a deaf gay male was a patient in the hospital, blood was drawn for an HIV test. When the results came back, no interpreters for the deaf were available. Because Kelly was adept at reading lips, he was given the test results directly. He was told that his results

28

were positive, meaning, of course, that he was HIV-positive. In deaf culture, however, "positive" means good and "negative" means bad. Kelly was relieved to hear that his test results were "positive"; that meant he was *not* HIV-positive! He went home and did not return for follow-up. What the nurse should have done was tell him that the results showed that he was, indeed, HIV-positive.

This incident was not unique. Carol Browner and her colleagues (2003) discovered that many Mexican-born pregnant women receiving genetic counseling misunderstood the term "positive" when given test results for fetal abnormalities. Rather than understand there was a problem, they thought it meant that everything was good; after all, the counselor said the results were "positive." It is important for health care providers to realize that some terms have a different meaning outside the context of medicine. The terms "positive" and "negative" as applied to test results can be confusing to anyone. It is important for health care professionals to clarify the significance of "positive" and "negative" findings. Paying attention to nonverbal reactions is also key; any misunderstanding of test results, for example, will often result in an inappropriate emotional response (such as relief).

Communication Style

Formal Versus Informal Language

The United States was founded in large part by British settlers who were escaping, among other things, the British system of nobility. The notion of equality became paramount in our national culture, as illustrated in the famous words of the Declaration of Independence: "We hold these truths to be self-evident, that all men are created equal." One manifestation of the importance of equality is the absence of a vocabulary that indicates status differences. At the same time, the westward movement embodied a greater informality, also reflected in our language. In Spanish, for example, different forms of the word "you" are used depending in part on the level of formality of the relationship to the speaker. When addressing one person, the speaker may use *tú* for a young person or for someone with whom he or she has a close relationship. Alternatively, he or she may use *usted* for a stranger or someone occupying a higher social position. The more formal *usted* is used when speaking to someone older or someone you don't know very well. The fact that some languages have formal and informal vocabulary, something that English lacks, can create problems. As you will read in the chapter on staff issues, young Filipino nurses may feel forced to resort to speaking in Tagalog in order to show respect to older Filipino nurses because Tagalog has a formal vocabulary. I have had several Nigerian students tell me they were offended by the "rude" behavior of young people who had the "nerve" to say "hi" to them. Why would they be offended by a friendly greeting? Because they perceived "hi" as rudely informal. Instead, they explained, young people should have the courtesy to say "hello" or "good day."

Tone of Voice

A famous anthropological linguist (John Gumperz of U.C. Berkeley) was called to a large company in England to deal with a problem they were having with the cafeteria workers. The company employees kept complaining that the cafeteria workers (who were all from India and Gujarati speakers) were rude. It turns out that the problem was that in English, we indicate a question by raising our voice at the end. In Gujarati, it is done by adding a word to the end of the sentence or phrase, not through tone of voice. So when they offered food, it would be done with a flat tone of voice, which the British perceived as rude. The linguist taught the Indian cafeteria workers how to change their tone of voice by raising it at the end of a question and this completely changed the way they were perceived. Now they were seen as friendly, not rude!

Directive Versus Nondirective Approaches

Different communication styles can also create misunderstandings. The current emphasis in medicine is on shared decision-making. The patient is seen as an equal partner in the health care interaction. However, not all cultures have this expectation, and it can sometimes backfire. Medical anthropologist Carole Browner and her colleagues did research on miscommunication between prenatal genetic service providers and patients born in Mexico (Browner et al. 2003). They point out that the nondirective approach taken in genetic counseling was interpreted by many of the patients to reflect a lack of concern about test results. They assumed that if their tests had indicated any serious danger, the clinician would have been more dramatic and directive in recommending amniocentesis. Thus, the standard nondirective style was misinterpreted to indicate that no intervention was necessary.

Personalismo

For many Hispanics, the establishment of personal relationships is extremely important. A health care provider who wants to develop a good relationship with a Hispanic patient will take the time to ask about the patient's family and interests before getting "down to business." Although this may seem to be a "waste of time," in the long run it will save time, as the patient will be more likely to open up more quickly to a trusted health care provider. Furthermore, it will improve the chances of the patient adhering to the health care provider's recommendations, because adherence becomes a matter of a "personal favor."

30   A middle-aged Hispanic woman had a very bad experience with a physician she saw for the first time. She complained that he didn't care for her as an individual; he wanted only to treat her disease. When asked why she felt this way, she explained that the doctor never bothered even to greet her. Furthermore, he stood in the doorway when taking her history. He was lacking in *personalismo,* and as a result, she felt isolated and did not trust him. Rather than return to him, she went to a *curandero,* a traditional healer.

In contrast, a pediatric nurse who described herself as having "lost touch" over the years with being sensitive and polite in her greetings changed her approach after learning about the importance of *personalismo.* She began to greet her Hispanic patients and their families with a simple "buenos dias" or "buenas tardes" and would make conversation about family life. For example, she would ask the ages of the children, or what plans the family had for the holidays. She found that family members exhibited much less reluctance when she had to insert an intravenous line or administer medications to their child. She said the family felt she was on "their side," and doing everything to help improve their child's health and well-being.

31   Stephanie's interaction with Juanita Rios, a forty-nine-year-old Mexican woman, illustrates how *personalismo* can improve patient outcomes through increased adherence to medical recommendations. Mrs. Rios was suffering from both renal failure and diabetes; her condition required her to be on dialysis while waiting for an organ transplant. Stephanie, her nurse, found that as she got to know Mrs. Rios better, making several home visits when she could not get a ride to the rural clinic, she began to open up more. When Stephanie learned that Mrs. Rios had left several of her children behind in Mexico, a necessity that caused her great sadness and periodic depression, Stephanie encouraged her to talk about her children and show her their photos. On Mrs. Rios's birthday, she arranged for her to call her sons from the clinic. As a result of Stephanie's display of *personalismo,* Mrs. Rios became much more adherent to diet and fluid restrictions. As Stephanie explained, "She knows we make these requests because we care about her."

Seeing a physician, especially when ill, can often be a source of anxiety for patients. Demonstrating a little *personalismo* can make an important difference. For example, taking a moment to ask patients a little about their family or children before going into surgery, and reassuring them that they will be with them again soon, can often help them relax and need less sedation medication, according to one nurse.

Personalismo can also sometimes turn difficult patients into cooperative ones, and spare a clinician from a lawsuit, as happened in the following case.

Dee was caring for Ramona Medina, a Latina with end-stage renal disease. She was number one on the liver transplant list. When Dee began her shift, the departing nurse warned her that she would be dealing with an extremely difficult family who had already lodged several complaints with the administration. Dee was in the middle of a cultural diversity class, and decided to apply the concepts she had been learning to this apparently difficult case. She obtained permission from the charge nurse to be flexible with the visiting hours. She invited the family to help her with hygiene care for the patient. She *talked* to them and developed a relationship with them. At the end of her shift, they requested that she care for their mother the next night. When she spoke with the oncoming day nurse, Dee tried to convince her to be flexible with visitation, but the nurse insisted on enforcing the restricted visiting rules. As a result, the day nurse experienced major conflicts with the family.

Mrs. Medina never received a liver transplant, and thus died. Afterward, the hospital held a risk management meeting. Mrs. Medina's family was suing the hospital; the lawsuit specifically named staff members the family felt were unprofessional and uncaring. The only two *not* named in the suit were Dee and one other nurse. Management spoke with both of them to see what they had done differently, what they had done right. Both had the same response; they talked with the family and kept them involved in the patient's care. In other words, they demonstrated *personalismo.*

Asking Questions

It's important for physicians to remember that doctors are held in very high regard in most cultures. This may make it difficult for patients to feel comfortable asking questions.

When Dr. Brandon came to see Marisol Moreno, a Latina in her sixties, only she and her husband were in the room. Although they spoke both English and Spanish, Spanish was their primary language. However, since they did speak English (with limitations), Dr. Brandon did not call for an interpreter. Later, one of their adult children called Mrs. Moreno's nurse, Tabitha. He was concerned because his parents told

32

33

him there were some changes on the CT scan and he wanted to know what they meant. When Tabitha asked him why he didn't ask his parents, he said that he had, but they weren't able to explain it to him. Tabitha then called the Dr. Brandon and asked him to call the son. He refused, saying he had already spoken with one of the family members, and didn't have time to call everyone. Tabitha then went to talk with Mr. and Mrs. Moreno to assess their understanding of what Dr. Brandon had told them. They understood very little, and had several questions. They complained that the doctor spoke too fast and seemed hurried, so when he asked if they had any questions, they both nodded, "No." They respected him and didn't want to take up more of his obviously limited time. Tabitha then called Dr. Brandon to tell him what she had learned. He responded defensively that they both were quiet and didn't ask any questions. When he asked if they had understood, they both nodded affirmatively. Tabitha then suggested that they schedule a family conference the next day when more family members could be present, and he could schedule his day around the conference and not be rushed. He agreed, and the next day, a very successful conference was held. Dr. Brandon took his time and practiced *personalismo* by asking them some nonmedical questions. He asked them about their concerns and fears (recall the 4 C's), and replaced medical jargon with clear and simple language and explanations. Fortunately, Dr. Brandon was open to changing. One would hope that in the future he—and all physicians— would take the time to explain things carefully in the first place and make sure the patient/family truly understand. It will save time in the long run.Lack of understanding often results in lack of adherence, so better patient outcomes will often result when questions are encouraged. Culturally competent clinicians will have patients demonstrate their understanding of any patient teaching, as well as ask patients what questions they have. Not "Do you have any questions?"—a question many patients will hesitate to respond to either out of respect for the physician's time, or for fear of appearing stupid—but "What questions do you have?" The tone should assume that *of course* they will have questions, and it is his or her job to be happy to answer them. Let them know that most patients have questions, and it will help you if they ask them now. In addition, it is always good practice for health care providers to ask patients what they understand about their condition.

In contrast to the patients who are uncomfortable asking questions out of respect for the physician are those that ask "too many" questions, usually of the nurse. It is not uncommon for family members from Middle Eastern cultures to ask a lot of questions, and the same question multiple times, sometimes to the same nurse, sometimes to different staff members. For nurses, this often feels like the family doesn't trust the staff. However, as one Iranian physician explained to a nurse, it has nothing to do with trust. Rather, it is a way for the family to feel safe, to feel a sense of control. Although from the nurse's perspective, the repeated questions may appear to be an information error that needs to be cleared up, from the family's perspective, it's more about gaining reassurance.

One final point regarding asking questions, this time directed at health care professionals. When you ask a question, *listen* for the answer. That may seem obvious, but oftentimes, patients will feel they must agree with what their symptoms are. The questions may be valid, but are too restrictive. It's important to ask more open-ended questions and let the story emerge, rather than be dictated, as we can see in the following case study.

Lotty Jefferson, an elderly African American woman, came to the Emergency Department complaining of chest pain. Georgianne, an RN, was at the bedside when Dr. Hanks was evaluating her. He placed his hand on the left side of her chest and asked, "Is this where it hurts? And does it feel like pressure?" Mrs. Jefferson nodded affirmatively. He then continued, "Are you having trouble walking?" She nodded again. The medical interview continued like that, with Dr. Hanks asking questions and Mrs. Jefferson nodding in agreement. When Dr. Hanks left, Georgianne began her assessment. She asked Mrs. Jefferson an open-ended question. "Tell me what you've been feeling and when it all started." What emerged from Mrs. Jefferson's story sounded more like epigastric burning pain. Although she did get short of breath with walking, that was not a new symptom associated with what brought her to the ED. Although cardiac issues should always be ruled out, assuming that it is a cardiac problem does not benefit a patient with gastrointestinal problems.

34

In a similar vein, Kohanya Scott, a middle-aged Anglo American woman, visited her ophthalmologist for an eye exam. As she sat in front of the phoropter to test her vision with different lenses while she looked at the eye chart, the ophthalmologist would ask, "Which is better, one or two?" However, rather than give her time to assess which was better, he would immediately follow up with, "One, right?" or "Two, right?" For whatever reason, perhaps she was unsure and unconsciously wanted to please him, she would agree. At the end of the exam, he wrote her a new prescription and she got new glasses that she couldn't see out of as well as she would like. A few weeks later she returned to the ophthalmologist to complain that she couldn't see very well. He tested her again. This time, she was more forceful in her assessment of "which was better, one or two?" and the resulting prescription was markedly different. The ophthalmologist, rather than assuming an error on his part, told her

35

that she should immediately see her physician to get checked for diabetes. It was the only reason he could think of for such a significant change in her vision in less than a month. Kohanya went to her physician the next day; the ophthalmologist had scared her because diabetes ran in her family. But her fasting plasma glucose test came out normal. She did not have diabetes. What she had was a health care professional who fed her answers, rather than listening to her responses. That was the last time she used his services.

36   When we were discussing the importance of really *listening* to what the patient says, Nancy shared an experience that occurred when she first began working in a psychiatric hospital. Her supervisor was observing her as she went through the intake questionnaire with a patient who had previously been admitted for suicidal ideation. At one point, she came to the question, "Do you still think about killing yourself"? The patient answered, "Yes." Rather than follow up on this very significant response, Nancy just said, "Okay," marked it down, and moved on to the next question. She was so intent on getting through the entire questionnaire that she hadn't really paid attention to what the patient was saying. This did not impress her supervisor, and had she not been in the trainee position with a supervisor there to back her up, could have had a disastrous result.

Asking Patients Questions About Their Culture or Religion

In order to provide culturally appropriate care, it's necessary to know something about the patient's ethnic and religious background. Some nurses have commented that there are patients who become upset when asked about their religious beliefs. There's also the danger of appearing intrusive. The key is in the way it is done. If you explain *why* you're asking such questions, people are more likely to give you answers. For example, "We're making an effort at our hospital to meet the needs of our diverse population. Knowing about your ethnic background, religious preferences, and sexual orientation can help us to provide better care, should you choose to share that information with us." Most people are delighted to be the "expert" about their culture with individuals who are genuinely interested.

First Versus Last Names

Americans tend to address each other by their first name. It is considered a sign of friendliness and equality. To use a first name for anyone other than a close friend, however, is both inappropriate and discourteous in most cultures, including European. In nineteenth-century English novels, even teenage girls referred to each other as Miss [last name] until they had been friends for at least a year. A mental health specialist said she often sees that when social workers or therapists try to engage Mexican patients by using their first name, it has the opposite effect. The patients often feel they are being disrespected. Hospital personnel should refer to all adult patients as Mr., Miss, Ms., or Mrs., unless instructed otherwise.

African Americans' sensitivity to perceived slights to their dignity is not surprising given their history in this country. It is therefore especially important to show them respect. Mary Washington, an elderly African American woman, was in the recovery room after surgery. To assess her condition, Cheryl, her nurse, spoke her name, "Mary." The patient slowly opened her eyes and turned her head but made no further sign of acknowledgment. Cheryl became concerned because most patients responded readily and clearly at this point. Shortly afterward Cheryl called the woman "Mrs. Washington." She then became alert, pleasant, and cooperative. She had perceived the use of her first name as a lack of respect and saw no need to respond.

Interpreters

In 2001, in an effort to improve access to care, quality of care, and ultimately, health outcomes, the U.S. Department of Health and Human Services, Office of Minority Health, published National Standards for Culturally and Linguistically Appropriate Services in Health Care, commonly known as "CLAS standards" (see National Standards 2001); they were updated and enhanced in 2013. Although most of the standards are recommendations, those requiring language access services are mandates, required for all recipients of federal funds. Thus, a section in this book on interpreters should no longer be necessary. However, the reality is that there are huge numbers of immigrants from a variety of countries, so it is not feasible to have interpreters for every language on staff 24 hours a day. Often, even if interpreters are on the hospital staff, they are not immediately available. Patients are often accompanied by family members, at least some of whom are usually bilingual. Therefore, the expedient choice often favored by physicians and nurses is to use family members. The case studies in this section illustrate why this is *not* a good idea.

I also want to mention that there are numerous telephonic services available, including some that use video phones. When used properly, these services work quite well. It is important, however, that speaker-phones be used, so that telephone receivers are not handed back and forth, making the process more cumbersome than needed. Even better than speaker phones are phones with two handsets, which both patients and physicians often prefer. There are times, however, when in-person interpreting is preferable, such as when a relationship needs to be built, when giving bad news, when the patient is hard of hearing, when mental health services are being provided, when communicating with children, or when visual information is central to the communication.

As a side note, for those who care about using correct terminology, the term "interpret" refers to spoken language; "translate" refers to written materials.

First, a case to illustrate the necessity of having interpreters available.

38   Pham Kim, a sixty-five-year-old Vietnamese patient, was diagnosed with poor nutrition and lower abdominal pain. Her refusal to eat was documented by the nurses: "No food intake, but only juice." When the interpreter finally spoke with her, three days post admission, she said she hadn't understood anything the doctor had said to her. When the physician asked through the interpreter why she hadn't been eating, she replied, "I do not like American food." He then asked if she had trouble chewing or swallowing food. "No." When the doctor explained through the interpreter that they were going to put a feeding tube through her nose to feed her, she quickly explained that her daughter (who also did not speak English) brought her rice and hot soup every night at 9:00 p.m. The nurses just hadn't seen her eat. If an interpreter hadn't finally been brought in, Mrs. Kim would have suffered a nasogastric tube, followed by a percutaneous endoscopic gastrostomy tube, all for no reason.

The next set of case studies illustrates the kinds of problems that can occur when family members are used as interpreters. It is particularly dangerous when children are used, yet they are most likely to be bilingual and, therefore, often the most expedient choice.

39   Hilda Gomez, a monolingual Spanish-speaking patient, came in to the clinic three days in a row to complain of abdominal pain. The first two times, the staff used her young, bilingual daughter to translate. They then treated Mrs. Gomez for the "stomach ache" she described. The staff didn't understand why she kept returning with the same problem. Finally, on her third visit, the nurse located a Spanish-speaking interpreter. It turned out that Mrs. Gomez needed treatment for a sexually transmitted disease, but was too embarrassed to talk about her sexual activity with her daughter as interpreter. It taught the staff an important lesson.

40   At least Mrs. Gomez was finally treated properly. Juan Vega had a less happy outcome when a family member was used to interpret a diagnosis

of HIV and a detailed explanation of the disease process and prognosis. The family member left the hospital immediately after interpreting, and never returned. Mr. Vega's family, who had been very supportive of him since he had become ill, abandoned him when they learned through the family interpreter that he was gay. After this unfortunate incident, the staff took the time to locate a professional interpreter when the patient did not speak English.

Joyce Kennish was a nineteen-year-old deaf girl admitted for threatened suicide. The emergency department staff relied on Joyce's parents to interpret, but she was withdrawn and refused to speak. When Daphne came on duty, she called for an interpreter who helped the psychiatrist conduct the interview. What emerged was that Joyce was upset with her parents because they were stricter with her than with her younger sister. They refused to let her go out with her friends. Her response was, "Well then I should just kill myself." This scared her parents and they brought her to the emergency department, saying she was suicidal. She had no history of depression or suicidal ideation. The psychiatrist determined that she was not a danger to herself and could be discharged. This was a case where an (unbiased) interpreter was essential, since the parents were the source of the patient's problem.   41

Maria Hidalgo was receiving home hospice care for metastatic breast cancer. She spoke only Spanish, so Patty, her hospice nurse, relied on family members to interpret. Maria was desperately fighting not to let her disease upset normal family routines. She was choosing to compromise her comfort in order to maintain her traditional role in the family as wife and mother; however, her exhaustion was making it increasingly difficult to do so. The rest of the family were having a hard time maintaining the illusion of normalcy, knowing that their lives were changing dramatically. In short, everyone was trying to protect everyone else but collapsing under the strain. It was not until Patty called in a bilingual/bicultural colleague that Maria was able to talk more openly about her need for pain medication. To discuss this through her family would have let down the pretense of normalcy.   42

An Arab woman had just given birth. Her Arab American mother-in-law was asked to translate the health teaching material to the new mother. All went well until the nurse reached the information on contraception. The mother-in-law refused to translate such information. She belonged to a culture that valued large families, and she wanted as many grandchildren as possible. In this case, the woman openly refused to translate. It is just as likely that she might have pretended to convey the information while actually talking about something else. It is important to remember that language is not the only issue involved in interpretation.   43

44   Helena became very frustrated while caring for Gwon Chin, a seventy-nine-year-old Korean man who had recently suffered a stroke. Her frustration and impatience were aimed at Mr. Gwon's wife and daughter. Since Mr. Gwon spoke only Korean, she had asked his bilingual daughter to tell her father not to get out of bed because his gait was unsteady. Helena was afraid he would fall and hurt himself. Throughout the day, however, Mr. Gwon continued to attempt to get out of bed. He became very agitated and his wife and daughter seemed almost afraid of him. When Helena questioned the daughter about it, she would only say that her father was "confused." Eventually Helena called on a Korean nurse to help her. When the nurse told Mr. Gwon not to get out of bed because he might fall, he asked in a surprised tone, "Why would I fall?" When the nurse explained that he was unsteady from the stroke, the patient was shocked. "I had a stroke?!" Helena was in disbelief. He had been on the unit for two days; how could he not know he had had a stroke? When she questioned Mr. Gwon's daughter about this, she explained that her brother has been out of town. He would be back today and tell him. When Helena, stunned by this, asked the daughter why *she* didn't tell her father, she replied, "I could never tell my father what is wrong with him and what he can or can't do. It would be disrespectful for me to do that when he has always told *me* what to do and what was wrong." Although Helena was angry that Mr. Gwon's daughter preferred having her father possibly fall and hurt himself than tell him why he was in the hospital and that he must stay in bed, Helena remained silent. She asked the Korean nurse to explain to the patient how the numbness on his left side would make walking difficult so he should remain in bed. She also added that his son would be in later that day and would explain everything to him. After that, the patient remained calm and stayed in bed.

          I had trouble deciding where to place this case, because it highlights several important points. It shows the hierarchical nature of communication patterns in many traditional Asian households. Parents tell children what to do; not the reverse. Sons have more status and authority than daughters. It is common for family members to try to protect loved ones from "bad news." And finally, it underscores the need to use professional interpreters rather than family members.

          It's often best to use a trained interpreter, even when the family doesn't request one.

45   Emilio Seine was a seven-year-old Hispanic boy with a recurrent intestinal obstruction. His physician, Dr. Harrison, wanted to operate, but needed the parents to sign informed consent. The parents were offered an interpreter, but the father declined, saying that he understood English. Dr. Harrison was explaining the risks of surgery, which included

the unlikely possibility that Emilio could die. At this point, Mr. Seine became hysterical and angrily shouted that he didn't want Dr. Harrison anywhere near his son. The nurse had to escort him out of the room. She convinced him to talk with Dr. Harrison again, this time, using an interpreter. With the interpreter present, it became clear that Mr. Seine had misunderstood the word, "risk," and thought the physician had said he was going to kill Emilio, not that death was a possible outcome.

Even though many hospital staff may speak a second language, it is still best to use professional interpreters.

Consuela was a medical technician from Mexico, and spoke Spanish 46 at home. She was also fluent in English. One would think that she would make an excellent interpreter, being bilingual and working in a hospital; however, when she took the test to become a certified healthcare interpreter, she failed it. She was unfamiliar with some of the medical terminology, and she incorrectly interpreted some of the terms she thought she knew. Although she eventually passed the certification exam, it was a good example of why it's best to use only trained professional interpreters. Patients cannot make truly informed decisions and give consent for tests or procedures without fully understanding the risks and benefits being explained to them. For that, they need a qualified and certified interpreter.

Although professional interpreters are generally a good idea, some- 47 times they can cause a problem, as in the following case.

Susana Ramos, a thirty-six-year-old Latina, brought her mother to the emergency department for evaluation and treatment. She was her mother's primary caregiver and expected to serve as interpreter. When told that it was hospital policy to use a trained medical interpreter, she became very upset. She was further distressed when told that confidentiality laws also prevented her from serving as her mother's interpreter. (As mentioned in Chapter 1, this is not necessarily the case, but that is how the hospital interpreted HIPAA.) Susana felt she was an ideal interpreter for her mother. As her mother's caretaker, she knew her mother's history. She felt her mother would be more comfortable having her as interpreter. She said the hospital policy made her feel like the staff were hiding something from her, and thus she did not trust them. She did not feel her mother would accurately express her needs or report her family history to a stranger. The nurse who reported this incident said that the rapport and care of this patient suffered as a result of the hospital policy.

What should the staff have done in this case? Under the circumstances, Susana would probably have been an appropriate interpreter. However, an even better approach would have been to explain that her mother's health was their shared priority, and because there might be medical terminology she was not familiar with, they wanted to use a professional medical interpreter. They could also have assured her that they would appreciate having her be part of the interview, once the interpreter ascertained that the patient *wanted* her daughter in the room. If Susana seemed offended by that, they could explain that in the past there had been problems when the patient did not feel comfortable being completely honest with the staff in front of family members, and although it was extremely unlikely in this case, wasn't it best to be sure? Susana would probably have been reassured by their concern that her mother get the best care possible.

Because the Latino population in this country is growing larger each year, many physicians are making an effort to learn some Spanish. Many feel that by talking directly to their patients, they can create greater rapport than they might have using an interpreter. Although that is probably true, it is often best to call for an interpreter anyway. Use the time you are waiting for the interpreter to arrive to develop *personalismo*, and save the medical content for the interpreter.

One final note on interpreters. It is essential that they be utilized properly. See Appendix 4, Tips for Working with Interpreters, developed by medical anthropologist M. Jean Gilbert.

Dealing with Silence

48   Ramona was trying to get a medical history from Mrs. Cata, a Navajo woman. After each question Ramona asked, there would be a long silence. When Ramona spoke, Mrs. Cata would often stare at the floor. Ramona assumed it meant that Mrs. Cata was shy and had trouble understanding her, but that was not the case. She was merely indicating in a culturally appropriate manner that she was paying close attention to Ramona. The Navajo value silence. A person who interrupts while someone is speaking is perceived as immature.

Most Americans are uncomfortable with silences and tend to fill them with words, making "small talk." The Navajo use silence to formulate their thoughts. Words should have significance. An anthropologist doing fieldwork among the Navajo commented that it took her a long time to get used to talking with them. She would ask a question and get no response. She assumed they had not heard or understood her. She was wrong. They were trying to give her the most complete answer possible, and that took consideration. Eventually, she became comfortable with long pauses in conversation.

When dealing with Navajo patients, if they seem slow to respond, be patient. Give them time to consider your question before answering. Don't make judgments based on the meaning of your own behavior.

Informed Consent

According to American laws, individuals undergoing surgery must sign a document of informed consent, indicating that they understand the procedure and its intended risks. It is consistent with the American value of autonomy that patients should make their own decisions regarding their health. However, it is not always a simple matter to obtain such consent, because not everyone values autonomy in that way. In addition, some patients may have issues with document signing based on past experiences. Or they may agree to sign without truly understanding what they are signing.

Mr. Fanous was a sixty-five-year-old man from the Middle East who had come to the cardiac cath lab for a heart catheterization. It was Nina's job to get him to sign an informed consent. He read the form, which described the various complications that could result along with the pros and cons of the procedure. After Nina went through everything with him, he refused to sign the form. He questioned why it was even necessary—why didn't they just go ahead and do the procedure? She explained to him that it was not ethical to talk someone into a procedure, and that it could not be done without his consent. After some discussion, Mr. Fanous finally signed the consent form.

Why had he been so reluctant to sign? Partly, it may have been because he did not want to be at the hospital in the first place; he had come only due to the urging of friends. From a cultural perspective, however, it may have been because many Arabs believe that because the doctor is the one with the knowledge and training, the doctor should be the one to make the decision. What did Mr. Fanous know about heart catheterization? Why was the hospital so unwilling to take responsibility for its actions? Although, as Nina suggests, there is probably no way to avoid this kind of cultural misunderstanding, just knowing what to expect might help.

Yea Samreth, an elderly Cambodian patient, had been severely burned on her back during a coining treatment when the alcohol being used caught fire. (See Chapter 12 for more information on coining.) This occurred while she was being treated by a traditional healer for diabetes. She spoke very little English. Before she could have a skin graft, she needed to sign informed consent. Rhonda, her nurse, had given Mrs. Samreth the form to sign, but she hadn't done so. Rhonda told Gillian, the nurse coming on shift, to be sure to get the document signed. When Gillian approached Mrs. Samreth with the document, she became agitated, and kept repeating, "Later, I sign later." Because Mrs. Samreth's language skills were minimal, Gillian was unsure as to how much she understood about what she was being asked to sign. This was

49

50

many years ago, and there was no interpreter available. Gillian later learned why the patient was probably so reluctant. During the Khmer Rouge war, signed life histories were required from those who were later executed. As a result, many older Cambodians are not comfortable signing written documents. A culturally competent health care provider would have made sure to have a family member available for support, a physician available to answer questions, and an interpreter available to explain the document to her. It would also have been helpful to ask the patient what concerns she had about signing.

51   Andrew Chan, the son of Wen Chan, a seventy-five-year-old Chinese man, was angry with his father's physician. His father was scheduled for an angiogram at noon. The nurse had explained everything to Andrew the day before, and he intended to come to the hospital that morning, speak to his father's physician, and help his father with the consent form. When he arrived at his father's room at 9:30 a.m., however, his father handed him the consent form, which he had already signed. Andrew walked over to the nursing station and furiously demanded to know who had made his father sign a consent form in English when he did not speak the language. After further discussion with Mr. Chan, it was determined that the physician had visited him at 8:00 that morning, and seeing the unsigned consent form on the bedside table, handed it to him to sign. The physician did explain the procedure to him, in English. He had no idea that Mr. Chan did not understand a word, because he was constantly nodding in agreement. Smiling and nodding is a common response in any language, when people do not understand. It is often done in an effort to be polite. Why did Mr. Chan sign a form he could not understand? Out of respect for the authority of the physician. Chinese culture is hierarchical, and physicians are held in high esteem.

There were a number of mistakes made in this case, beginning with the nurse explaining the procedure to the patient's son rather than using an interpreter to explain it to the patient. In addition, the physician should have taken the time to question the patient about his understanding of the procedure. If he had done that, it would have been clear that the patient did not speak English. Fortunately, there were no adverse health effects from the errors.

52   Diego, a bilingual surgical nurse, was reviewing Carlos Herrera's consent for surgery and asked Mr. Herrera to explain in his own words what type of surgery he was going to have done. He responded in Spanish that he was going to "have his back lasered to relieve his pain." Diego noted from the consent form that Mr. Herrera was in fact going to have a lumbar decompression and fusion. Diego asked who had explained this to him, and he replied that the surgeon had told him and his family

about it, but they had not understood what he had said. Diego asked who had been the interpreter, and Mr. Herrera responded that it was a family member who was with him at the bedside. At this point, Diego called in the surgeon to explain the surgery again, with Diego acting as interpreter. (Ideally, a professional interpreter would have been called in, but in this case, it worked out.) The surgeon was annoyed, because this meant a delay in starting the surgery. But Diego was firm in insisting that the patient was not well informed about the procedure. When the surgeon came in to explain it again to Mr. Herrera, it became clear that the patient had no idea that there would be a large incision and screws and plates would be implanted in his back. He kept asking, "But will you do it with a laser?" Mr. Herrera hadn't realized that the surgery would be so involved, and wanted more time to think about it. The surgery was then canceled and in the end, the surgeon thanked Diego. He said he was glad that Diego had made him explain it again to the patient, because had Mr. Herrera gone through with the surgery without understanding what was involved, it would not have been a good outcome. One of the most surprising things about this case is that Mr. Hererra had seen at least three nurses and two physicians prior to seeing Diego, and yet no one had realized that he hadn't understood what the surgery involved. It is essential that professional interpreters be used when obtaining informed consent, and critical that the patient be able to explain back their understanding of the procedure.

Nonverbal Communication

Eye Contact

Ellen was trying to teach her Navajo patient, Jim Nez, how to live with his newly diagnosed diabetes. She soon became extremely frustrated because she felt she was not getting through to him. He asked very few questions and never met her eyes. She reasoned from this that he was uninterested and therefore not listening to her.

53

Rather than signaling disinterest, however, Mr. Nez's behavior demonstrated a respect for the nurse's authority. His lack of eye contact probably reflected the Navajo belief that the eyes are the windows to the soul. To make direct eye contact is disrespectful and can endanger the spirits of both parties. Thus his lack of eye contact actually displayed his concern.

A former student of mine said she automatically rejected job applicants who did not make eye contact on the basis that they could not be trusted. In fact, there may be good cultural reasons why eye contact is purposely avoided.

Many Asians consider it disrespectful to look someone directly in the eye, especially if that person is in a superior position. Most Asian cultures are hierarchical; men are considered superior to women, parents to children, teachers to students, doctors to nurses, and so forth. Looking someone directly in the eye implies equality. An Asian patient may avoid eye contact out of respect for the "superior status" of the doctor or nurse, rather than for reasons of disinterest or dishonesty. A Korean nurse shared that when she scolded her children, she would get angry if they had the nerve to look her in the eye. She instructed them to show respect by looking down.

54 Angela, a nurse case manager, was doing patient teaching with Cha Xeng, a fourteen-year-old Hmong girl who had just delivered a premature baby. Cha Xeng had been in the United States since she was six years old and spoke English fluently. Angela was disturbed because Cha Xeng avoided making eye contact with her and spoke in a soft, timid voice. She immediately assumed that the young mother was hiding something from her, that she was having trouble bonding with the infant or was not interested in her child's special needs. The nurse even suspected her of using illegal drugs, all because she would not make eye contact.

In reality, Cha Xeng was showing Angela respect by avoiding contact. She kept her voice low to avoid appearing rude. She did not ask for further explanations, not out of lack of interest, but to avoid appearing stupid or implying that Angela was doing a poor job of explaining. Hmong culture, like most Asian cultures, is hierarchical. Cha Xeng's respect for Angela's higher status led Angela to make many incorrect assumptions.

Direct eye contact is also avoided in Nigeria to show respect. Rather than make eye contact with a physician, the Nigerian patient will probably look down.

Many Middle Easterners regard direct eye contact between a man and a woman as a sexual invitation. Female doctors or nurses dealing with Middle Eastern men must be aware that their eye contact may be interpreted not as directness but as seductiveness. In general, eye contact should be avoided with Middle Easterners of the opposite sex. Medical personnel should be aware of the meaning of eye contact in their patients' cultures and make sure the appropriate communication is both transmitted and received.

Touching

It is considered very poor taste in most Asian countries for people to touch in public. Men and women should not hug, kiss, or hold hands.

It is, however, common for individuals of the *same* sex to hold hands or walk arm-in-arm. It merely indicates that they are close friends or relatives.

Juen, a former student from mainland China, told me that when she first came to the United States she was staying in the home of an American family. One evening, a male friend of the family came to visit. When he left, he lightly kissed everyone good-bye, including Juen. She was completely shocked, and said, "When he kissed me, it made me feel so uncomfortable, just like you ate a fly!"

Health care workers should be advised that many Asian coworkers and patients will not be comfortable with the casual touching and hugging that many Latinos and Americans do without even thinking. Observe their behavior (and that of their families) to see what they are comfortable with.

When my mother was hospitalized, a rabbi associated with the hospital came to visit her. My husband and I were in the room at the time. We both introduced ourselves to the rabbi. My husband went first, and offered his hand, which the rabbi immediately shook. When I offered my hand, however, it hung in the air as the rabbi pointedly ignored it. After a moment I realized that he must be Orthodox and was thus forbidden to touch me. I've been told that other Orthodox rabbis *will* shake hands with a woman, rather than cause her embarrassment; this particular rabbi was from Chabad, one of the more ultra-Orthodox sects. If the rabbi were more culturally sensitive, he would have explained his actions. I felt uncomfortable by his rejection of my hand, even though, as an anthropologist, I understood it. The same rule against touching holds true for Muslims. Whenever possible, same-sex caregivers should be assigned to Orthodox Jews and Muslims, and opposite-sex touching should be avoided.

55

Gestures

56

Other forms of nonverbal communication can be equally problematic. An Anglo patient named Jon Smith called out to Maria, a Filipina nurse: "Nurse, nurse." Maria came to Mr. Smith's door and politely asked, "May I help you?" Mr. Smith beckoned for her to come closer by motioning with his right index finger. Maria remained where she was and responded in an angry voice, "What do you want?"

Mr. Smith was confused. Why had Maria's manner suddenly changed? The problem was that the innocent "come here" gesture is used in the Philippines (and in Korea) only to call animals, and in a sense Mr. Smith had called Maria a dog. To summon a person, Filipinos motion with the whole hand, palm in, and fingers down.

57   Unfortunately, many Americans are confused as to whether this gesture means "come here" or "go away," as Teresa, a Filipina nurse, discovered when she tried to call Nancy, an Anglo American nurse's aide, to assist her with a patient. She motioned to her, palm in, fingers down, to come over. Rather than move nearer to Teresa, Nancy merely smiled and waved back, using the same gesture. At the time, Teresa was confused and a bit hurt over Nancy's refusal to help her. She later learned that Nancy simply thought she was waving goodbye.

Problems such as this can best be handled through in-service education classes. If hospital personnel from other cultures are taught the different meanings of gestures, they might not take offense. Maria might have responded to Mr. Smith's request and then politely explained how she felt about the gesture. Mr. Smith would have learned something important about cross-cultural communication and probably refrained from using that gesture with a Filipino again.

There are other seemingly innocuous gestures that can create misunderstandings. The "V" made with the index and middle fingers (used in the U.S. to signify either peace or victory), has a very different meaning in British speaking countries such as Great Britain, South Africa, Australia and New Zealand. When done palm in, it has the same offensive meaning as a raised middle finger in U.S. culture. There is a story told that President George Bush senior unknowingly offended protesting farmers while in Australia by giving them what he thought was the "peace" sign, palm inward. That was not how the farmers interpreted it.

In Brazil, the "okay" sign (thumb and index fingers together in a circle, other fingers straight up) is a crude sexual invitation. I was giving a talk at a conference years ago, and when I mentioned that gesture, a clergyman in the audience raised his hand and shared an incident that occurred when he was doing missionary work in Brazil. He had finished his service and was packing his suitcases to leave. Two nuns entered his room and asked if he needed any help. He shook his head "no," and gave them what he thought was the "okay" sign, to signal that he was fine and didn't need any assistance. Needless to say, the nuns were quite offended. A man of the cloth was crudely inviting *nuns* to have sex!

"Thumbs-up" in Iran, like the "V" held palm in, is an insulting gesture similar to the raised middle finger in U.S. culture. If an Iranian patient ever asks how his test results came out, refrain from giving him a thumbs up.

Body Language

Body language is another form of nonverbal communication fraught with the possibility of unintentional messages. I first learned about this when setting up a demonstration regarding interpreters in one of my classes. I had arranged myself and two other students in a triangle; I was the patient, one of the other students was the physician, and the other was the interpreter. I then asked the class what was wrong with the picture. My intention was to illustrate that the triangle was a poor set-up, since it led to a lack of eye contact between the health care provider and the patient. However, that is not what the first volunteer commented on.

My student from Ghana noted that I was challenging the physician with my posture. "What posture?" I asked. She indicated the fact that my arms were folded in front of my body, a position I had put them in because I didn't have any pockets and didn't know what to do with my hands. She explained that in Ghana they should be kept behind the body to show respect, "unless," she added, "you're being yelled at, in which case it is okay to keep them in front."

At that point, one of the Vietnamese students joined in the discussion, saying that in Vietnam it is a sign of disrespect to keep your hands in back. The same is true in Korea and the Philippines, according to other students from those countries. The Asian students all agreed that hands should be kept folded in front. In Vietnam, they should be at waist level; in the Philippines, they can be down. Once again, the same gesture can have very different meaning, depending on where you are.

Although there will be times when you inadvertently offend someone with a gesture or body language, the best thing to do when you notice their reaction is to apologize and ask what it means in their culture. These can be excellent opportunities to exchange information about different cultural customs.

Time Orientation

As explained in the previous chapter, time orientation can refer to two different aspects of how people relate to time. One aspect involves whether they are oriented toward the clock or to activities. Conflicts can occur when someone who is clock oriented interacts with someone who is activity oriented. Another aspect of time orientation is more global, and relates to whether people tend to focus on the past, present, or future. The health care culture, as a subculture of American culture, tends to be future oriented, even though many of the patients it serves are present oriented.

Clock Time Versus Activity Time

Cultural differences in clock time versus activity time become particularly significant in health care clinics, which tend to be run on clock time and are often frequented by people operating on activity time. The following two cases illustrate the problem.

58   Mr. Jacinto, a middle-aged Filipino patient new to the clinic, arrived thirty minutes late for his appointment. The front clerk asked him to reschedule, because he was too late to be seen. Mr. Jacinto was very upset, complaining that in the Philippines his doctor would see him even if he were an hour late. He didn't realize that there would be a problem. He was adamant that he be seen right away for the physical exam he needed to obtain a license from the Department of Motor Vehicles. Araceli, a Filipina nurse, was called over to talk with Mr. Jacinto. Knowing the importance of respect in Filipino culture, she used the words *po* and *opo*, both words of respect in Tagalog. She explained in their mutual native language that according to clinic policy, a patient will be asked to reschedule an appointment if he or she arrives fifteen minutes after the scheduled time to avoid creating a long backup in the clinic. Araceli then found him an appointment for the next day, and emphasized the need to arrive on time. Mr. Jacinto was mollified, and thankful both for the respect he had been given through her use of *po* and *opo*, and for the explanation. Most people will be reasonable if they are treated with respect and are made to understand why things are being done the way they are. Too often patients are simply told the rules, without the reasons behind them, and treated in a curt manner, because health care professionals are often overworked with very little time for the "niceties." However, taking a moment in the first place can ultimately save a lot of time and aggravation. (When you read Chapter 13 on Improving Adherence, keep in mind the importance of explaining the rationale for things.)

59   It is possible to work with people's time orientation. Juanita Avelar was a forty-nine-year-old Mexican woman with kidney failure and diabetes. She relied on her niece and nephew to drive her to the clinic and was often late. In Mexican culture, the needs of the family typically take precedence over those of an individual. The nurses learned to take this into account when scheduling her appointments, and they allowed plenty of time for the family to discuss Mrs. Avelar's condition as a family. When certain tests and medications required specific timing for accuracy and effectiveness, they stressed the importance of clock time.

People from developing countries often have a present time orientation. These cultures are usually based on agriculture, which does not require adherence to a clock. It is only in industrialized nations that clock time is important. Because the performance of everyone's job depends on all others doing theirs, it becomes necessary to adhere to a standard of time. Health care professionals can do little about the present time orientation of patients. It is difficult for people who are not used to running their lives by the clock, who think it is rude to interrupt one activity to start another, or whose poverty makes it difficult for them to adhere to other people's schedules, to change their ways. The best health care professionals can do is to stress how important it is that patients show up on time for scheduled appointments. But they should be prepared for patients to be late, or better yet, design more flexible scheduling if the patient population warrants it. See Chapter 14 for what some clinics are doing to resolve the conflict of time orientations in scheduling.

Sometimes it is important that medication be taken on a specific schedule, for example, one time daily in the morning. If the patient is not oriented to the clock, it can be helpful to find out the patient's routine and incorporate it into his or her schedule. For example, if the patient watches the news every morning, tell them to take the medication when the news comes on. But be sure the patient clearly understands what you mean. I was on a panel at a conference, and one of the other speakers shared a story of a Mexican patient who was told to "take his medication with food." The patient thus took the bottle of pills to work every day in his lunch box. He never actually swallowed the medication, but was quite compliant in literally "taking them with food."

Past, Present, and Future Time Orientation

As discussed in Chapter 1, a present time orientation can conflict with the future time orientation of the health care profession, often resulting in lack of adherence to medical recommendations. Although people living in poverty or coming from developing countries often have a *present* time orientation, it may be hard to predict. One way to begin to assess patients' time orientation is to listen to the types of questions they ask and statements they make. Such questions as, "Does the pain in my finger mean I'm developing arthritis?" "How will this medication affect my life expectancy?" and statements like, "I want to lose 20 pounds by next year" indicate a *future* time orientation. Questions like, "I know you want me to take this medication so I don't have a heart attack, but how will it affect my sleep?" and statements such as, "I only take my blood pressure pills when my blood pressure feels high" and "I'll deal with that when it happens" indicate a *present* time orientation. Statements like, "I drink tea with honey and lemon when I have a sore throat; that's what my nana always gave me" indicate a *past* time orientation.

Jaime Ortega, a middle-aged Latino patient, suffered from congestive heart failure and hyperkalemia. He was readmitted to the hospital only two weeks after being discharged. Celia, the admitting nurse, discovered that Mr. Ortega had neglected to take the lasix and potassium the doctor

60

had ordered. Why? Because he felt much better; he no longer had any shortness of breath or swelling in his leg. Because his symptoms had disappeared, he stopped taking the medications. After a few days, fluid began to build in his system, necessitating a return to the hospital. Rather than look ahead to the long-term consequences of his condition and need for medication, Mr. Ortega focused on the present. As soon as he felt well, he discontinued the medication.

Physicians are unlikely to change the time orientation of their patients; however, adherence is often key to positive outcomes. Understanding the time orientation of your patient can be important in patient teaching. It may be necessary for physicians to spend extra time with patients who have a present time orientation, in order to make sure they clearly understand the reason for following medical advice, and the consequences of lack of adherence. It might be helpful to tie long-term measures or preventive medication to concrete outcomes of values the patient holds, for example, "If you want to see your daughter get married . . ." or "If you want to hold your grandchild. . . ."

Keep in mind that all patients, even those with a future time orientation, are more likely to adhere to medical recommendations if they understand the reasons. How many half-full bottles of antibiotics sit in medicine cabinets around the country?

Summary

Miscommunication between health care professionals and their patients often has nothing to do with ethnic background. A common problem is the use of medical jargon, for example, "voided" instead of "peed" or "myocardial infarction" instead of "heart attack." Patients may lack the technical vocabulary to describe their symptoms in a way physicians can understand. Some patients may be very forthright, whereas others may need probing; a health care provider must be sensitive to different communication styles. Patients may be too embarrassed to discuss certain problems, particularly those of a sexual nature. A health care provider needs excellent communication skills to be able to handle sensitive issues.

When the health care provider and the patient are of different ethnic backgrounds, there are numerous additional opportunities for misunderstandings. Communication styles and time orientation vary considerably from culture to culture, causing confusion and sometimes annoyance for hospital personnel. As a further complication, people from different cultures may behave in similar ways for different reasons. Understanding why people communicate (or do not) in the way they do, however, can help relieve the frustration of health care workers and perhaps contribute to better patient care.

Key Points

- Avoid using idioms.
- Avoid using the terms "positive" and "negative" with respect to test results in order to avoid confusion with the lay meaning of those terms.
- Pay attention to patients' nonverbal reactions.
- Avoid asking "yes" or "no" questions with Asian patients; it is generally better to ask open-ended questions with *all* patients.
- *Listen* to the responses your patients give you; don't direct them what to answer.
- Realize that some patients prefer shared decision-making, while others prefer a more directive approach. Be flexible and match your approach to the expectations of your patient.
- Some patients expect a more personal relationship with their health care providers.
- Encourage patients to ask questions. Ask, "What questions do you have?" not, "Do you have any questions?"
- Ask patients what they know about their condition.
- Ask patients about their ethnic and religious background, and explain why you are asking.
- Use professional, trained interpreters. Use telephone interpreters if live ones are not available. Avoid using family members, especially children, whenever possible.
- Understand that lack of eye contact means different things in different cultures. Avoid using gestures; they can mean different things in different cultures.
- People from lower socioeconomic strata often have a present time orientation. They may need additional patient teaching when it comes to preventive medicine, and outcomes should be attached to things they value.

For additional issues related to informed consent, see Chapters 6 and 7.
For additional issues related to language and communication, see Chapter 8.

Chapter 3

Pain

An important health care issue is the treatment of pain. Untreated pain can interfere with the healing process, both by reducing the amount of movement that is comfortable for the patient and by compromising the immune system. Before it can be treated, however, it must be properly assessed. This can cause confusion for health care providers who are unaware of cultural differences in response to pain, particularly in how it is expressed. Some patients come from cultures that encourage emotional expressiveness. Others come from cultures in which stoicism is valued, thus masking any visual signs of pain patients might be experiencing, as well as inhibiting requests for pain medication. Also crucial are cultural variations in attitudes toward the use of pain medication.

Expression of Pain

Although the physical experience of pain is a human universal, there is tremendous variation in the way pain is expressed. Although there are, of course, individual differences, cultures also influence whether or not people will be stoic or expressive in response to pain.

61   Differing responses to pain are well illustrated in the cases of Mr. Wu and Mr. Valdez. Bobbie, the nurse, had two patients who had both had coronary artery bypass grafts. Mr. Valdez, a middle-aged Nicaraguan man, was the first to come up from the recovery room. He was already hooked up to a morphine PCA (patient-controlled analgesia) machine, which allowed him to administer pain medication as needed in controlled doses and at controlled intervals. For the next two hours, he summoned Bobbie every ten minutes to request more pain medication. Bobbie finally called the physician to have his dosage increased and to request additional pain injections every three hours as needed. Every three hours he requested an injection. He continually whimpered in painful agony.

Mr. Wu, a Chinese patient, was transferred from the recovery room 62
an hour later. In contrast to Mr. Valdez, he was quiet and passive. He,
too, was in pain, because he used his PCA machine frequently, but he
did not show it. When Bobbie offered supplemental pain pills, he
refused them. Not once did he use the call light to summon her.

This is an instance of two patients with the same condition, yet vastly
different ways of handling the pain. Nurses usually report that "expressive" patients often come from Hispanic, Middle Eastern, and Mediterranean backgrounds, while "stoic" patients often come from Northern
European and Asian backgrounds. As a young Chinese man told me,
"Even since I was a little boy, my family watched dubbed Chinese mov-
ies, and by watching many of the male protagonists state 'I'd rather shed
blood than my tears,' it is imbedded in my mind that crying or showing
pain shows my weakness." However, simply knowing a person's ethnicity
will not allow you to predict accurately how a patient will respond to
pain; in fact, there are great dangers in stereotyping, as the next case
demonstrates.

Mrs. Mendez, a sixty-two-year-old Mexican patient, had just had a fem- 63
oral-popliteal bypass graft on her right leg. She was still under sedation
when she entered the recovery room, but an hour later she awoke and
began screaming, "*Aye! Aye! Aye! Mucho dolor!* [Much pain]." Robert, her
nurse, immediately administered the dosage of morphine the doctor
had prescribed. This did nothing to diminish Mrs. Mendez's cries of
pain. He then checked her vital signs and pulse; all were stable. Her
dressing had minimal bloody drainage. To all appearances, Mrs. Mendez
was in good condition. Robert soon became angry over her outbursts
and stereotyped her as a "whining Mexican female who, as usual, was
exaggerating her pain."

After another hour, Robert called the physician. The surgical team
came on rounds and opened Mrs. Mendez's dressing. Despite a slight
swelling in her leg, there was minimal bleeding. However, when the physician inserted a large needle into the incision site, he removed a large
amount of blood. The blood had put pressure on the nerves and tissues
in the area and caused her excruciating pain.

She was taken back to the operating room. This time, when she
returned and awoke in recovery, she was calm and cooperative. She complained only of minimal pain. Had the physician not examined her
again and discovered the blood in the incision site, Mrs. Mendez would
have probably suffered severe complications.

Despite the fact that Mexicans are generally expressive of their pain,
it does not mean that every Mexican patient will be, or that there is not
a legitimate basis for their cries. Oftentimes, recent immigrants from
Mexico are quite stoic, especially the males, according to one nurse.

The generalizations in this chapter (and book) are meant to be only generalizations; beware the dangers of stereotyping—it can have disastrous consequences.

64   One case involving cultural differences in expressing pain had a tragic ending. The Irish mother-in-law of one of my nursing students was in the hospital. She was scheduled for surgery at the end of the week. (This happened many years ago, before hospital stays became more limited.) Her family became very concerned when she suddenly started complaining of pain. They knew Mrs. Carroll was typically Irish in her stoicism. They spoke to her doctor, who was from India. He was not worried. In his country, women were usually vocal when in pain. He ignored their requests that the surgery be done sooner, thinking it unnecessary.

When he finally did operate, he discovered that Mrs. Carroll's condition had progressed to the point that she could not be saved. My student, a nurse, felt that if he had recognized her expressions of pain as a sign that something was very wrong and had operated sooner, she might have lived.

65   Serena received Maria Messina, an elderly Italian patient, from triage. The triage nurse warned Serena that Mrs. Messina was "very dramatic." Fortunately for Mrs. Messina, Serena had been taking a course in cultural diversity. She realized that Italian culture encourages emotional expressiveness. She spoke very calmly to Mrs. Messina and her family and explained what would happen to her while she was in the hospital. She then administered some non-narcotic pain medication. Within ten minutes, Mrs. Messina had calmed down and reported a significant lessening in her pain. She thanked Serena effusively for her wonderful care. It can take so little to turn a difficult patient into a grateful one.

A classic study done in a New York hospital in the early 1950s sheds some light on Mrs. Messina's behavior. Mark Zborowski's project (1952) focused on three groups: Jews, Italians, and "Old Americans" (White Anglo-Saxon Protestants, or WASPs). These groups were selected because Jews and Italians had a reputation for "exaggerating" their pain, whereas the behavior of "Old Americans" was consistent with the values of the medical system; they were stoic and undemanding.

Although Jews and Italians reacted similarly to pain—loudly—they did so for different reasons. The Italians complained because the pain hurt. Pain medication usually satisfied them. This remedy was rarely effective with Jewish patients, however. In addition to everything else, they would then worry about becoming addicted. Their primary concern was not the pain sensation but the meaning and significance of the pain. How would it affect them and their families? The next case exemplifies this finding, and the one after typifies the "Old American" response.

Jane Stein's pinky finger hurt. Not enough to need an aspirin, but   66
enough to cause her worry for the entire summer of her thirty-fifth year.
She was concerned because her grandmother had suffered from bad
arthritis. Did the slight pain in her pinky signal oncoming arthritis?
Would her hands be gnarled by the time she was forty, and would she
be unable even to walk by the time she was fifty? Fortunately, the pain
eventually went away, and Jane is fine. But she is a wonderful example
of how the concern of many Jewish patients is more for the meaning
and significance of the pain than it is for the pain itself. Compare Jane's
experience with that of young Heather Brady.

Mimsy Brady took her young daughter Heather to see the doctor. This   67
Anglo American girl was suffering from a very painful condition that
caused her to grow nerve tumors. While the physician poked and prod-
ded Heather, she stiffened, but never cried out. The doctor gave them
some bad news about Heather's condition, but both mother and daughter remained stoic. When the physician left the room, Heather burst
into tears. When Mrs. Brady asked her why she didn't tell the doctor
how much it hurt, she said, "I didn't want to seem like a baby in front
of him." Mrs. Brady waited until she was alone to cry.

Zborowski observed that Jews and Italians have a similar socialization
process. Children are warned to avoid injury, colds, and fights. Crying
elicits sympathy, concern, and aid. The more they complain, the more
attention and sympathy they receive. In many Jewish families, even a
sneeze is seen as illness, thus predisposing children to become anxious
about the meaning and significance of any symptoms. Jewish and Italian
children are praised for avoiding physical injury and reprimanded for
ignoring bad weather or drafts, or for playing rough games. Although
this may not be as true today as it was at the time of the study, the
behavior of older patients may still reflect this upbringing.

In contrast, WASP children are encouraged to participate in sports.
Boys are taught to "take pain like a man" rather than "cry like a sissy"
when injured. The body is seen as a machine, which when not working
(that is, when ill or injured) should be taken to a specialist (a doctor)
and treated with as little fuss as possible.

Given their upbringing, it should not be surprising that adult Jews
and Italians complain and desire attention when ill, while WASPs tend
to be "easy" patients. When they are ill, most people revert to childhood
behavior, even if the desired results are not forthcoming. If, like the
Jewish patient described earlier, they were rewarded for complaining as
children, they will complain as adults. If they were taught to lie quietly
and not make a fuss, they will probably do the same when they grow up.

Many nurses find it difficult to care for patients like Mrs. Messina who
are expressive of their pain. Nurses often prefer stoicism and compliance. When they do not get it, they tend to do as little as possible, and

a new nurse is assigned to such patients each day. However, as many of the examples in this book show, a little patience and understanding can make a huge difference. The important thing is to figure out the source of the patient's concern; this is something that can often be ascertained simply by asking. Once you understand the source, it is much easier to address.

Why are people from some cultures generally more expressive of pain than those from others? One theory I would offer is that it has to do in part with the weather and degree of crowding. If it is cold, or heavily populated, such that large numbers of people are forced into close contact for long periods of time, it is generally advantageous to have people control their emotions. Otherwise, fights and general chaos are likely to result. In such cultures, such as those in northern Europe (cold weather) and Japan (crowding), individuals are socialized to control their emotions. The British (who live on a small island where the climate is often cool), for example, take pride in having a "stiff upper lip." In warmer and less crowded conditions, if there is conflict, people can leave the scene. There is less inherent danger of chaos and, thus, no cultural "selection" for controlling one's emotions.

68   A triage nurse working in the emergency department of a major urban medical center stated that part of her job is to pay attention to who "looks sick" in the waiting room. After taking a course on cultural diversity, she began looking at the whole picture, rather than being influenced solely by how expressive the person is. She now recognizes that the Chinese woman with abdominal pain, sitting in the corner and quietly rocking back and forth, may be in much more acute distress than the Mexican patient with abdominal pain who is yelling one moment, and laughing with his family the next.

Pediatrics

It should be noted when dealing with very young children that their expressions of pain are very similar. Differences arise around school age, when they tend to take on the behaviors they've learned from their parents. As one pediatric nurse observed, some young Hispanic males will attempt to be "brave, quiet and uncomplaining," but when assessed and observed for nonverbal cues, are clearly suffering. Mirroring the variation among adult males, others will be quite expressive. Another nurse noted that Middle Eastern children tend to be very expressive, regardless of gender. In contrast, Vietnamese children, like their parents, are often very stoic. It shouldn't be surprising that children learn how to respond to pain from adults, and carry that behavior into adulthood, passing it on to their own children.

Paj Khab, a sixteen-year-old Hmong girl, was suffering with Ewing's   69
sarcoma, a very painful bone cancer. She never asked for pain medication or complained about pain. When Karen came on shift, she entered
Paj's room. The girl was silent, but had tears rolling down her face.
When Karen asked her to rate her pain, she rated it a 10 out of 10, the
worst pain imaginable. On earlier visits, when her demeanor was quiet
and calm with no outward signs of pain, she had rated it a 7 or 8 out of
10. Karen noted that they had difficulty with pain control because both
Paj and her parents would usually refuse any pain medication until the
pain reached a 10.

Although the patients described thus far fit the cultural generalizations for response to pain, remember that there is always variation.

Evie Scott, a five-year-old Jewish child, had to have a urinary catheter   70
inserted for the first time. This is an unpleasant procedure, yet Evie
said she was going to be "very, very brave and not be a baby." True to
her word, she was wide awake and aware through the procedure and
thanked Amelia, her nurse, when it was done. Evie didn't cry, but Amelia did.

Pain Medication

Requesting Pain Medication

There is a general assumption on the part of most health care professionals that if someone is in pain, they will ask for pain medication.
Unfortunately, that is not always the case.

Some patients tolerate even the most severe pain with little more than   71
a clenched jaw and frequently refuse pain medication. Osito Seisay, a
Nigerian farmer who had been injured by a charging bull, was in the
United States for arthroscopic knee surgery. His nurse waited for him
to request pain medication, but he never did. She learned the reason
when his sister-in-law came to visit and spoke to Mr. Seisay in his native
language. Mr. Seisay was Muslim, and he was enduring the pain as an
offering to Allah in thanks for the good fortune of being allowed such
specialized surgery.

Vickie, a research nurse dispensing experimental analgesics, noted   72
that an elderly Filipino patient named Fernando Abatay had not
received any pain medication following his shoulder repair. When she
asked him how much pain he was experiencing, he replied, "A lot."
Vickie then questioned why he had not taken any medication. Mr. Abatay explained, "No one asked me if I wanted a shot and I didn't want to
bother the nurses." The regular nurses assigned to him claimed that

they could not tell he was in pain, and because he did not request any pain medication, they saw no need to give him any.

Mr. Abatay's behavior can be explained in part by the Filipino concept of *Bahala na* (God's will). Filipinos may appear stoic because they believe pain is the will of God and thus God will give them the strength to bear it. Besides, one cannot change it. This attitude is reminiscent of the fatalistic Hispanic concept *Qué será, será*. A second explanation relates to Filipinos' respect for authority. Mr. Abatay did not want to bother the nurses. A professional's time is valuable and, unless one's problem is very serious, it is better left unmentioned. I know of at least one hospital in which the policy is to only administer pain medication when the patient requests it. Patients like Mr. Abatay would certainly suffer under such a policy. It is extremely important that nurses inquire about a patient's pain levels and not wait until the patient brings it up.

73   Keisha handled a similar situation somewhat differently, applying cultural competence skills. Bjung Hsu, an Asian patient, never requested postoperative pain medication. Keisha, his nurse, realized that he might be practicing stoicism. She therefore looked beyond the absence of complaints and noted his elevated vital signs. She then took the time to educate him on the importance of pain management. She explained that it would reduce recovery time and the risk of postoperative complications. Mr. Hsu then accepted pain medication and recovered comfortably, without incident.

His attitude is very different from that of most American patients. The Chinese are taught self-restraint. Assertive and individualistic people are considered crude and poorly socialized. The needs of the group are more important than those of the individual. Inconspicuousness is highly valued and in recent history has proved necessary for survival. It is best not to call attention to oneself.

One other factor that may be involved in Asians' refusal of pain medication is courtesy. They generally consider it impolite to accept something the first time it is offered. Several nurses from mainland China said they often went hungry during the first few weeks of their stay in the United States. Whenever someone asked them if they wanted something to eat, they politely refused, awaiting a second offer. It rarely came. They soon learned that in America, if one does not accept something the first time, there may be no second chance. Hospital nurses are so busy that they seldom offer something more than once. They should be aware of Asian rules of etiquette when offering pain medication, food, back rubs, or other services.

The safest approach for the health care professional is to anticipate the needs of an Asian patient for pain medication without waiting for requests. If patients are told that their doctor ordered the medication—

and why, they will be less likely to refuse on the grounds of courtesy. Asians tend to respect the authority of the physician. But if patients continue to refuse medication, their wishes should be respected.

Attitudes Toward Pain Medication

Use of pain medication is a somewhat controversial topic due to a widespread and somewhat misplaced fear of drug addiction.

Kari, a nurse from India, recounted the story of her aunt who recently had a total knee replacement. She went to visit her two days after she was discharged from the hospital. Kari noticed that her aunt seemed very tense. She asked her when she had last taken her pain medication. Before her aunt could answer, her son, a physician, responded, "Oh, Mom had her last pain medicine yesterday and she really does not need any more medicine. After all, we don't want her to get too used to taking the pain medication." In this case, reducing the pain medication had a negative impact on her aunt's health. She had stopped using her passive range-of-motion machine because it was too painful. By doing so, she risked not regaining full movement in her knee. It was important that her aunt take her pain medication as prescribed so she could become more mobile as well as more comfortable.

The potential problem might have been avoided if the health care provider had explained the rationale behind the use of pain medication. Its purpose is not merely to make her feel better, but also to allow her to do the rehabilitation exercises necessary for recovery.

It is important that education regarding pain and pain control be done with the family of the patient present. Many patients have misunderstandings regarding the importance of pain medication to recovery, as well as the dangers of addiction. Family members who are not educated in the reality of pain medicine may put pressure on the patient to avoid using it. Sometimes having a social worker present when discussing it with the family and patient can be helpful.

It is also important for patients and providers to understand the nature of addiction. It is largely a psychological and behavioral disorder rather than a physical dependency. When properly prescribed, patients, unlike addicts, do not need increasingly large doses to treat pain because they do not develop a tolerance for it. If higher dosages are needed, it is usually because an inadequate dosage was prescribed in the first place.

There has been a movement in the past few decades to educate health care professionals about pain medication and to combat the general prejudice against using high dosages. This is especially important for

74

dying patients, since many have suffered needless pain due to physicians' fear of overmedication. Perhaps this is part of the legacy of our Puritan forebears, the belief that pain should be stoically borne. But given the advances in pain medication, except under the most unusual circumstances, there is no reason for anyone to die in pain.

Drug Seeking

It is not uncommon to hear a physician or nurse remark about a patient—usually a minority patient or someone who appears to be living on the street—"Oh, he's just seeking drugs." The response is usually to withhold such drugs from the patient, whom they see as a "drug addict" whose addiction should not be supported. However, as one renowned emergency department physician noted, you can't ever truly know who is in pain and who is not.

The Form of Medication

Medication can be administered in many forms, including orally, intravenously, and intramuscularly via a "shot." Although one might assume that the least painful form would be preferred, that is not always the case.

75   Mr. Hassan was an eighty-one-year-old Egyptian patient suffering from advanced lung cancer with bone metastases. Pain control was achieved with long-acting oral morphine. He was receiving hospice care from a home health agency. According to the hospital discharge planner, his pain was well controlled with two narcotic analgesic tablets twice a day; however, when the hospice nurse did her initial evaluation, she found that the patient was requesting intramuscular or intravenous medications, despite the absence of pain between dosages. She explained to him that oral medications were preferable, but he was not satisfied. Two days later, he was readmitted to the hospital, where he happily received an intravenous morphine infusion.

Why did he want intravenous medication or even shots when the oral medication was doing its job? Because he is from a culture in which many people believe that the more intrusive the procedure the better it is for them, just as it has been found that many Americans think medicine has to "taste bad" in order for it to be effective. There is a lesson from this example: it is best to ask the patient what type of medication is preferred, rather than assuming it should be the least invasive form.

Instructions on the Use of Pain Medication

It is essential that you carefully explain the use of pain medication, and the reasoning behind it, lest a situation like the following occurs.

Jesus Garcia, a middle-aged male Hispanic patient, was admitted to   76
the hospital following an overdose of pain medication. He had no history of depression or suicide attempts. It turned out that the overdose
was accidental. He had been told to take up to six tablets of pain medication a day. Since his pain was unbearable, he took all six tablets at once,
figuring it would be more effective.

It took a meeting with the hospital psychiatrist, who confirmed the
facts of the situation with the patient's wife, to understand what had
happened. Once it was understood, a nurse spent time going over the
protocol with Mr. Garcia. Had she done that in the first place, she could
have prevented a near accidental death.

Terminology

Be careful about the terminology you use with your patients, even if they   77
are English speaking. Hilda, a nurse working at a cancer center, had a
patient with unrelated leg pain. Mrs. Patterson, the patient, was referred
to the pain team at the center. Hilda was becoming a bit frustrated with
Mrs. Patterson because she kept canceling and rescheduling her
appointments, while continuing to complain about her pain. When
Hilda finally asked her why she wasn't keeping any of her appointments
with the pain team, Mrs. Patterson replied that she had already suffered
enough pain. She didn't need a team to provide her with more!

Once Hilda explained that the pain team would only assess her pain
and prescribe pain medication, that there was no pain involved in the
process, Mrs. Patterson kept her appointment and stopped calling to
complain.

The Influence of the Health Care Provider

It is important for health care providers to be aware of their own cultural
and personal biases and how they may affect their response to patients
in pain. According to Davidhizar and Giger (2004):

- If they expect patients to be stoic, they might over-react to patients
  who are expressive, or ignore them because they are "difficult"
  patients. If they expect patients to be expressive, they might ignore
  patients who are stoic.
- If they believe that pain is a part of life and to be endured, they may
  take a less aggressive approach to pain management than someone
  who believes pain can be managed and should be avoided.

- If they believe that pain is part of the childbirth experience, they may believe it doesn't require as much intervention as the laboring woman does.
- If they are concerned with drug addiction, they may hesitate to provide narcotics.
- If they are fearful of respiratory distress, they may be hesitant to provide a terminally ill patient with enough pain medication to ensure comfort and will thus cause the patient to suffer unnecessary pain.

78   Cecilia was a Filipina nurse in one of my classes. One day we were discussing the tendency of Filipino nurses to undermedicate their pain patients. If the physician prescribes a range of dosages, they will often administer the lowest dose. When asked about this, Filipino students have given a number of explanations. Pain medication is scarce in the Philippines, so they are trained not to use too much. One nurse said that in the Philippines families pay for the medicine they get in the hospital. Many can't afford it, which is one reason nurses use the lowest dosage prescribed. Other reasons mentioned include that addiction is highly feared; stoicism is valued; and, for Catholic Filipinos, there is virtue in suffering. After a few minutes, I noticed tears falling from Cecilia's eyes. When I asked her what was wrong, she explained that a year earlier her mother had died of cancer. The doctor had prescribed high dosages of pain medication in the months before her death. Cecilia administered the medication to her mother, but had cut each dosage in half before giving it to her mother. She did not want her mother to become addicted, she explained. Now, in class, she realized that she had allowed her mother to suffer needlessly. She was dying; what would it matter if she became addicted to the medication? The important lesson here is that caregivers must examine their own attitudes toward the use of pain medication and not let them affect the way they administer it to patients.

Summary

Pain is an unrelenting fact of human life. Although nearly all people experience pain sensations similarly, there are vast cultural differences in the expression of pain. Some cultures encourage the open expression of pain, while others socialize their members to be stoic. Although it is helpful at times to know these generalizations, inaccurate stereotyping can seriously compromise a patient's life. Treat each patient as an individual. The family can also be helpful in letting you know if the patient's behavior is typical or abnormal.

With regard to pain medication, it is often best to anticipate a patient's pain needs, since cultural or religious reasons may inhibit a patient from requesting pain medication even when it is medically necessary for recovery. Also realize that not every patient will share a desire for the least intrusive medication possible. When alternatives are available, it is best to check with the patient; which form would he or she prefer?

Key Points

- Culture influences whether a patient will be stoic or expressive in response to pain.
- Do not base your assessment of pain on the patient's expression of pain.
- Anticipate a patient's pain needs; do not wait for him or her to request pain medication, because cultural factors may inhibit them from asking.
- Address the patient's concerns regarding pain; for some it may be the pain sensation, for others, the meaning and significance of the pain.
- When alternate forms of pain medication are available, ask the patient what kind he or she would prefer.
- Address patient and family member concerns about addiction and explain the importance of pain medication to healing.
- Give clear instructions on the use of pain medication and explain the reasoning for it.
- Examine your own biases and make sure they do not affect your response to patients in pain.

For labor pain, see Chapter 9.
For more on medication, see Chapter 12.

Chapter 4

Religion and Spirituality

Religion is rarely a topic of conversation in hospitals, but religious beliefs and spiritual practices are common sources of conflict and misunderstanding. Patients' exercise of their beliefs can sometimes result in interference with medical care. This chapter examines religious and spiritual beliefs that can create conflicts, misunderstandings, or worse. It also looks at several cases where a culturally competent approach on the part of health care providers made a positive difference for patients.

Religious Practices

Buddhist

79   A twenty-year-old Buddhist monk from Cambodia was in same-day surgery for a hernia repair, accompanied by his mother, aunt, and male cousin. When Lisa, his nurse, entered the room, she greeted him, put her hand on his shoulder, and directed him to a chair across the room. The patient suddenly jumped from her in horror. His mother and aunt lunged at Lisa, shouting at her in Cambodian. Lisa fled the room and called a "code gray," which summoned all male hospital personnel to the area.

When everyone arrived, the cousin was in the corner comforting the patient. Security questioned the patient, but he did not speak enough English to respond. His cousin explained that the patient was a monk and could not be touched by a woman. Should it happen, he was not to look at her, move, or respond in any way. Even a slight tensing of the muscles would be interpreted as showing desire and a breaking of his vows. Because of the incident, he would have to do great penance.

Sadly, this incident could have been avoided. Apparently, the need for strict sexual segregation had been thoroughly discussed with the physician prior to admission. The doctor assured them that there would be no problem. However, he neglected to convey this information to the staff. The hospital made arrangements to assure that thereafter the patient would have contact only with males, but the damage had already been done.

Although this is an unusual case, it highlights the importance of sexual segregation found in many religious and ethnic groups.

Catholic

Hilda Romero, an elderly Spanish-speaking Hispanic patient, was brought into the recovery room following a laparoscopic cholecystectomy. Rita, her nurse, was told Mrs. Romero had requested to be seen by a Catholic priest in the pre-op holding area, but they had been unable to accommodate her request due to time constraints. Rita thought that even though the surgery was over, she should still try to fulfill her patient's request. She called the chaplain's office and asked for a Spanish-speaking priest to come to the recovery room. When the priest arrived, Rita drew her curtains for privacy. Mrs. Romero and the priest spoke a while, and he said a prayer. When Mrs. Romero told her family what Rita had done, they all thanked her profusely. Later that week, Mrs. Romero and her family sent Rita a touching thank-you note and a box of chocolates (which she shared with the staff). Rita then realized the impact that a simple call to a priest had had for the patient.

80

Christian Scientist

Betty Williams, a sixty-five-year-old Anglo American woman, came to see a physician specializing in diseases of the colon and rectum. Although Christian Scientists generally take a spiritual rather than physical approach to healing, using their own practitioners, they are allowed to see a physician, and Mrs. Williams made that choice when she began experiencing rectal pain. She was diagnosed with a rectal tumor. The physician, Dr. James, recommended surgery. She refused, despite the fact that it was a resectable tumor and there was no apparent spread. Dr. James saw her over the next six years. In that time, the tumor grew. Mrs. Williams began to experience bleeding and discomfort. She finally agreed to a colonoscopy, but not to a resection of the tumor. Dr. James operated on her. She was "clean" inside. The tumor had not metastasized. If she had allowed the surgeon to resect the tumor, she would have been cured of colon cancer. But her religious beliefs did not allow her to go that far. She would only allow palliative intervention. She died two years later, after the tumor did metastasize. I spoke with one of Dr. James's partners and asked how the physicians felt about the situation.

81

"Sad," he replied. "We could have saved her, but she chose another path." In this case, the physicians acted with cultural competence. Although Mrs. William's actions conflicted with their own beliefs, they accepted her decisions, and did what they could to help her while staying within the bounds of her beliefs.

This case is also interesting as an illustration of the range of beliefs within a religion. One of the basic tenets of the Christian Science Church is that God's creation of man and the universe is perfect. Disease is thus a "misunderstanding." Further, all reality is thought to be ultimately mental/spiritual, not material/physical. Illness, therefore, is of mental, not physical origin and can be cured through proper mental processes. Treatment consists of prayer and counsel with the sick person, and involves three phases. In the first phase, the practitioner tries to remove the sick person's belief in suffering; in the second, the practitioner tries to convince the patient that he or she is well and knows it; in the final phase, the practitioner focuses on his or her own thoughts to free the afflicted person of the belief in sickness. Due to their beliefs, Christian Scientists will rarely seek out medical care. They have seen the effectiveness of spiritual healing. Yet, as in this case, they are free to choose medical intervention. Mrs. Williams even agreed to a colostomy, but drew the line at surgery to remove her tumor, a decision that ultimately cost her her life but preserved her spiritual integrity. Presumably, Mrs. Williams sought the assistance of a Christian Science practitioner at the same time that she saw Dr. James. Dr. James's associate expressed some small surprise that her tumor went so long without metastasizing. Perhaps spiritual healing kept it at bay.

Indian Orthodox Christian

The following case study is not one that will be experienced frequently, but it contains many interesting aspects.

82   His Holiness, the spiritual leader of an Indian Orthodox Christian church, became a patient in an American hospital when he fell ill during a visit to an American diocese. His condition required cardiac catheterization and open-heart surgery. Because it was determined that despite the extraordinary precautions taken his body had become contaminated during the first procedure, there was a ten-day delay during which he had to undergo a purification ceremony before he could have open-heart surgery.

How had he become contaminated? First of all, the surgical team members had allowed non-Orthodox Christians to do the electrocardiogram and blood withdrawal and to shave the groin on His Holiness. Second, priests and bishops in this church must avoid exposing their bodies to any female in order to maintain purity. Although there were no female members directly caring for His Holiness, the director of the catheterization laboratory was a female. Even though she was in the back room, operating the x-ray machines, this was a breach of sexual segregation: His Holiness's private parts had been exposed to a woman.

Although he had not received any food prior to surgery—as is common when anesthesia is used—the medical team allowed him to receive Holy Communion the morning of his heart catheterization. Unfortunately, this led to a cardinal sin. After surgery, His Holiness vomited and the medical team discarded the emesis. The bread and wine of Holy Communion are the blood and body of Jesus Christ; when he vomited, His Holiness was in essence vomiting Christ. The hospital staff should have saved the emesis to be drunk by the priests and bishops there to take care of His Holiness. Drinking the emesis is considered a very holy act that will wash away one's sins.

The cardiologist in charge of the surgery, himself a member of the church, was held responsible for the breaches of purity. He has been socially isolated from the church as a result. His Holiness's party members, also complicit in the contamination, have probably been banished to remote church monasteries simply because a highly qualified woman was allowed to work the x-ray equipment in the back room and because the hospital staff discarded some vomit.

Although routine sexual segregation is a common practice in many cultures, it is important for health care providers to realize that in some religious contexts it is not just a preference but a mandate. If that rule is to be violated in any way—such as allowing a woman to work the x-ray equipment—this should be discussed beforehand. Had the cardiologist realized the strength of the church's requirements in the matter, he probably would not have had her at that job. Second, it would be a good idea to go over all possible complications (such as vomiting) to discuss any rules in that regard. Recognizing that rules for religious leaders may be much more stringent than those for others, and ascertaining them in advance, will avoid most of the problems.

Muslim

Maggie answered the call light and heard a panic-stricken voice saying, "Please come to my room. My neighbor collapsed on the floor and is lying there, muttering. I think he had a seizure." She ran to the room with the charge nurse and discovered Ali Saeed on the floor behind the curtain, praying. Mr. Saeed did not speak English, and his bilingual son had left the room. When Mr. Saeed knelt on the floor to pray, his neighbor had no idea what he was doing and no way to ask. Concerned, he summoned the nurse with the call light.

83

Devout Muslims believe they must pray facing toward Mecca, the Holy city, five times a day. They pray on the floor, with their forehead on the ground to show submission to Allah (God). Traditionally, they pray on a prayer rug placed on the floor. Though most Muslims in the United States use prayer rugs only in the privacy of their homes, devout Muslims in the Middle East may take them when they travel. Because Mr. Saeed was scheduled for surgery the next day, he thought it was especially important to pray. Culturally sensitive health care providers will learn on admission about such practices and arrange for privacy during those times. Some culturally sensitive hospitals provide prayer rugs for their Muslim patients (see Chapter 14).

Jehovah's Witness

Most people are aware of the Jehovah's Witness prohibition about accepting blood transfusions. They believe that blood represents life and is therefore sacred. They base this belief upon several sections of the Bible, including Leviticus 17:10: "Whatsoever man . . . eateth any manner of blood; I will . . . cut him off from among his people"; Leviticus 17:11: "For the life of the flesh is in the blood"; and Acts 15:20: "Abstain from . . . things strangled and from blood." They have no problems accepting any other form of medical treatment, and will use non-blood expanders. Blood is the only medical issue, as in the following case.

84   Susi Givens, a thirty-seven-year-old woman with two children, was horseback riding one day when a snake startled her horse. She was thrown off and landed on a stump, resulting in massive internal injuries. She was rushed to the hospital, where the surgical team discovered that there was a large amount of blood in her abdomen and that she needed to have a kidney removed.

Mrs. Givens had a medical alert card identifying her as a Jehovah's Witness and stating that under no circumstances was she to receive blood. Her physician knew this but felt impelled by his oath to save lives to give her a blood transfusion. The hospital was unable to locate her husband, so the physician decided to transfuse her.

His actions saved her life; however, she was not grateful. She sued her doctor for assault and battery and won a $20,000 settlement. She was a competent adult and had made a decision that her physician chose to ignore. In a study done of Jehovah's Witnesses in the 1980s, two-thirds of those polled said they would sue if transfused against their will. Many feel that this is the only way that others will be protected and have their beliefs taken seriously. A physician in a position like that of Dr. Andrews should realize the possible ramifications (including legal ones) of violating the patient's express wishes in order to fulfill his own beliefs (Hippocratic oath) and make a conscious, fully informed decision.

Sometimes a Jehovah's Witness will reconsider at the last minute. For example, a twenty-seven-year-old woman who began bleeding heavily several days after giving birth required a hysterectomy. After the operation, she urgently needed blood but refused it. Two days later, when she developed acute respiratory distress and had to be placed on a respirator, she agreed to the blood transfusion. It saved her life.

Many health care professionals have strong moral difficulty in respecting the Jehovah's Witness position. The conflict lies in two areas: values and worldview. Jehovah's Witnesses believe that when Armageddon comes, 144,000 of those who have followed God's laws will rise from the dead to spend eternity in heaven. Those who have followed God's laws but do not go to heaven will spend eternity in a paradise on earth. All those who have violated God's laws (e.g., had a blood transfusion, placed themselves above God by celebrating their own birthdays, or worshipped idols by saluting the American flag) are doomed to spend eternity in nothingness.

Suppose for a moment that they are correct. Choosing to have a blood transfusion can be interpreted as giving up the chance to spend eternity in heaven or paradise in exchange for a few more years on earth. In this scenario, it is not very rational to have the transfusion. Few health care professionals are Jehovah's Witnesses. They do not believe that the fate of their soul rests on whether they have a blood transfusion. Thus the worldview of Jehovah's Witness patients comes into direct conflict with that of most clinicians.

Most health care professionals value the life of the physical body. In refusing blood, the Jehovah's Witness is valuing the life of the soul over that of the physical body. The question is, does any group have the right to impose its values and beliefs on others? Can we be so arrogant and ethnocentric as to be sure we are right and they are wrong?

The issue is most difficult when children are involved. Do their parents have the right to choose for them? This question is not easily answered. In an extreme case, parents abandoned their child after he had been given a blood transfusion under court order.

Finally, there are social issues. If an individual who is a member of a very tightly knit conservative group of Jehovah's Witnesses accepts blood, the act might lead to rejection by his or her entire social network. A few more years of life may not be worth that price.

Why do some members change their minds and accept blood at the last minute? Obviously, not all members of a religion are equally devout. Many people have doubts about their beliefs. When it is a matter of life and death, faith is often not strong enough to dictate the giving up of life.

Dealing with a Jehovah's Witness patient can be very difficult if the need for a blood transfusion arises. Doctors and nurses often feel helpless and frustrated. They value life so strongly that they find it hard to understand why some people willingly choose to give it up. They should try to see the situation from an emic perspective and consider the possibility that the Jehovah's Witnesses are right. They should also acknowledge the role Jehovah's Witnesses have played in the pioneering of bloodless surgeries.

86   Matthew Granger was rapidly losing large amounts of blood as a result of gastrointestinal bleeding. He was unresponsive, and unable to make decisions regarding his care. The situation was particularly complicated because he was a Jehovah's Witness. And he desperately needed blood. His wife, who was also a Jehovah's Witness, understood how critical his condition was, but would not allow the staff to administer a blood transfusion. Many Jehovah's Witnesses do, however, allow the use of albumin, a protein made by the liver and released into the blood, as an alternative. It is generally considered a personal decision. The physicians who spoke to Mrs. Granger emphasized how important it was that they give her husband albumin, but she still refused. Michael, a nurse currently in a course on cultural competence, decided to take a slightly different approach with Mrs. Granger. He began the conversation by telling her that he respected and understood her beliefs, and then continued by explaining why treating her husband with albumin might be beneficial. This time, his wife agreed to the procedure. Simply acknowledging her beliefs, something the physicians neglected to do, made all the difference.

Jewish

87   Jews also have blood beliefs, in their case with implications for burial, as outlined in the following case study. The incident involved Sarah Weinberg, a four-year-old Orthodox Jewish girl who was hit by a car and sustained fatal injuries. A paramedic team rushed Sarah to the hospital emergency room, after performing several resuscitation attempts en route. She was still alive when they reached the hospital, but died on the operating table. When Mr. Weinberg was notified of his daughter's death, he approached Robert, one of the nurses who worked on her. Mr. Weinberg accepted Robert's condolences and then asked him for his scrubs. Robert did not understand the request; why would the bereaved father want his clothing? Mr. Weinberg explained that, according to Jewish tradition, the individual must be buried whole. Since Sara's

blood was on Robert's scrubs, they had to be buried with her. Although Robert was unfamiliar with this custom, he immediately complied. Fortunately, this case was easily resolved.

Another case involving the death of a Jewish patient was also resolved   *88* due to the cultural competence of the nurse. Matthew Goldstein, the son of an Orthodox Jewish man, requested that he stay with the body of his deceased father until the mortuary service came to pick the body up. According to Reyna, the nurse, hospital policy does not allow that, because it sometimes takes hours for the service to arrive and hospital beds are in great demand. However, because Reyna was taking a class in cultural competence at the time, she was especially sensitive to meeting Mr. Goldstein's needs. Therefore, she arranged for his father's body to be moved into a little-used and secluded area so he could stay with him until the mortuary service arrived the next morning. Reyna reported that she felt very good about being able to accommodate him. "It required very little work on my part and the family was allowed to practice their religious customs."

It is a Jewish custom that the body of the deceased is not to be left unattended. To do so is a sign of disrespect. The custom evolved from early times, in which people went to great lengths to guard the deceased from ghosts and spirits—or body snatchers.

Every religion has days that are considered holy and on which behav-   89 ior is often strictly proscribed. Sol Meyers, an Orthodox Jew, created a problem for the nursing staff when he tried to observe the Sabbath. Mr. Meyers brought his wife to the hospital in active labor at 8 P.M. on a Friday. When she gave birth at midnight, the nurses suggested that Mr. Meyers accompany her to the postpartum unit and then return home to rest. He thanked them but explained that he could not drive home because it was the Sabbath. The nurses understood and arranged for him to stay in his wife's room.

In the morning, Mr. Meyers asked the nurses for breakfast. They explained that the hospital provided food only for patients; he would have to buy his breakfast in the dining room. When Mr. Meyers told them he was forbidden to ride in an elevator or handle money, one of the nurses offered to get him food. But Mr. Meyers had no money with him. Frustrated, the nurses finally ordered extra food for his wife to share with him. At lunch, Mr. Meyers once again requested food. This time the nurses suggested that he call a friend or relative to pick him up. Mr. Meyers replied that he could not use the phone on the Sabbath, and even if he made a call, no one would answer because all his friends and relatives were Orthodox. By this time, the nurses were losing patience. If Mr. Meyers could drive to the hospital, why couldn't he drive home? If he knew he would have to stay at the hospital, why had he not brought food with him?

The answers can be found in the Torah. One of the most important laws of the Torah states that Orthodox Jews must observe the Sabbath. It is a time to be with one's family and to worship God. The Sabbath begins at sundown Friday and ends at sundown Saturday. During this time, work of any kind is prohibited, including driving, using the telephone, handling money, and even pushing an elevator button. (A large Jewish hospital in Los Angeles features a few elevators that automatically stop on every floor on Saturday.)

The only law higher than the law of the Sabbath is the law that demands one do everything possible to save a life. Mr. Meyers could drive his wife to the hospital on the Sabbath because her life and that of their child were at stake. He could not drive home, however, because a life was not threatened. Mr. Meyers did not bring food with him because it is forbidden to travel with food on the Sabbath (unless it is milk for a baby). Very little else could have been done in this situation other than to charge extra food to the patient's bill.

Sikh

90   Raj Singh, a seventy-two-year-old Sikh from India, had been admitted to the hospital after a heart attack. He was scheduled for a heart catheterization to determine the extent of the blockage in his coronary arteries. The procedure involved running a catheter up the femoral artery, located in the groin, and then passing it into his heart, where special x-rays could be taken. His son was a cardiologist on staff and had explained the procedure to him in detail.

Susan, his nurse, entered Mr. Singh's room and explained that she had to shave his groin to prevent infection from the catheterization. As she pulled the razor from her pocket, she was suddenly confronted with the sight of shining metal flashing in front of her. Mr. Singh had a short sword in his hand and was waving it at her as he spoke excitedly in his native tongue. Susan got the message. She would not shave his groin.

She put away her "weapon," and he did the same. Susan, thinking the problem was that she was a woman, said she would get a male orderly to shave him. Mr. Singh's eyes lit up again as he angrily yelled, "No shaving of hair by anyone!"

Susan managed to calm him down by agreeing. She then called her supervisor and the attending physician to report the incident. The physician said he would do the procedure on an unshaved groin. At that moment, Mr. Singh's son stopped by. When he heard what had happened, he apologized profusely for not explaining his father's Orthodox Sikh customs.

The Sikh religion forbids cutting or shaving any body hair. Orthodox Sikhs always carry a short sword with them as a representation of their duty to stand up to injustice. The *kirpan* (sword) is considered one of the five articles of faith. The others are *kesh* (wearing hair and beard unshorn); *kanga* (comb to keep hair clean and tidy); *kachera* (under-shorts worn to remind them of the need for self-restraint over passions and lust); and *kara* (steel bracelet worn on the right wrist to remind them of their vows). These articles of faith reflect the Sikhs' military history and reminds them of their commitment.

Many of the procedures medical professionals consider necessary may not be. Shaving to reduce the risk of serious infection, for example, *may* be valid in some cases; however, a review article on reducing surgical site infections found that preoperative hair removal did *not* reduce the risk of infection, and in some cases, increased it due to microscopic cuts (Reichman and Greenberg 2009). If new evidence emerges to support decreased infection risk with shaving, the patient could be presented with the statistics and allowed to decide whether to take the additional risk. Physicians should make every effort not to impose their own theoretical concerns (such as the belief that shaving reduces the risk of infection) on patients, and to let patients make the informed choice to take risks when the medical evidence conflicts with their beliefs.

In a similar situation, Griselda avoided a potential problem when she had to shave a Sikh child to prep him for an appendectomy. Knowing that traditional Sikh religion forbids cutting or shaving hair, she told the patient and his mother that she understood the prohibition against shaving and assured them that only the surgical site would be shaved. She explained that the purpose was to create a sterile field free of germs and microorganisms that could cause an infection. As stated above, there is some question as to whether this is actually true and based on scientific evidence. However, the approach Griselda took in acknowledging the patient's beliefs and explaining why they wanted to violate them was a good one. In this case, the family chose to allow the child to be shaved, and any potential problems were avoided.

Sacred Symbols

Catholic

Religious and spiritual symbols are not always obvious to members of other religions; this can lead to problems. However, culturally competent health care personnel can truly make a difference. It was a set of rosary beads that offered Ariadne the opportunity to demonstrate cultural sensitivity and flexibility. Celia Montes, an elderly Latina patient, asked that she be able to wear her rosary beads into surgery. Her request was denied. When Ariadne later spoke to her about it, Celia was distraught. She explained that the beads would bring strength to the surgeons and protect her during the surgery. She was afraid to have the surgery without them. Understanding how important they were to her, Ariadne spoke to Ettie, the charge nurse in the operating room. Ettie was hesitant to accommodate her request, explaining that the policy existed because too many things had been lost during surgery; if they didn't allow personal effects into surgery, nothing could get lost. Ariadne assured the Ettie that she would label the beads, and again emphasized their importance to the patient. Ettie finally relented. When Ariadne told Mrs. Montes that she would be allowed to wear the rosary beads into surgery, her relief and gratitude were palpable. Policies often exist for the convenience of the hospital and staff, but accommodating the needs of the patients should be primary.

93   Disrespect for the Catholic scapular (two small, usually rectangular pieces of cloth, wood, or laminated paper, joined by two bands of cloth and containing religious images or text) caused a family to request a transfer to another hospital. Felisa Arogetti, an elderly Italian woman, was wearing a scapular attached to her hospital gown. When the gown became soiled, it was thrown into the laundry without removing Mrs. Arogetti's scapular, which was then lost.

Mrs. Arogetti's relationship with the nurse and hospital might have survived the incident, had the nurse bothered to apologize to Mrs. Arogetti. However, she did not. By discounting the patient's symbol of hope, the nurse caused the family to lose faith in the health care team's ability to help Mrs. Arogetti. Due to this loss of trust, the family requested she be transferred to another hospital. The situation could have been avoided by paying more careful attention to Mrs. Arogetti's religious symbol. It could have later been recovered with a sincere apology that acknowledged the importance of the symbol. Unfortunately, neither was done.

94   Silvia made a positive difference for a Mexican patient named Juan Robles. Prior to her being assigned to him, he was having conflicts with several of the nurses over the religious statues he kept in his room. One of the nurses told him point blank that he had to get rid of the statues because they were in the way and were interfering with his treatment. He was very upset and angry over this. Silvia took the time to sit down with Mr. Robles, and ask him about the importance of the statues to him. He explained that he was Catholic and that the images of the saints would help in his healing. Seeing how important they were to him, Silvia raised the issue at a staff meeting. She suggested that they change their unofficial policy and allow patients to keep statues in the room. The initial response to her suggestion was quite negative. But Silvia persisted, emphasizing how important they were to patient comfort. She then suggested that the nurses tell the patients that they would have to move them while they were working with the patient, but would return them to their place once they finished. They agreed to this. It made for a little more work for the nurses but greatly increased the comfort of patients like Juan Robles.

Sacred symbols for people of one religion can cause problems for   95
people of other religions. Rao Chean, a seventy-two-year-old Cambodian woman, was admitted to a Catholic hospital following a motor vehicle accident. Amanda, her nurse, found her unresponsive during the assessment. She noted that Mrs. Rao kept staring at the wall. She assumed it was due to the shock of the accident. Amanda turned to Mrs. Rao's daughter to request that she ask her mother how she was feeling. The daughter then asked Amanda to please remove the crucifix from the wall, because it was bothering her mother. Mrs. Rao was a Buddhist. Amanda quickly removed the crucifix and put the Bible in the bottom drawer. As a result, Mrs. Rao appeared to relax and became more talkative. When Amanda later asked her about the crucifix, she felt it made her feel she was being proselytized to worship a God she does not recognize.

Mormon (Church of Jesus Christ of Latter Day Saints)

Grace Kettering, a Mormon woman, was admitted to the hospital for   96
facial surgery. Before entering the operating room, she was told to remove all her clothes except the hospital gown. She refused to remove her long underwear, and the surgeon refused to operate unless she did.

Very devout Mormons who have attained adult religious status in the church wear "the garment." It resembles short-sleeved long underwear and ends just above the knee. Although not exactly magical, it is considered sacred and is generally worn except when it is being cleaned or while one is bathing, swimming, or exercising. Although most Mormon patients will have no trouble removing it for exams or procedures, having to remove the garment associated with God's protection could be very distressing for some, as it was for Mrs. Kettering.

Eventually, Mrs. Kettering's surgeon relented. In such cases, an understanding attitude and a discussion of the options beforehand are advisable. For example, the lower half of the garment could be pulled down to the patient's ankles in the event of abdominal surgery.

Native American

Abby, a nurse who worked at a hospital close to the Hoopa Valley Indian   97
reservation in Northern California, told of an elderly Native American

man in intensive care. His granddaughter brought in an object consisting of a circular frame with feathers hanging from it. The object fits the description of a "soul catcher." She asked if she could hang it on the wall. Fortunately, Abby was quite understanding and hung it from the intravenous hook above the patient's bed instead. The granddaughter was both relieved and grateful. It was a small concession on the part of the nurse but provided tremendous psychological comfort for the patient and his family.

Cambodian

98   A Cambodian infant was brought into the hospital diagnosed with severe dehydration and vomiting. Mona, the nurse, examined the child's extremities, looking for a vein in which to start an intravenous line. She finally found one on the baby's arm. At that point, she noticed several strands of dark brown strings, about one-half inch wide, on both wrists. Mona prepared to cut the strings with scissors, since it would have been difficult to disinfect the skin, tape the IV, and stabilize the arm without removing the strings. Mrs. Tep, the baby's mother, walked in at that moment, looked horrified at what Mona was about to do, and began speaking loudly in her native tongue. Mona assumed she was upset because the infant was crying. But Mrs. Tep kept pointing to the strings; it was obvious that she did not want them cut. Mona did not understand what the problem was, but communicated through gestures that she would not cut the strings.

What was the problem with the strings? They are known as *baci*. It is a tradition believed to have originated with the Lao culture, but is practiced by Mien and Cambodians as well. The strings are tied around a person's wrists at important occasions—birthdays, promotions, weddings, and so forth. They are believed to "tie in the soul" so it doesn't get lost. They should never be cut off; they simply wear off in time. The Teps believed that if Mona had cut the strings, she would have jeopardized the infant's life.

Unfortunately, the only alternative—putting the IV line in the infant's scalp—also caused a great deal of distress for the parents. When Mona started an intravenous line in the infant's scalp, Mrs. Tep began to cry. While it is upsetting for any parent to see intravenous lines put into their child's scalp, for many Southeast Asians it is especially traumatic. As the Teps explained through an interpreter, the head is thought to be the seat of life. By introducing holes into it, the nurse had made an easy exit for the child's soul.

What Mona might have done is acknowledge their concern about putting a hole in their child's scalp, assure them that it would be as small as possible, and explain why it was necessary, given their child's condition. If the Teps were convinced that Mona respected their beliefs and was only doing what was necessary to help their child, they might have been less upset.

Chinese Buddhist

Bao Chin, a Chinese Buddhist patient, was being prepped for surgery. All was going well until Donna told her to remove her bracelet. Mrs. Chin refused. Donna explained to her and her family that the policy at that hospital requires that all patients entering a sterile surgical suite remove all personal belongings and don a hospital issued gown and socks. All clothing and jewelry items are to be placed in a belonging bag. All items that have potentially come in contact with germs from the outside are forbidden to enter the operating room to reduce the patient's risk of infection. Donna told her that the policy is based on infection control, although as in case study #92, concern for liability for lost items may have also played a role in the hospital's policy. Mrs. Chin's daughter understood the policy, but the patient did not. She asked her daughter to take her home. Since Mrs. Chin was asking to cancel a major surgery, Donna had to call the department manager. The department nurse manager and the director of the anesthesia department both came and talked with Mrs. Chin. They explained to her and her daughter about the importance of infection control and sterility, and added that her wrist would be restrained during surgery and they didn't want to risk injury. But Mrs. Chin was adamant; no bracelet, no surgery. It was a special protection bracelet, and she didn't feel safe going into surgery without it. She wanted her daughter to take her home. After another hour of discussion, they came to a compromise. Her bracelet would be put into a sterile specimen bag and placed in the front pocket of her gown. Mrs. Chin then agreed to the surgery, and all went well. When the hospital made the usual 48-hour postoperative courtesy call, Mrs. Chin's daughter expressed how grateful she was that her mother was able to go into surgery in good spirits, knowing she had her bracelet to protect her.

Since Donna had run across similar situations with other Chinese Buddhists, she spoke with her manager and the director of anesthesia about developing a policy for such situations. The decided that in the future, patients would be allowed to take religious items with them into surgery, as long as the patient agreed to have the item cleaned with a disinfectant wipe and placed in a sterile bag. Nonmetal items could then be placed in the patient's gown; metal items could be placed underneath the gurney. Although it requires a bit more work, the difference it can make to the patient's state of mind is enormous.

Hindu

100   Fortunately for Arden Patel, Carrie Ann was taking a course in cultural competence when he was assigned to her. Mr. Patel, a Hindu patient from India, was dying, and in the process, becoming extremely bloated. His abdomen was distended and he was suffering from severe edema in his arms. A Filipino nursing assistant was about to remove a string tied around Mr. Patel's wrist because it was cutting off his circulation. Carrie Ann stopped him, and asked him to wait until the patient's daughter arrived. She knew that Hindus sometimes wore sacred threads around their necks or arms, and felt that since the patient was near death in any case, cutting it off without permission might be more harmful than leaving it on. When Mr. Patel's daughter arrived, Carrie Ann explained her concerns. His daughter agreed to allow the strings to be cut, and thanked Carrie Ann for her sensitivity.

A general rule of thumb is to assume that a patient who is wearing anything that looks unusual may be doing so for religious or spiritual reasons. Hindus may wear sacred threads around their necks or arms; Native Americans may carry medicine bundles; Mexican children may wear a bit of red ribbon; Mediterranean peoples may wear a special charm on a chain, such as a mustard seed in a blue circle or a ram's horn, to ward off the evil eye. If an item must be removed to perform a medical procedure, the reason should be explained to the patient and the family. The item should be removed gently and respectfully and placed in contact with the patient's body if possible.

Spiritual Beliefs and Practices

For many people, spirituality is an integral part of their life. Spiritual needs become even more important when people are ill, but these needs often either are ignored or receive low priority from health care professionals. This can create even greater distress for patients who are already stressed from trying to cope with illness, as the next case illustrates.

101   Marietta Amador, a Filipina woman and nurse, felt she was a "victim of cultural ignorance" when her six-week-old daughter Emilita fell ill with sepsis. Emilita was hospitalized for ten days so she could receive massive doses of antibiotics. Fearing that her child would not survive, Marietta asked the nurse to send a chaplain or other religious person to bless or baptize her daughter. She waited for three days, completely distraught, until the nurse sent someone. Marietta had very strong religious values, and spiritual healing was very important to her. Nurses

should make every effort to meet patients' spiritual needs as well as their physical needs in a timely manner.

Prayer

A seventy-five-year-old African American woman named Agnes Jones was *102* in the hospital recovering from a heart attack. Mrs. Jones was very religious and spent most of her time praying. Her "brothers and sisters" from the church visited daily, and she appeared closer to them than to members of her family.

During her hospital stay, Mrs. Jones consented to only the procedures and medications she believed were ordered by God because, according to her worldview, only God could make her well. While the nurses bathed Mrs. Jones, she preached to them about Jesus. Before too long, the hospital staff began to avoid her.

For many African Americans, religion is an essential and integral part of life. God is viewed as the source of both good health and serious illness. God can cure any disease, but to be cured one must pray and have faith. This worldview, like all effective ones, is internally consistent: if a patient is not cured, it is not because God failed but because the patient lacked sufficient faith.

The hospital personnel did not handle Mrs. Jones's case well. Rather than avoiding her, they should have had a team conference to discuss her beliefs and perhaps have invited a minister from her church to attend. The minister might have convinced Mrs. Jones to be more cooperative, and the staff might have learned to be more understanding and tolerant of her beliefs.

An excellent example of how to handle this kind of situation is one *103* involving a diabetic Hispanic woman named Elena Montoya, who had stopped taking her medication because she was told by a *curandera* (a traditional healer) that God had taken away her diabetes. She returned to her physician when her symptoms—excessive thirst and frequent urination—returned, but she was reluctant to go back on her medication. The wise health care practitioner, rather than contradict her, suggested that God might have taken away her diabetes for a while, but that it had returned and perhaps He had brought her to the doctor so that it could be treated with medicine. He encouraged her to continue to pray, but got her to agree to allow him to monitor her condition before stopping her medication again.

Karin's sensitivity and flexibility led to a very positive colonoscopy *104* experience for Laura de la Cruz, an elderly Mexican patient, and her family. When she came in for a pre-procedure assessment—accompanied by 13 family members—Mrs. de la Cruz's son commented that the outcome of the procedure "was in God's hands" and requested that they be allowed to pray before their mother's procedure. Although this was not normal procedure, Karin recognized the importance of the family's religious beliefs, and allowed them to pray together in private before the colonoscopy. The family were effusive in their gratitude, and shared that their previous requests to pray had always been denied by health care staff. It took very little to make the experience a much more positive one for both the patient and her family.

105   Emilin was caring for Maria Garcia, a fearful Hispanic patient who had had a very severe reaction to a narcotic medication, a reaction that further escalated her fear and anxiety. She was very emotional, vocal, and loud and kept asking for her eldest son. Once Emilin identified the son, she asked him to explain to his mother that because of the reaction she had had, she couldn't give her any medication. In trying to come up with a way to calm her down, Emilin noticed a cross around Mrs. Garcia's neck and encouraged the family to pray with her. As she began to pray, Mrs. Garcia slowly calmed down and relaxed. Emilin left the room for a while, and when she returned, Mrs. Garcia gave her a giant smile and held out her hand. When Emilin went over to her, Mrs. Garcia grabbed her hand and kissed it; in return, Emilin asked if she could give her a hug. Mrs. Garcia agreed. Emilin later remarked that it was the first time in a long time that she felt she had bonded with a patient. Utilizing her patient's religious beliefs to help control her anxiety was inspired.

Evil Spirits

106   Lhee Pha, a sixteen-year-old Hmong patient, was brought to the emergency department with abdominal pain. She was diagnosed with appendicitis, and it was determined that surgery was necessary. Her father, however, refused to allow the surgery. Within a few days, her appendix ruptured, and she became septic and died. Cheryl, her nurse, was very frustrated by the situation. Lhee could have easily been saved had her father allowed her to have surgery. Several days later, Lhee's sister came in to the emergency department on another matter. She thanked Cheryl for the care she had provided for her sister. Cheryl asked her if there were anything they could have done differently, or anything they could have said to make Lhee's parents see how serious the situation was, and how necessary the surgery. Lhee's sister explained that her parents knew that Lhee might die without surgery, but they did not want to risk her living with an evil spirit. Cheryl learned that they believed that not only could an incision create an opening for her soul to leave, but it could also create an opening for an evil spirit to enter. Her parents did not want to risk this, even if it meant their daughter's death. Lhee's sister

said her family thought the hospital staff had handled the situation well, and were grateful that they had made an exception to visiting rules and allowed all thirty members of her extended family to be in the room with Lhee as she died. Sometimes, cultural competence involves truly accepting other peoples' beliefs, even when they contradict the highest value of medicine—saving life.

Soul Loss

This next case is an old one, but still makes an important point. For those unfamiliar with a Polaroid camera, it was a camera that produced an instant photograph on paper from the camera itself. This case could easily be updated by replacing "Polaroid" with "digital" and "offer(ing) him the photograph" with "deleting the photo."

Melissa was working in a busy pediatric intensive care unit the day she inadvertently jeopardized Jimmy Hosea's life. Jimmy was a twelve-year-old Navajo post-op patient. The day he transferred into Melissa's unit, the staff had just been given a new Polaroid camera. She gathered Jimmy and two other children together for a photo. Because her attention was on the two others, who happily mugged for the camera, Melissa never noticed the look of horror on Jimmy's face until she saw the photo. He had disappeared while it was developing.

When Melissa found him, Jimmy was sitting on the edge of his bed, gazing at the floor and looking as though he were ready to die. When she asked him what had happened, he carefully responded, "I've lost my soul." Melissa had no idea what he was talking about. He explained that pictures took the soul out of the face captured on the photograph. Melissa was astounded. How could he believe that?

She told him how sorry she was and offered him the photograph. He took it, saying that his family could help him get his soul back with a "sing," a religious ceremony.

This case is a good example of how important it is to know about the spiritual beliefs of those for whom you are caring. Although it is obviously unrealistic to expect to know everything about every culture, just having an awareness that your patients' beliefs may be different from your own may help you to be more sensitive and aware. Melissa certainly is.

Blood Beliefs

Earlier in the chapter the blood beliefs of Jehovah's Witnesses and Jews were addressed. Other groups also have beliefs about this vital life force.

107

108   This case relates to both Mien attitudes regarding blood and the issue of soul loss. Saelee Mui Chua, a forty-two-year-old Mien man, arrived at the clinic with his twelve-year-old son, who acted as interpreter. The son explained that his father had seen a traditional healer the previous week, but the healer had been unable to cure his father's symptoms: weakness, fatigue, increased urination, and thirst. The symptoms suggested diabetes to the physician, and he ordered a blood glucose test. When Shawnee, the nurse, came to draw the blood, Mr. Saelee fearfully yelled, "No!" His son told Shawnee that his father refused to have his blood drawn. When she asked for an explanation, all he would say is, "My father does not want the test."

The staff assumed that Mr. Saelee was afraid of the needle. However, it is more likely that he was concerned about having his blood drawn. There is a Mien legend about an evil bird that brought bad fortune and death by drinking a person's blood. This is probably connected to the Mien belief that losing blood saps strength (Mr. Saelee was already feeling weak) and may result in the soul leaving the body.

The staff tried to "educate" Mr. Saelee about the procedure of drawing blood, and explained its importance in diagnosing his symptoms, but their efforts were to no avail. He would not give his permission for the procedure and simply left the hospital.

What could have been done? Although there are no guarantees that any intervention could have changed Mr. Saelee's mind, they might have explained that the amount of blood needed was extremely small, and that new blood would be made to replace it. If possible, perhaps the traditional healer could have been involved in the procedure. They might have also spent more time explaining why the tests were so necessary. The connection between his symptoms and his blood is not immediately obvious. Having a trained interpreter, familiar with Mien culture, might have also been helpful. The following case study illustrates a more culturally competent approach.

109   When Leslie admitted a seventy-eight-year-old Cambodian woman who had just suffered a myocardial infarction, she realized that the blood sample she was going to have to draw prior to cardiac catheterization could be traumatic for her patient. She therefore took the time to explain to the woman's daughter why it was necessary to draw blood, and assured her she would take the minimum amount necessary. The daughter then explained it to her mother, and stood by her side while the blood was drawn. The patient remained calm and cooperative. Although Leslie did not find out whether her patient shared traditional Cambodian blood beliefs, if she did, the short time it took to explain things may have saved her patient significant distress. And if she didn't, well, it is a good idea to provide patients with explanations in any case.

Blood beliefs are common throughout rural Southeast Asia. Some Hmong may not want blood drawn due to the beliefs that blood is a life force and the body has a limited amount of blood that it cannot replenish. Repeated blood sampling, especially from small children, may thus be thought to be fatal.

Summary

Although conflicting belief systems can be a source of frustration, confusion, and misunderstanding, most can be dealt with successfully. One must understand the patient's beliefs and be willing to respect them. When health care personnel work *with* the patient's beliefs, rather than against them, the outcomes are usually more successful, measured not only in patient satisfaction but also in ease for the medical team in managing the patient and family.

Key Points

- Honor patient requests for same-sex providers whenever possible.
- Provide clergy when requested.
- Respect your patients' religious beliefs, even when they conflict with your own.
- Realize that rules for religious leaders may be much more stringent than those for others. Ascertain them in advance to avoid problems.
- Allow patients privacy for prayer.
- Remember that individuals will vary in their degree of adherence to religious practices.
- Be aware that different religions have different holy days. It is Friday for Muslims, Saturday for Jews, and Sunday for Christians.
- Allow patients to make informed choices regarding risks when medical procedures conflict with their religious beliefs.
- Learn what symbols are sacred to those you treat, and respect them. They can provide tremendous psychological comfort to your patients. Do not cut or remove anything without first discussing it with the patient.
- Recognize that many Southeast Asian patients may have beliefs about blood that will make them reluctant to have it drawn. Ask their concerns and provide clear explanations for the need to draw blood.

Chapter 5

Activities of Daily Living and the Body

There are some basic activities that patients must perform each day, including eating, bathing, using the bathroom, and caring for their hair. Not surprisingly, these activities are influenced by culture and thus a potential source of conflict in the hospital. A second topic concerns the concept of body image. The ideal image varies considerably from culture to culture and may affect patients' attitudes toward specific treatments.

Eating

Dietary practices are an important issue for hospitals. Patients who do not eat are often a cause of concern for physicians and nurses. Is there a gastrointestinal problem? Is the patient suffering from depression? The food is bad, but not bad enough to explain it. The problem may in fact be a religious or cultural one. Issues around diet may also arise when families bring in traditional foods for patients, which may in fact be harmful to their health condition. Knowledge of cultural differences in dietary rules and food preferences is essential in terms of both patient satisfaction and health.

Religious Restrictions

Islam prohibits eating from sunrise to sunset during the month of Ramadan. Judaism requires its members to fast from sundown to sundown during Yom Kippur, the Day of Atonement. Both forbid the eating of pork, and Judaism has other restrictions that will be discussed below. Hindus are forbidden to eat meat, as are Seventh Day Adventists. Although alcohol is not generally served in hospitals, dietary departments should be aware that the very devout members of religions that forbid it, including Muslims, Mormons, and Seventh Day Adventists, consider vanilla extract alcohol. The latter two are also prohibited from caffeine. The body is seen as a gift from God or as a holy temple that should not be polluted by drugs or alcohol. Not every member of these religions will necessarily follow the food prohibitions, but it is important to ask.

Muslim: Ramadan

Mona Azula was an older Egyptian Muslim woman who came to Juliana's clinic for management of diabetes and hypertension. It was late November, the time of year when staff and patients brought in sweets and other foods in celebration of the holidays. Juliana said that she often walked around the clinic eating and offering food to the patients. Because she was taking a class on cultural diversity, seeing Mrs. Azula reminded her it was Ramadan. She immediately apologized for eating in front of her during Ramadan. Juliana reported that this simple statement opened a line of communication she had been trying to establish with the patient for the past six months. Mrs. Azula then began to talk to her about the spiritual and physical significance of fasting. Juliana learned that during the month of Ramadan, followers of Islam are forbidden to eat from sunrise to sunset in order to detach themselves from material cravings and focus on the spiritual. It is thought to help the rich empathize with the suffering of the poor. Although for many Muslims illness provides an exemption from the rules, they are obligated to make it up when they are in good health, a time when it will be more difficult because they will be doing it alone.

Through their discussion, Juliana became much more open about her concerns regarding Mrs. Azula's medical treatment. Although she was still taking her medications, she was fasting during daylight. She was suffering from cold sweats, fatigue, headaches, lightheadedness, and dizziness, along with anxiety and hand tremors. Juliana and Mrs. Azula then developed a treatment plan for the month of Ramadan that involved taking her diabetes medication only at dinnertime. Juliana went over the symptoms of hypoglycemia with her, and asked Mrs. Azula to let her know if she felt any better after adjusting the medications as they had discussed. Two days later, Mrs. Azula returned to the clinic to thank Juliana and tell her how much better she felt. This is an excellent example of how a little cultural competence—this time, in the form of some knowledge of an important religious holiday—led to greater trust and openness and resulted in the improved health of the patient.

It is important to remember that not all Muslim patients are from the Middle East. Juana had a patient from the Philippines who kept getting into conflicts with the Filipino nurses because she refused to eat during the day, would not take her medications at the assigned time, and kept

110

111

requesting time for prayer. The nurses didn't take the time to ask her *why*; they merely grumbled about her noncompliance. It wasn't until Juana asked Emilita Jacinto why she wasn't eating that she explained she was Muslim and it was Ramadan. Juana then notified the physician to change her diet and adjust her medications to fit her religious needs. Once Juana's coworkers understood the situation, they realized they had stereotyped Mrs. Jacinto as Catholic because she was from the Philippines, and viewed her simply as noncompliant. This case is instructive as a reminder to (1) avoid stereotyping; (2) ask about patients' religious practices on admission; and (3) try to understand patients' behavior from their point of view. Noncompliance (or, rather, nonadherence) is often a result of cultural misunderstanding. The case is also a good example of cultural competence on the part of Juana.

Jewish: Kosher Dietary Practices

112

Why would a fifty-four-year-old man burst into tears when served roast beef, milk, and a roll with butter on the same lunch tray? What would cause an eighty-seven-year-old woman to refuse beef and chicken, even though she was not a vegetarian? Why would the mother of a two-year-old patient refuse to use the flatware provided and instead insist on plastic utensils? All these individuals are Orthodox Jews following the kosher dietary laws. These laws forbid eating pork and shellfish and non-kosher red meat and poultry. They also prohibit mixing meat and dairy products, either in the same meal or by using the same plates, pots, or utensils for both.

As with most cultural and religious laws, there is both a practical and an ideological basis for their origin. The overriding ideology behind the kosher laws is humaneness. The practical reasons are generally associated with health.

Shellfish are to be avoided because they are scavengers. They can pick up diseases and transmit them. Pork, if not properly cooked, can cause trichinosis. Furthermore, as cultural materialist Marvin Harris (1974) points out, raising pigs in a desert environment is not a wise ecological choice; pigs are not thermodynamically adapted to arid environments. In order to regulate their body temperature in environments over 84 degrees, where mud is not readily available, pigs will wallow in their own urine and feces. The more scarce water and shade, the greater the luxury it is to raise pigs. Furthermore, since they eat the same food as humans—scraps may not have been plentiful in those times—it didn't make ecological sense for the prehistoric Hebrews to raise pigs in large numbers, and small-scale production would only increase temptation. (Pigs taste good!) Thus, according to Harris, it became taboo for the Jews—and their Muslim neighbors—to eat them. Pigs require shade, water, and human food. In the desert environment it is not a good idea to raise animals that compete with humans for scarce resources. The last two points might explain why Muslims also forbid eating pork. An alternative explanation suggests that because pork and shellfish were dietary staples in the lands where the Jews lived at different points in their history, the prohibition was designed to prevent the Jews from assimilating. Another practical reason for the kosher laws is that for meat to be considered kosher, animals must be killed with a single blow and not strangled. The pain and suffering an animal experiences between the first and final blows or during the time it takes to die from strangulation can stimulate the release of hormones detrimental to humans. Finally, a common supposition is that if meat and dairy products are combined, bits of meat may lodge in a wooden or pottery bowl, mix with the dairy products, and in the desert sun provide an ideal breeding ground for bacteria.

Again, the notion of humaneness underlies most of the kosher laws. One can get milk from a living cow or goat, eggs from a living chicken, and wool from a living sheep, but pigs are useful only when dead. To raise an animal strictly for slaughter is considered cruel and inhumane, as is mixing the meat of a calf with the milk of its mother. Finally, the most humane death is one that is instantaneous.

The practical reasons for most of the kosher laws no longer exist. Yet Orthodox Jews continue to uphold the traditions. The behavior of the patients described earlier becomes clear in light of these laws. All these situations can easily be avoided through knowledge of these laws and the use of readily available frozen kosher meal trays and nonreusable paper plates and plastic utensils.

Hindu: The Sacred Cow

Christy, an Anglo nurse, took pity on an elderly man in the emergency room. He had been there for hours and appeared hungry. She went out of her way to get him a hamburger. When she gave it to him, his son, rather than appear grateful, was angry. His father was Hindu, and therefore forbidden to eat beef. Although she meant well, she would have been wise to offer a few alternatives prior to getting him food. 113

Cultural Restrictions: Hot and Cold

Nonreligious food restrictions can also create problems. Mina Asami, a sixty-seven-year-old Pakistani woman, was hospitalized with tuberculosis. When Rachel, her nurse, noticed that Mrs. Asami's appetite was poor, she became concerned. Wanting to make sure her patient received 114

enough protein, she made a concerted effort to feed her meat and potatoes with gravy. Mrs. Asami, however, was uncooperative, eating only
fruit and Jello.

When Mrs. Asami's son Davi came to the hospital, he provided information that resolved the problem. Rachel, it appears, was trying to feed
Mrs. Asami foods that Pakistanis normally avoid during the summer.
Foods are considered either "hot" or "cold." These are qualities, not
temperatures. In the summer, Pakistanis avoid "hot" foods like beef
because they "make our insides hot." In winter, they avoid "cold" foods
that make their insides cold. Beef, pork, potatoes, and whiskey are considered "hot" foods and are avoided in summer; in winter, Pakistanis
refrain from eating "cold" foods such as chicken, fish, fruit, and beer.
Once Rachel understood this, she ordered the appropriate foods for
Mrs. Asami, who suddenly developed a much heartier appetite.

115   It is best to ask about food preferences during the admission interview
or to arrange for a family member to bring food in for the patient. The
latter approach was taken by the family of Chi-Wa Koo, a Chinese patient
with lung cancer. A complete Chinese kitchen was laid out on a hospital
serving cart. Mr. Koo refused to eat anything prepared by the hospital,
consuming only items brought and prepared by his family.

Mr. Koo's family regarded his lung cancer as a *yin*, or "cold," condition. To restore balance to his system, it was necessary to give him *yang*
or "hot" foods. Without knowledge of yin and yang, it would be impossible for the hospital to serve Mr. Koo the appropriate foods. Furthermore, in China the family traditionally supplies a patient's food.
Fortunately, this incident occurred in a national medical center that is
used to treating patients from all over the world. The staff willingly
accommodated Mr. Koo's needs by allowing his family to bring in his
food.

116   Adhering to the rules of hot and cold was compromising the condition of Juanita Palacio, a forty-nine-year-old Mexican woman with kidney
failure and diabetes. She considered her kidney problem a "hot" condition that she treated with "cold" food and drinks. Unfortunately, many
of the fruits, vegetables, and dairy products she considered "cold" and
thus good for her disease contained large amounts of phosphorus and
potassium, dangerous for someone on dialysis. Rather than telling her
not to eat these foods, an injunction that would have led to decreased
trust and probably been ignored, the nurses emphasized eating large
amounts of the "cold" foods that are lower in dangerous minerals, while
eating small amounts of the foods that are high in them. They also made
adjustments to her dialysis to remove these minerals and waste products
from her blood more efficiently. And they frequently monitored her
blood chemistry and medications. Although it made more work for the

health care providers, the payoff was substantial. Juanita's condition became stable and she was able to follow her cultural traditions. This is an excellent example of cultural compromise.

Food Preferences

Each ethnic group has its own food preferences. Filipinos, for example, like rice with every meal and may feel deprived without it. They sometimes say it is a great comfort to eat rice when they feel ill. Japanese may prefer small amounts of beef or chicken, mixed with vegetables and rice or noodles. Food preferences should be ascertained when a patient is admitted and checked throughout hospitalization because they can have an important psychological effect. Simply discussing the daily menu with the patient can make a significant difference in the patient's attitude and recovery.

Mrs. Bae, a sixty-two-year-old Korean woman, had been admitted to the telemetry unit two days earlier for exacerbation of congestive heart failure. Her adult daughter, Angela, was at the hospital and served as her interpreter. Micky, a nurse on the unit, used the opportunity to interview her for a class assignment. Micky was concerned about Mrs. Bae because she had eaten very little. When she asked one of the other nurses why Mrs. Bae hadn't been eating, the nurse responded, "I don't know; she probably isn't hungry." During the course of the interview, Micky asked her why she hadn't been eating. She didn't answer right away. Mrs. Bae's daughter said that Micky was the first person to ask her why, and she was embarrassed to tell her. Micky reassured her that it was okay to tell her anything. Finally, Mrs. Bae explained that she wasn't accustomed to eating the type of food she was being served. It was bland and unappealing. Furthermore, she explained, she could not eat in bed and preferred to eat with her family. She said that she was willing to wait until she got home; she would eat then. Micky explained how important nutrition was to her recovery and that they needed to work together to come up with a solution. Mrs. Bae asked her daughter to stay with her while she ate, and Micky suggested to her daughter that they talk with the dietician and physician and figure out which of the foods she normally ate would be acceptable. Angela could then bring them in for her. Micky also suggested that she ask her nurse to let her sit in a chair at mealtime. Mrs. Bae was quite pleased with the solution and soon began eating.

Giang Hoa, a sixty-four-year-old Vietnamese refugee, was dehydrated and malnourished. She was receiving palliative care for lung cancer. She ate little and did not use the dietitian's recommended liquid supplement. While interviewing Mrs. Hoa regarding her condition and health

117

118

care practices, Martha, the home health nurse, learned that she was not taking the supplement. Martha realized that it was in the form of a sweet-tasting shake, agreeable to the Western palate but not to her client. She spoke with the dietitian and obtained a nonsweet substitute, which Mrs. Hoa found much more to her liking. She said the taste was similar to that of rice-water. It is important to realize that people of different cultures prefer different "tastes"; nonadherence may simply be a result of unpalatable flavors.

Another kind of dietary problem may result from the intersection of food preferences and belief systems, as illustrated in the following case.

119   Sophia, an American nurse working in Saudi Arabia, encountered a potentially life-threatening dietary problem involving many of her hemodialysis patients. Dates, a favorite food of many Arabs, are very high in potassium, which must be strictly limited in someone suffering from kidney failure. Sophia could not always find an interpreter to explain the situation clearly and convincingly to patients. The situation was further complicated, first, because in Saudi Arabia, food deprivation is thought to *cause* illness. From an Arab perspective, the nurses were helping bring on illness by depriving patients of dates. Second, dates are considered a special food by many Muslims. It is the first food generally eaten to break their fast during Ramadan, and was one of the Prophet Mohammad's favorite foods. Finally, Muslims believe that Allah (God) is all-powerful. Neither dates nor potassium would influence their health; rather, it was God's will. If Allah meant them to die, so be it. If not, they would survive. Beyond patient teaching, there is little one can do in such a situation.

Dietary Problems

Lactose Intolerance

Some ethnic groups cannot tolerate certain foods. According to some studies, most adult Asians, Africans, African Americans, and Native Americans are lactose intolerant, and milk products give them gas and diarrhea. Calcium needs should be considered, however, in planning meals for pregnant women, whether in the hospital or at home. Calcium supplements may be necessary. Other foods such as tofu, collard greens, bok choy, and sardines, all high in calcium, should be emphasized.

Ethnic Diets

Typical ethnic diets must also be taken into account when discharging patients with special dietary requirements. Asian diets are generally very high in sodium but low in fats. Mexican Americans tend to use a lot of salt and fats in their cooking. These cooking styles could prove problematic for hypertensive patients. It may be unrealistic to expect someone to change cooking and eating styles completely. Teaching sessions or adjustment of medications may be necessary. The family cook should be included in all discussions. Fortunately, there are many cookbooks and online recipes that adapt traditional recipes to the needs of diabetic and hypertensive patients. Hospitals should keep some of these cookbooks and links to websites on hand to help with patient teaching.

It is common for nurses to educate patients and family on what foods interact with the medications prescribed for them. However, as Libby realized when taking a class on cultural diversity, the kinds of foods she usually covered were probably not the ones her patients were eating. She gave the example of Pepe Acab, a Filipino patient who was being discharged on Coumadin, a blood thinner, to prevent clotting. Vitamin K reverses the effect of the drug and must be avoided. Normally, Libby would tell such patients to avoid foods like liver, broccoli, brussels sprouts, spinach, Swiss chard, coriander, collards, cabbage, and any green, leafy vegetables. She suddenly realized, however, that there might be other foods he should avoid. She spoke with Mr. Acab and his wife, and got a list of foods he commonly ate. She then did some research and discovered that two foods on the list—soybeans and fish liver oils—are very high in Vitamin K. She was then able to educate him properly on what to avoid. There is an important lesson here—you must find out what the patient normally eats before you can give appropriate advice on dietary issues.

Bathing

Niki's eyes rolled when she saw her patient, Mr. Johnson. "Another street person," she thought. It wasn't that she had anything against the homeless; the problem was that they just didn't like to bathe. As a nurse, she thought cleanliness was next to godliness. Sure enough, when she tried to bathe Mr. Johnson, he became visibly upset. "No, no!" When she asked him why, he explained that the layer of dirt would help to protect him from illness. Although this belief is in direct contradiction with Western medicine, it is easy to see why it would be adaptive for people living on the street to develop a belief consistent with their circumstances—specifically, greatly reduced access to bathing facilities.

Niki wished she could just force him to bathe, but she knew she couldn't; it was a matter of patients' rights. Only if he had to have surgery could she make him take a shower. She sighed and reminded herself that it was a question of beliefs and values, and she shouldn't impose hers on others.

As an interesting note, not all countries that practice Western medicine share our custom of bathing patients daily. In France, according to Lynn Payer in her book *Medicine and Culture* (1996), patients are typically bathed weekly. The difference in frequency can be explained by a difference in cultural beliefs regarding the cause of disease. In the United States, germs are thought to be the primary cause, and great efforts are made to destroy them. Bathing is one way of accomplishing that. Although the French see germs as a source of disease, more important to them is the *terrain*—roughly the equivalent of the immune system. Payer describes how the French would be more likely to give patients a tonic to build up their immune system, than antibiotics to kill germs. I can recall being in France and seeing dogs in restaurants, and going into wonderful pastry shops in which the apple tart they are going to sell you is buzzing with flies. Such violations of "cleanliness" never seem to bother the natives, only the American tourists.

Using the Bathroom

The need to eliminate body waste is a human universal. What is not universal, however, is the way it is done. Such variations can create cultural conflicts and misunderstandings, as the following cases illustrate.

Asian Toilets

122   Mr. Abatay, a fifty-eight-year-old Filipino patient, created a problem for the staff with his bathroom habits. The nurses, housekeepers, and his two former hospital "roommates" complained that the lid of the toilet was always dirty, and that there were shoe marks and water all over the toilet seat. Although he was suffering from dizziness and placed on strict bed rest, he refused to use the bedpan or bedside commode. One night the nurse responded to the emergency call light from Mr. Abatay's room and found him with his feet on the toilet seat, squatting over the toilet. He had to be helped back to bed. This explained the mystery of the shoe marks on the toilet seat. But why would he do that, and why was there water all over the seat as well?

Mr. Abatay had been raised in a farming village in the Philippines. His only "bathroom" was a *kasilyas*, or "dig-in-the-pit" toilet. It is necessary to squat over them to use them. Since bathrooms are considered dirty, the *kasilyas* is generally located in the backyard, away from the house. There is no water there; people carry a bucket of water with them. People do not use toilet paper; it is thought to cause irritation and mild bleeding and to be rather ineffective at cleaning the area. Water is used instead to rinse off the area. People do not worry about spills; the water dries on its own. And although homes are meant to be kept spotless, because *kasilyas* are thought to be dirty, no one thinks of cleaning them. Mr. Abatay did not want to use the bedpan and "dirty" his bed.

It is unlikely that hospital staff will be able to "train" patients to use a toilet in a way different from the way they have grown accustomed. It is important to realize that not all toilets are designed the way American toilets are. In this case, what could have been done is twofold. First, the staff could have been educated on the differences in toilets in various parts of the world, and second, Mr. Abatay could have been provided with clean towels, a wastebasket, and disinfectant spray to use after he went to the bathroom.

In an interesting postscript to this case, I was contacted by the safety director for a small manufacturing company. Employees come from all over the world. He had received numerous complaints about employees' bathroom habits, which resulted in messy, wet toilet stalls. He was stunned to read the above case study, for it helped explain what was going on. He was feeling frustrated, however, because despite issuing memos on the importance of having their backside as close to the seat as possible, and providing seat covers in all the stalls, the toilets were still a mess. He was hoping that I could direct him to an adult training program on "American" toilet etiquette.

I told him that I was unaware of any such programs, but I suggested that someone from his human resources department lead small group discussions in which information is presented regarding toilet habits in different countries due to differences in such things as plumbing. In countries where toilets are essentially a hole in the ground, people are used to squatting. In the United States, they may adapt by squatting with their feet on the toilet seat. In other countries, the plumbing cannot handle toilet paper, so it is put into a wastebasket next to the toilet.

A friend of mine was teaching kindergarten in a Mexican neighbor-   123
hood. She said she was going to have to give her students a lesson in hygiene because they kept throwing their used toilet paper on the floor next to the toilet. I suggested to her that the problem might be one of plumbing rather than hygiene. I suspected that no one had told their parents that the plumbing is better in the United States and can handle toilet paper. Their parents probably had a wastebasket by the toilet at home. Because there were no wastebaskets in the toilet stalls at school, her students were throwing the toilet paper on the floor. I've noticed that in the downtown Los Angeles shopping area frequented by many

Mexicans, the bathroom stalls often have waste baskets filled with used toilet paper next to the toilets.

More than once I have had the experience of going into a public restroom, checking the floor of the stalls for an empty one, and, having found it, opened the door to find an Asian woman with her feet on the seat, squatting over the toilet. It is biomechanically easier to move the bowels in this position and is common in many parts of the world where Western plumbing is not found—and, occasionally, where it is. In a museum in southern France several years ago, I went to use the restroom, but once inside, could not find the toilet. Finally, someone pointed out a hole in the ground. There were depressions on either side in the shape of footprints. I had to overcome a great deal of ethnocentrism before I was able to use it. The experience did, however, help me be more understanding when I open a stall door to discover a woman with her feet on the toilet seat.

Arabs and the Left Hand

124   Conflicts can also occur due to different customs for cleaning oneself after using the toilet. Issam Khattab was an Arab student at an American university. He had a perforated colon and needed a temporary colostomy. Sylvia was the nurse assigned to teach him how to use the pouch applied over the surgical opening on his bowel. Sylvia was surprised to find Issam noncompliant when it came to learning how to perform his self-care with the pouch. The main problem is that he would only use one hand to open and rinse out the pouch; he refused to use both hands. Because this task was extremely difficult to do one-handed, he would always call Sylvia to empty the pouch. Sylvia warned him of the dangers of having the unemptied pouch burst, but he still refused to empty it. Finally, to "teach him a lesson," she let it burst. Issam, now covered with his own feces, was angry and embarrassed, but at last began to care for himself.

Why was he so stubborn? Probably because in the Arab tradition one uses one's right hand to eat and one's left hand to clean after going to the bathroom. Because food in much of the Middle East is traditionally eaten with one's hand out of a communal bowl, it is an important hygiene measure that people use different hands for eating and cleaning. Most likely, Issam was avoiding using his right hand to clean his pouch. It is unfortunate that he did not explain the situation to Sylvia; she could have used disposable pouches that he could change using one hand. Since that incident, she has done just that with her patients who are reluctant to perform the necessary maintenance of their pouches.

Hair

Many cultures have prohibitions against cutting hair, as was illustrated in the case involving Mr. Singh, the Sikh patient in Chapter 4. The biblical tale of Samson, who lost his strength when his hair was cut, reflects a similar prohibition.

Native Americans

A Native American woman named Estelle Begay brought her fifteen-month-old granddaughter Elena into the emergency room. The child was suffering from severe dehydration and fever. To restore fluids intravenously, the nurse shaved Elena's right temple and inserted an intravenous line. Mrs. Begay was busy completing admitting papers while this was done. When she reached the unit to see her granddaughter, she became very anxious and upset. The nurse tried to reassure her that the intravenous lines were temporary and that as soon as the problem was corrected, the child would be fine. Mrs. Begay responded with sorrow and resignation. "She's going to die." The nurse tried to reassure her, but Mrs. Begay would not leave Elena's bedside.

At one point, Mrs. Begay did leave for a few hours. She returned with two relatives and a "medicine bundle," which she tried to put on Elena's bed. This was against hospital policy and was not permitted. The nurse said she could leave it by the window, if she desired. Mrs. Begay and the other relatives, who were no longer permitted in the unit except during limited visiting hours, kept a vigil outside the door. The next day, despite Elena's improvement, Mrs. Begay insisted on taking her home against medical advice.

The following day, her mother readmitted Elena. She was still feverish and would not eat. A small bundle was attached to the child's shirt. As the nurse started to remove it, the mother stopped her. "Please let her keep it. It is our custom." She went on to explain why Mrs. Begay had taken the child home against medical advice. She was afraid Elena would die.

"In our culture, it is taboo to cut a child's hair. Long, thick hair is a sign of a healthy child. To cut or shave it means the child will become sick or die." Mrs. Begay had obtained a medicine bundle to counteract the effect of violating the taboo, but was not permitted to put it next to the child. It was useless sitting by the window. Mrs. Begay had no recourse but to take Elena home, where she could use the curative charm. This time, the nurses agreed to let the medicine bundle be placed next to Elena. After four days, her condition improved and she was able to go home.

125

This example illustrates two important points. The first is the same discussed in the previous chapter with respect to religious and spiritual symbols: do not remove them. The second is that hair may have important significance beyond aesthetics for the patient and should not be cut or shaved without prior discussion.

The Body

Scars

126 Most Americans are concerned with their appearance. Surgeons therefore try to leave as small a scar as possible. This effort had a negative effect with forty-one-year-old Nigerian patient Osito Seisay, who was introduced in Chapter 3. He had come to the United States to have his brother operate on his knee, which was injured when a bull charged him. His nurse was concerned when he did not request pain medication following surgery. He was Muslim and was enduring the pain as an offering to Allah.

The next cultural incident occurred when Mr. Seisay's brother, the surgeon, came to remove the bandages. He was very proud of his work and pointed out how small the surgical scar was. Mr. Seisay, however, did not share his brother's happiness. He was disappointed over the small size of the scar. He felt that without a large scar to mark the surgery, the other members of his tribe would not believe he had suffered very much. What kind of offering to Allah would that be?

His surgeon brother had obviously shed most of the old ways. He could not believe Osito still held these beliefs and tried in vain to convince him otherwise. At this point, nothing could be done. One would think that Mr. Seisay's brother, being aware of tribal customs, would have anticipated Osito's response. He did not. He was too westernized. Surgeons, however, should be aware that all patients do not share the same ideal body image and should discuss such things in advance.

Fat

Mention of body image brings up the subject of fat. American culture values thinness and views obesity as a disease. Many cultures, however, see thinness as a problem and plumpness as the ideal.

127 Jane, a nurse, was about fifty pounds overweight. She was embarrassed about her size and eventually managed to lose most of the excess weight. She related an incident that occurred when she was at her heaviest.

Her Panamanian boyfriend, Mario, brought her home to meet his family. When they saw her, they were delighted that she was so fat. They told her this several times during the evening. Jane was totally humiliated by their remarks. She was already nervous about meeting Mario's family, and now they were insulting her. Yet they seemed so friendly.

Near the end of the evening, Mario, sensing her discomfort, took her aside and explained. In his culture, fat is seen as healthy. A fat woman can have lots of babies. All his other girlfriends had been far too thin to suit his family. At last he was going out with a "real woman." They had not been insulting her by calling her fat; they were bestowing a great compliment. His explanation made Jane feel a little better, though their repeated comments about her size continued to disturb her.

Although this incident did not take place in the hospital, it illustrates a problem that could arise there. Many Latin Americans and Eastern Europeans, among others, share Mario's family's view of body size. Advice that a patient lose weight might not be followed because it would create a negative body image. Imagine a slim American woman being told she should gain twenty-five pounds for the sake of her health. How willing would she be to trade her "attractive" figure for one that she sees as too fat? Health care professionals should be aware of possible resistance and be prepared to deal with it.

An article in the *New York Times* (LaFraniere 2007) focused on the efforts the Mauritanian government has been making in recent years to promote a healthy lifestyle. They are fighting an uphill battle, however, because it is a culture that sees fat as attractive in women, so much so that women go to great lengths to put on as much weight as possible. A 2001 government survey showed that 20 percent of the women between ages fifteen and forty-nine had been deliberately overfed, and nearly 70 percent of these had no regrets. Obesity is culturally associated with family wealth and epitomizes ideal female beauty. In addition to purposely overeating, many women also take a steroid hormone that can cause weight gain. Others take prescription antihistamines because they make them drowsy, and thus less active and more likely to put on weight. One can only imagine the difficulties a physician might face in trying to convince a woman with such beliefs that it is important to lose weight.

Summary

There are many potential sources of conflict within the hospital. Those that involve activities of daily living have the potential to occur on a daily basis. Awareness of potential areas of conflict can go a long way toward avoiding them. The most common source of problems is diet. Food is essential to health, yet the traditional diet of many patients may conflict with standard hospital fare. As a result, patients may refuse to eat, which can both compromise their health and confuse their diagnosis. It is advisable for health care personnel to have some knowledge of traditional diets, in terms of both content and preparation, and to involve the patient or family in designing meals. In an era of increasing competition between hospitals for patients, it is the savvy hospital that will make accommodations to the patients' preferred diets.

It is also important to understand that toilets take very different forms in different parts of the world; sitting on a toilet seat may not come naturally for many people in developing countries. Some may prefer washing themselves off to using toilet paper.

Hair is another potentially sensitive issue. Do not expect to cut or shave hair without discussion, especially if the patient is a Sikh or Native American.

Finally, remember that the Anglo American view of the body, where the goal is to be thin and free of scars or other marks, is not necessarily shared by all. In many countries, it is seen as healthier and more attractive to be a bit plump. In others, scars may represent an offering of suffering to God.

Key Points

- Ask about food preferences and religious restrictions on diet during the admission interview.
- Involve the patient and/or family in choosing meals when possible.
- Take ethnic diets into account when discharging patients with special dietary requirements. Heart-healthy ethnic recipes are available online.
- Learn about your patient's toilet habits and try to accommodate them.
- If your patient comes from a culture or religion that forbids shaving or cutting hair, do not do so without discussing it first with the patient.
- Realize that not everyone values thinness and unblemished skin.

Chapter 6

Family

When asked to name their most common problem in dealing with non-Anglo ethnic groups, most nurses respond, "their families." This is understandable, given cultural differences in a number of issues related to family, including decision-making and the role of family members when someone is ill. However, the application of cultural sensitivity can make the hospital experience less stressful for patients, family members, *and* health care providers.

Decision-Making

Family as Decision-Maker

In U.S. culture the *individual* is the primary unit, and autonomy and independence are highly valued. As such, we expect individuals to make their own decisions regarding health care, as long as they are mentally competent. Many other cultures, however, see the *family* as the primary unit, and family *inter*dependence is valued over independence. Usually such cultures are agriculturally based, since subsistence farming requires the coordinated efforts of a large family, the larger the better since that means more (unpaid) hands to do the work. Even when they are no longer farming, they may continue traditional patterns of decision-making. What affects one person, affects every member of the family. Unfortunately, health care providers are often ill prepared to deal with patients who refuse to make decisions until they consult with family members.

Mrs. De Luiz was a Latina woman in her late fifties, suffering from diabetes. She and her husband lived with their son and his family. Her physician, Dr. Moustafa, found that the oral medication she had been taking was not doing enough to control her blood sugar levels and wanted to put her on insulin. He expected Mrs. De Luiz to comply;

128

however, she said that she would first have to consult with her family. This both annoyed and confused him. This was *her* health; why did she need to consult with her family? It is actually somewhat surprising that Dr. Moustafa did not understand, since he was Egyptian and family decision-making is common in that culture. However, he was only in his thirties and may have adopted more American attitudes. At the same time, because the physician's authority is paramount in Egypt, he may have been disturbed by the fact that Mrs. De Luiz did not immediately accede to his recommendation, thus undermining his authority. Somewhat annoyed, he told Mrs. De Luiz to return the next day with her husband or son.

When Mrs. De Luiz returned the next morning with her husband, Dr. Moustafa explained to them the importance of keeping her blood sugar under control. Mr. De Luiz said that he was concerned that if his wife went on insulin, she would be unable to care for their grandson and that if she followed a special diet, she would not cook the foods he liked.

This case highlights the fact that in most traditional Hispanic families, the needs of the family take precedence over those of the individual, and important decisions are made by the family, not the individual. It also emphasizes the importance of asking the patient what concerns she or he might have in following the physician's recommendations. In this case, the patient's husband was forthcoming, but in others the likely outcome is that the patient would simply not adhere to the physician's recommendations and the physician would have no clue as to why. At least by asking, the physician can have an opportunity to address the patient's concerns.

Although the nurse who reported this case did not report on the outcome, the clinical implications are clear. When treating Hispanic patients, try to involve the family as much as possible. Understand that what affects one individual affects the entire household. This point is true for all families, not just Hispanic ones. Finally, ask about their concerns regarding treatment. One way to ask is to simply say, "I know that patients sometimes find it hard to follow all my recommendations. What problems do you think you might have in following them?" Compromises can be made, particularly with regard to diet. There are ways to adjust traditional ethnic diets to conform to the needs of patients with diabetes and heart disease; it just takes more time and patient education on the part of the clinician.

Health care providers must be aware that making your own decisions about your own health care is very American and reflects our strong value of independence. It is good practice to ask a patient, "Is there anyone you would like to consult with before making a decision?" Keep in mind that even many Americans may want to consult with family members.

Authority Figures

In Chapter 7 you will read about cases in which the husband is the authority figure in the family and responsible for making the major decisions, even those regarding the health of his wife and children. However, in some cases, it may be the grandparents or other family members who are in charge, as with the following case.

Ricardo Gallegos was a twenty-two-year-old Mexican patient who needed a kidney biopsy. Carmen, a bilingual nurse, acted as interpreter when Swan, his regular nurse, needed him to sign informed consent. They were both surprised when he refused to sign, since they thought he understood the need for the biopsy. He explained that he could not make the decision; that was the job of his eldest brother, since his father, who would normally make such a decision, was in Mexico. Carmen and Swan insisted that he was old enough to make his own health care decisions. Furthermore, the doctor had advised him to have the procedure as soon as possible. It was Friday, and if he didn't have it done immediately, he would probably have to wait until Monday. But his brother was at work and couldn't make it to the hospital until later that evening.

Fortunately for Ricardo, consent could be obtained over the phone with a doctor's order and two nurses witnessing and signing consent. But the situation could have easily been avoided had staff thought to ask Ricardo on admission if there was anyone he wanted to consult with before making decisions. He had been in the hospital for two days already, and his brother had been there, signing consents and making medical decisions. This specific consent could have been signed earlier. But everyone involved had made the incorrect assumption that because he was twenty-two years old, he would make his own decisions.

In many cultures, including Romani (Gypsy), Asian, Middle Eastern, and Hispanic, males are traditionally the authority figures. Unless they are very acculturated, it is often best to consider them the spokespersons for the family. They are often the ones who will make the decisions. This recommendation may be difficult for those with feminist leanings, but it is likely to be the most productive approach. Age is also a sign of authority in Gypsy and Asian cultures, so initial conversations should be addressed to the eldest male.

It is unwise, however, to assume that males are always in charge. In matrilineal societies such as the Navajo, where descent is traced through the female line, the eldest women may have the greatest authority and decision-making power. Even in male-dominated cultures, women may have authority.

130   Julia was treating Mrs. Torres, an elderly Hispanic patient who was intubated. When she needed information, she would direct her questions to the eldest son. She assumed he would be the family spokesperson. However, he rarely had an answer for her. While in many cases the eldest son would be the decision-maker, in this case he was not. The youngest daughter held the durable power of attorney for medical decisions. It was several days before anyone even thought to ask the family who held power of attorney. The staff had made the mistake of stereotyping. Once Julia learned that the youngest daughter was responsible for making medical decisions for her mother, such decisions were reached more quickly and without unnecessary strain on the rest of the family.

Female authority in the home is especially common when it comes to children and health issues. I was talking with a pediatrician at a large county hospital that serves a sizeable Mexican population. She said that when a child needs to continue treatment in the home—for example, when a child has asthma—she will ask the mother who gives her advice about child rearing, and if that person lives with them. Often that person will be the grandmother. She said she would then include that person in any teaching, because she has learned through experience that if she can get that authority figure on board with her treatment plan, it has a much greater chance of being successful.

131   Ricky, a five-year-old African American male with asthma, was supposed to take a controller medication (asthma inhaler #1, Steroid) twice a day as a preventative measure. When he was wheezing and/or having breathing problems, he was supposed to take asthma inhaler #2 (Albuterol) as an emergency medication. Dr. Arabel felt that she had given very clear instructions on how to use the two inhalers, but Ricky's mother kept bring him back to the clinic with a lot of wheezing; his asthma was obviously not being well controlled. As it turned out, Ricky had not been using the inhalers as directed. His mother, who was enrolled in school, was overwhelmed and did not understand the significance of his asthma and the need to use the two inhalers properly. On one of the visits, Dr. Arabel learned that Ricky's grandmother had accompanied them to the clinic. She brought the grandmother into the exam room and explained everything to her. Once the grandmother became involved, everything changed. There were no more emergency room/urgent clinic visits and Ricky's asthma was much better controlled. He only rarely needed the "emergency" Albuterol compared to earlier. Involving the grandmother had made a tremendous difference.

As a general practice, health care providers should *ask* their patients if they would like to consult with any other family members when decisions need to be made, and expect that the responses will vary along both cultural and individual lines. (It should also be noted that in the case of gay and lesbian patients, the person might be outside the "traditional" family structure.) Much time will be saved if such questions are asked on admission, rather than when the need for a decision arises.

The Role of the Family

Another important issue involves the role of the family when a member is ill. The general expectation of the health care system is that families will be there—during visiting hours only—to visit with the patient. Ideally, they will make no demands on the doctors or nurses but will help out as requested. That is not the way many families behave in reality. Problems with too many visitors are a common nursing complaint. However, a little cultural competence can make a huge difference.

What Constitutes Family?

Before we get into the question of the role of the family, we need to define family. Many hospitals distinguish between "immediate family" and "extended family." Immediate family generally refers to the spouse, parents, siblings, and children of the patient. However, in many cultures, relations between cousins can be closer than those between siblings in American culture. Plus there is the issue of gay and lesbian families, in a country in which there is still much prejudice and state-to-state variation in whether marriages are recognized.

The police officer burst through the ambulance bay doors carrying a limp child and attempting to perform mouth-to-mouth resuscitation as he rushed in. Following the officer and the medics was a woman, soaking wet and hysterical. The woman, Hannah, had been working on her computer while Elle, her two-year-old daughter, was playing. Deb, her partner, came home and asked where Elle was. When they noticed the open sliding glass door, they both panicked and ran outside. It was then that they noticed their young daughter at the bottom of the pool. Deb ran to call 911 while Hannah jumped into the pool, retrieved their daughter, and began CPR.

Hannah stood by her child, stroking her face and praying to God while the staff tried to resuscitate her. An admitting clerk came in and asked if the child could have another visitor. Since hospital policy allowed only parents at the bedside during a code, the nurse answered,

132

"Only if the visitor is the father." The clerk replied that it was the mother, to which the nurse said, "But the mother is already here." Another staff member told Hannah that there was another woman outside claiming to be the child's mother and asked if she knew who it could be. Hannah shouted, "It's her mother. We're lesbians!"

Deb was then escorted into the room. When she saw their child, she gasped, let out a subdued scream, and then ran to Elle, quietly sobbing. Hannah stepped back to allow Deb to kiss and stroke Elle's hair. Then Hannah and Deb turned to each other for comfort.

Fortunately, the staff was able to revive Elle; she had a strong heartbeat and began to regain some color. This case took place many years ago; as time goes on, treating gay and lesbian families will become a common occurrence and hopefully not cause the kind of confusion found in this case.

Gay and lesbian couples should be encouraged to fill out a Durable Power of Attorney for Health Care form in which each designates the other as patient advocate. This will allow the patient advocate to make medical decisions on behalf of the patient in case of emergency, authorize a medical provider to give medical information about the patient to the patient advocate, and authorize the patient advocate to sign documents on the patient's behalf.

Visitors

133   Reggie was working in the critical care unit when he was assigned Concepción Rios, a fifty-seven-year-old Hispanic female with new-onset chest pain requiring cardiac intervention. The nurse who took the phone report laughed when she warned Reggie that twenty or thirty very emotional family members were accompanying the patient onto the unit. As a precaution, security had already been called.

Fortunately for Mrs. Rios, Reggie used this situation as an opportunity to apply what he had been learning in his cultural competency class. He immediately called for an interpreter and discussed his plan with her before talking with the family, to make sure his ideas were communicated properly.

He and the interpreter greeted the family in the critical care waiting room. The men were huddled together talking while the women were crying loudly. Mrs. Rios had thirteen children, and members of each of their families were in attendance. Reggie told everyone that although hospital policy allowed a maximum of two visitors at a time for up to ten minutes until 9:00 P.M., he understood how important family was to them. Therefore, he would bend the rules and allow one family member to stay at Mrs. Rios's bedside at all times to assist him in caring for her, and that two other family members could rotate visits throughout the night. One of the younger daughters was selected to assist Mrs. Rios, and the patient's husband volunteered to be the family spokesperson. Mr. Rios then hugged Reggie and told him that he felt comfortable leaving his wife with their family and "such a nice man."

Reggie included the daughter in as much of the routine care as possible, as she was very eager to assist. Grateful family members visited throughout the night. The daughter kept her father informed of her mother's condition, and he in turn, let the rest of the family know. The daughter expressed her appreciation to Reggie many times.

The entire experience was positive for everyone involved. A potentially hysterical crowd became calm and comfortable during what could have been extremely trying circumstances. Contrary to expectations, security was *not* needed to clear out the room. The patient did well and the family was grateful. It was wonderful PR for the hospital. In order to provide culturally appropriate care, all it took was a little knowledge of the importance of family in Hispanic culture and the willingness to be flexible with the visiting rules. Of course, a private room is essential in such a situation.

Terry, a labor and delivery nurse, has found a similar approach to be successful in dealing with large numbers of visitors. She finds that most family members just want to help, so she puts them to work. She'll give the grandmother a rocker at the bedside; her job is to "be there" for the laboring woman. Sisters are given the job of massaging feet, hands, and back. She'll put the husband in charge of applying cool cloths to the forehead, fetching ice chips, and letting her know when the IV bag is down to 100cc. The mother of the patient is put in charge of pericare. If the father of the patient is there, she puts him in charge of the family—making sure the noise level is kept down, the door kept shut, and the television on the station of the patient's choice. If any children are there, their job is to make sure grandma has everything she needs, from coffee to blankets. *134*

Terry's experience is that big families, rather than creating problems, can actually be helpful if you put them to work. After about an hour or so, she will suggest they take a break or go to lunch, since she'll "be needing them later." Often they take a break on their own. She finds that this approach earns her a lot of positive feedback from her patients.

Clay utilized his knowledge of Mexican family dynamics to deal with the problem of too many visitors in Mrs. Canul's room in the emergency department. He noticed a fifty-ish man standing stoically by the door, introduced himself, and asked the man how he was related to the patient. When he answered that he was the patient's eldest son, Clay asked for his help in dealing with a problem. He explained that they all *135* wanted Mrs. Canul's family to be at her side to support her in her time of need, but that the room couldn't accommodate more than two people at a time. Clay asked him to be in charge of the room and decide which two family members could be with her at which time. He accepted the responsibility, and after that the problem of too many visitors ended. Understanding the importance of family dynamics can help eliminate the conflict between the patient's cultural values and the needs of the hospital. But, recall case #130 above, family dynamics may not always be what you expect.

Asian patients will also often have family at the bedside day and night. The custom in both China and Japan is for the family to take care of the patient's personal needs. The medical staff is there to practice medicine. Both respect and obligation require that children minister to their parents. The Asian value of respect for parents can be illustrated by the famous hypothetical riddle. You are in a boat with your mother and your child when the boat capsizes. You can save only one person. Whom do you save? Most Americans would respond, "My child," reasoning that their mother had lived her life whereas their child's was just beginning. Most Asians perceive the situation differently. They would more likely respond, "My mother," explaining that they can always have another child, but they can have only one mother. (Nigerians ask a similar question, but the boat's occupants are your mother and your *wife*. The culturally "correct" response is the same as that described for Asians.)

The different perspectives also reflect a difference in family relationships. Traditionally, most Asians lived in extended family households and tended to value the family of orientation (the individual, parents, and siblings) above the family of procreation (the individual, spouse, and children). Sons generally lived with their parents until they died, and thus that long-term relationship took precedence over any other. In contrast, Americans usually live in nuclear family households. Ties to parents are weakened after marriage, while those to spouse and children are strengthened. The choice of whether to save the mother or child reflects the traditionally stronger familial tie.

One reason large numbers of ethnic family members who visit patients and often remain twenty-four hours a day create significant difficulties for hospital staff is that hospitals in the United States were built to suit Anglo American culture. Anglo Americans tend to have small families and live in nuclear family households. Privacy is a major value. Generally few family members live near enough to the hospital to visit very often. When they do, they usually stay for only a short period of time because they feel the patient should be left alone to rest in order to get well. Therefore, hospital rooms rarely have more than one visitor's chair per bed and visiting hours may be extremely limited. In addition, Anglo Americans value money as well as privacy. Hospitals are a business. If there is room for another bed, it should be for a patient, not for a family member who wants to sleep over.

Nurses who have worked in or visited hospitals in other countries describe very different situations from those in the United States. For example, one student of mine reported that at a hospital in Thailand, families would often sleep under the beds (tables with plastic covers), on the floor, or even in the bed with the patient. A nurse who worked at a Thai hospital told her that family members would often provide meals for the patient because it would be embarrassing for the patient if the family didn't "care enough" to bring food. A nurse who visited a hospital in Spain reported that it had rooms situated around a large patio, where family members relaxed and cooked food for the patients. Families were there around the clock and helped bathe and feed patients. The physicians and nurses provided only medical care. This arrangement helps make sense of the next case.

Betsy Sanders, a former student of mine, broke her leg in a skiing   136
accident in Spain. The doctor at the clinic told Betsy that her ligaments were shredded but that he could correct the condition with surgery. When Betsy awoke from surgery, she was nauseated and in terrible pain but could not vomit. She was too embarrassed. There were ten people in the room waiting to see her. She was in a large private room, and a couch had been turned into a guest bed. All her friends in Spain had gotten together and decided Betsy should never be left alone. They worked out a visiting schedule. One friend even took a leave of absence from work to be with her.

Although Betsy appreciated their concern, their solicitousness made her uncomfortable. All but one of her friends were male. She was in bed with her leg in the air for two weeks, wearing nothing but a hospital gown. She had to be washed in bed and use a bedpan. She could not wash her hair or even brush her teeth. She looked awful and felt worse. All she wanted was to be left alone.

Her situation was the reverse of the non-Anglo in an American hospital. The hospital staff expected her to have visitors around the clock and provided a bed for that purpose. Her friends assumed she would want company and ignored what they interpreted as her polite protestations that she would be fine if left alone. She did not have any family in Spain, so they were filling in. They would have wanted the same attention had the situation been reversed. In this case, however, what the patient longed for was some privacy.

I understand the way people from many of these traditional cultures   137
feel, coming from one myself (Sephardic culture). When I had my first mammogram, the radiologist found a lump. It turned out to be benign, but when I went to the hospital for the surgery—a 12-minute outpatient

procedure—I was accompanied by my husband, my parents, my brother, two aunts, and a cousin. And, truthfully, I was a little hurt that more relatives didn't show up!

In summary, then, hospitals are designed with the needs and values of the culture in mind. Problems arise, as they did with Betsy, when the patient is of a different ethnic group. In a country like the United States, with its huge population of non-Anglo residents, this is frequently the case. It is important to remember that the patient is not just an individual but also a member of a family. When one member is ill, the entire group is affected. Ideally, the family can help care for the patient, freeing the staff for more technical medical care.

Familismo

138   The concept of *familismo*, or the importance of the extended family support system, is essential for understanding Hispanic families. Knowledge of it can help increase patient satisfaction, as the following case illustrates. Charisse, an RN, worked in the department of the hospital where patients and families came to express their complaints. One afternoon, Sonia Sanchez came to her office, accompanied by an older woman and two children. Normally, Charisse said, she would have greeted Mrs. Sanchez, suggest that she and her family be seated, and then listened to her concerns. On the surface, this appears to be an appropriate way to deal with complaints. However, after taking a course in cultural competence, Charisse had new tools to use in the situation. Applying the concept of *familismo*, she first introduced herself to the angry Mrs. Sanchez, and asked about her companions. As Mrs. Sanchez introduced her to her mother and children, Charisse greeted each one individually and then proceeded to inquire after Mrs. Sanchez's concerns. At this point, Mrs. Sanchez visibly relaxed. While Charisse acknowledged that Mrs. Sanchez's change in attitude for the better may have been due to the time she gave her to calm down, it is more likely that it was due to the attention and respect Charisse paid to her family. She reported that the interaction was a positive one, and that she felt Mrs. Sanchez left feeling that her concerns had been heard. It was a small gesture on Charisse's part, but it may have made an essential difference in their communication.

Self-Care

Another problem often stems from the fact that in many cultures *interdependence* is valued over *independence*, as can be seen in the following cases.

139   Tome Tanaka, a Japanese man in his sixties, was a patient in the rehabilitation unit. A stroke had left him with significant weakness on his left

side. Self-care was an important part of his therapy. He had to relearn to feed himself, dress, shave, use the bathroom, and do other daily activities. Kathy, his nurse, spent a great deal of time carefully explaining to Mr. Tanaka how the staff would work with him on these tasks. The patient and his wife listened passively; his children and grandchildren appeared more interested. Several hours later, when Mr. Tanaka's children and grandchildren left, Kathy came into the room and discovered Mrs. Tanaka waiting on her husband as though he were an invalid.

She was not alone in impeding his progress, however. He refused to do anything for himself and continually barked commands at his wife. Rather than use the toilet, he insisted that she hold the bedpan for him. He refused to brush his teeth, shave, or dress, demanding that his wife do everything for him.

Mr. Tanaka attended physical therapy and occupational therapy sessions each day and did quite well. He learned to walk with a cane. He needed minimal assistance with self-care activities. Despite his progress in therapy, however, as soon as his wife or one of his children arrived, he regressed. He was discharged after four weeks, almost as dependent as when he first came.

Kathy and the other nurses were frustrated over Mr. Tanaka's dependency, especially when they saw that he was capable of taking care of himself. They took his "failure" personally, as though they were not doing their jobs properly. What might the nurses have done differently? First, they needed to understand that patients and their families do not always have the same goals as health care personnel. Second, they might have allowed the family to observe Mr. Tanaka during physical and occupational therapy sessions. Unlike most hospitals, this one barred families from such sessions because of the potential distraction for the patient. In this case, the rule might have been waived.

Juan Martinez, a thirty-six-year-old Mexican man with second-degree burns on his hands and arms, posed a similar problem. The skin grafts had healed, and there was now danger that the area would stiffen and the tissue shorten. The only way to maintain maximum mobility was through regular stretching and exercise. The nurses explained to Mr. Martinez's wife that feeding himself was an essential therapeutic exercise. The act of grasping the utensils and lifting the food to the mouth stretches the necessary areas. Mrs. Martinez seemed to understand the nurses' explanation, yet she continued to cut her husband's food and put it in his mouth.

When Linda, one of his nurses, observed this, she took the fork out of Mrs. Martinez's hand and told Mr. Martinez to feed himself because he needed to exercise his arms and hands. Linda again explained to Mr.

140

Martinez's wife how important it was for him to do it himself. Mrs. Martinez appeared skeptical but did not argue. Mr. Martinez looked at Linda peevishly and made a feeble attempt at eating. His wife watched with pity. Linda knew from seeing Mr. Martinez when his wife was not around that he was perfectly capable of feeding himself. Linda left the room. When she looked in five minutes later, she saw Mrs. Martinez once again cutting her husband's food and putting it in his mouth.

Failure to care for oneself is common in cultures that emphasize the family over the individual—in other words, almost all cultures other than Anglo American. Self-care is important to Americans in part because we value independence so highly. In contrast, Asian and Hispanic cultures emphasize family interdependence over independence. For them, self-care is not an important concept.

In many cases, Americans' ethnocentrism blinds them to the fact that life in a typical Asian or Hispanic household may be different from that in an Anglo one. Self-care may be a practical necessity in the Anglo home, where there may be no one to help the former patient with such tasks. In contrast, many Asians and Hispanics live in large extended family households, where someone is usually at home to care for the patient. If they don't live in the same home, they will often live on the same block or at least the same neighborhood. The same is true in many other cultures. One of my cousins married into a large Persian family. They all live in the same small community. The sisters and sisters-in-law are together most of the time. My cousin commented that one of the great things about being part of a Persian family is that you never have to worry about being alone, especially when you are old or ill.

Another significant factor is the difference between egalitarian and hierarchical cultures. In an egalitarian culture such as our own, everyone is thought to be equal—in theory, if not always in practice. No one in the family is considered subservient to anyone else. In hierarchical Asian cultures, some members of the family are clearly dominant (males and elders) while others are clearly subordinate (females and children). The case study involving the Tanakas illustrates the proper roles of wife and children in hierarchical cultures. It is their duty to obey and care for the dominant family member—the husband and father. An additional element when dealing with elderly Asians is the notion that old age is a time for rest, reflection, and being cared for by loved ones after a lifetime of labor. It is seen as inappropriate to insist on self-care when family members are available to assist.

In the situation with the Martinez couple, duty plays a less prominent role. It is of greater importance that when a family member is ill, love and concern are demonstrated through care and attention. The nurses might have instructed Mrs. Martinez to help her husband in ways that would not hinder his rehabilitation. For example, they could have shown her how to massage lotion onto his hands.

I gained some additional insight into the dynamic when my father, a seventy-one-year-old Sephardic man, was dying from complications related to diabetes. He was in the hospital for the last four months of his life. I remember bringing him some watermelon on one of my visits. I had removed the seeds and cut it into bite-size pieces. I handed him the container of watermelon along with a fork so he could eat it. He insisted, however, that I feed it to him. I was shocked. My father had always been a very strong, tough man. We used to joke that if the doctors would allow him, he would perform surgery on himself. Although his legs had been amputated, his arms and hands worked just fine. Why was he insisting that I feed him? At first I saw this as a sign of weakness on his part, but as I sat there feeding him, I asked myself, who is in charge here? It clearly was not me.

I believe that control may also play a role in the failure to care for oneself. Each of the situations described above involved a man whose culture clearly acknowledged his power and authority. All these men, however, were reduced to a state of physical weakness by their medical condition. Ordering people around and having them wait on one's every need are ways of demonstrating dominance. It may masquerade as helplessness, but it can be an important way of maintaining control.

The wise health care provider will acknowledge the powerful role of family in such cultures. When appropriate, patient teaching should involve all members of the patient's family. They are the ones who will likely be caring for the patient at home.

Demanding Families

The hospital staff often has conflicts with family members over issues other than self-care or too many visitors. In some cultures, part of the "job" of the family is to make sure that the nurses are spending enough time caring for their loved one. Unfortunately, given the huge demands placed on nurses, this is not always possible.

Before taking my course in cultural diversity, Jennifer, like all the nurses on her unit, tried to avoid taking care of Naser Assharj, a middle-aged Iranian Muslim patient, because the entire staff found his family to be very "uptight and demanding." The nurses rotated care for this patient, because no one was willing to care for him more than one day at a time. When Jennifer learned a bit about Muslim culture, however, she understood why his family kept demanding a private room and made such a fuss over his meals. It was their way of showing love and care for their family member. He needed a private room so that, as

141

142

devout Muslims, the family could pray together five times a day as commanded by Allah. It was also important that his food be *halal*, or follow the Muslim laws of what is permissible (see Chapter 5). Once Jennifer realized this, she contacted her supervisor and arranged to have the patient moved to a private room and spoke to the dietician regarding his food. The family members were very grateful for her efforts, and became much easier to deal with.

143   A speaker at a workshop I attended on cultural diversity told an interesting story that shed some light on why many Iranian patients' families are always on top of the staff and constantly questioning everything and advocating (to use a nice word) for their family member. He said that the medical system in Iran, particularly during the time of transition to the Shah, was quite poor. Unless family members kept constant watch, patients could die. When his grandmother was in the hospital, his mother kept watch over her. One night around 2 or 3 A.M. his mother noticed that her mother was no longer getting oxygen. She ran down to check on things and discovered that the man in charge of changing the oxygen tanks had fallen asleep. If she hadn't woken him up to do his job, her mother might have died. With experiences like that, how could you *not* be constantly watching for mistakes? Plus, given all the bad press about medical errors, it's not surprising that people would be concerned—and not necessarily a bad idea.

A social worker attending the workshop had an excellent strategy for dealing with loud, difficult, demanding family members. She sits down with them to figure out exactly what they want. Then she talks to them about different strategies that can be used to accomplish that: "You've tried yelling and screaming at the nurses, and that hasn't worked out for you so far. The nurses are very overworked, and when they're yelled at, they feel angry and unappreciated. This makes them less likely to do what you want. Why don't you try this strategy . . . ."

As someone who has had family members hospitalized, I can well understand the frustration of having someone you care for be seriously ill, yet lacking the medical skills to do anything to help the patient. Staying "on top of" the nurses allows you to feel that you're doing something for your loved one. Although this example focuses on a Middle Eastern family because their culture allows them to be more openly verbally aggressive, families from any ethnic background can be demanding.

144   My brother spent the last week of his life unconscious in the ICU. My large extended Sephardic family filled the small waiting room. I observed that with some nurses we were difficult, demanding family members, constantly inquiring as to my brother's condition. With other nurses we were easy. What made the difference? A few minutes of time

at the beginning of a shift. Some of the nurses came and asked us questions about my brother—"what is he like, what is he interested in?" For these nurses, we were easy because we believed they cared about my brother as an individual. What can you do to ease the concern of family members and reduce your own stress? Do as those nurses did.

At the beginning of the patient's hospitalization, spend a few minutes with the family, asking questions about the patient:

- Show that you care.
- Tell them that you will be happy to talk with them on a regular basis (set up a schedule that you feel comfortable with) so you can update them on the patient's condition and they can share their concerns. Explain that if you don't update them at the time you arranged, it's because you're taking care of their loved one, and will talk to them as soon as possible. (And, obviously, follow through.)
- Give the family small, helpful tasks they can do, such as massaging lotion into the patient's hands or feet, so they can feel they are doing something for the patient.

Often, families become demanding because they feel helpless and out of control. By following these suggestions, you can help to alleviate some of their frustration.

Protective Families

Knowing something about a patient's culture can help health care professionals provide more culturally appropriate care. Doreen was caring for a sixty-two-year-old Korean patient, Su Jo. Doreen had learned that Korean culture is hierarchical, and that negative diagnoses may be withheld from the patient. So, rather than assume that Mr. Jo was aware of his cancer diagnosis, she asked his son what his father knew about his medical condition. She also asked the son who was the family spokesperson. The son then told her that his father *was* aware of his condition, but asked that she not tell his mother. He also asked that any questions be directed toward him, as he was the spokesperson for family. Things went much more smoothly than they might have, due to Doreen's cultural competence skills. She said that she now asks this question (how much does the patient know about his or her condition?) with all her patients. However, as will be discussed in Chapter 10 (End of Life), it would be even better to ask the *patient* what he knows about his condition, along with how much he *wants* to know.

A nurse who worked in a hospital in Africa for a few years said that they rarely gave detailed information to patients about their diagnosis

145

or treatment. Such information was usually given to the family, who would then tell the patient. It was felt that having the family relay such news would help to prevent a severe emotional breakdown.

146   An extreme example of the lengths people will go to protect family members was the case of a Pakistani woman. Her son, who was living in the United States, had died of cancer at fifty. She was old and in ill health, and her family was afraid the news would kill her. They even went to the extent of having her son-in-law call her in Pakistan, pretending to be her son. She died presumably not knowing her son had predeceased her.

Once again, because you cannot know how much a patient truly wants to know about their condition, it is always wise to ask. (For more on this subject, see Chapter 10.)

Gifts

147   Mrs. Cato, a fifty-five-year-old Japanese woman, was admitted for uncontrolled diabetes mellitus. She was second generation Japanese and was fluent in English. She made beaded jewelry for a living and while in the hospital, wore her beautiful bracelets and necklaces with her hospital gown. On discharge, the physician asked Aly to go over the use of a glucometer with Mrs. Cato. Aly spent at least 20 minutes showing Mrs. Cato how to check her glucose level with the glucometer. To show her gratitude, Mrs. Cato handed Aly one of her beautiful beaded necklaces, "as a gift." Aly thanked her, but refused because it was against hospital policy for nurses to accept gifts from patients. Mrs. Cato was clearly hurt. Aly remembered learning in class that reciprocity is important in many Asian cultures. When someone does something for another, something is owed in exchange. If the exchange is not completed, the person receiving the kindness is in the other's debt. Because this is an uncomfortable position to be in, it is extremely important not to let such indebtedness occur. A gift to the nurse satisfied the reciprocal obligation. So Aly was caught in a bind. What she did was explain the hospital policy, and then offered Mrs. Cato an alternative. She told her that filling out a "gratitude card" would be acceptable to the hospital, and that she would appreciate it tremendously. Mrs. Cato quickly and eagerly filled one out. Mrs. Cato was satisfied and Aly was pleased to have reached a cultural compromise.

The families of Jewish patients also often give nurses gifts while the patient is in the hospital. It is not done so much through a feeling of obligation and reciprocity, however, but as a way of ensuring good care.

If food is offered, it should be accepted. Even if you don't want the food, thank the patient and say you will share it with the rest of the staff.

One nurse found out the hard way when she refused the offer of candy from a Middle Eastern family because she was on a diet. She said she could immediately tell from the look on their faces that what she had done was very impolite and hurtful.

Whatever the reason for gift giving, when a family member presents a gift to the nurse or doctor, refusing it will likely create a great deal of awkwardness. The solution most commonly practiced is for the health care provider to share the gift with the other staff members. If the gift is inappropriate (e.g., too expensive or too personal), then the physician or nurse should do his or her best to refuse it graciously and if possible, offer an alternative as Aly did (above).

Summary

Family structure and relationships are not the same in every culture. In many cases accommodation will be difficult, if not impossible, given hospital architecture, American medical values, and the American legal system. At the very least, however, greater understanding of the ways of other cultures may have a positive effect on the attitudes of those providing patient care. Culturally competent practices will include involving the family in patient care, both in the hospital and at home.

Key Points

- In cultures where the family, rather than the individual, is the primary unit, decisions are often made by the family. In such cultures, interdependence is usually valued over independence.
- When medical decisions need to be made, ask patients if there is anyone they would like to consult with before making a decision. Ideally, they should be asked before the need arises, such as when they are first admitted or become your patient. Expect that the responses will vary along both cultural and individual lines.
- Be sure to ask patients if they have any concerns regarding your recommendations.
- Males are traditionally the authority figure in most cultures and often act as spokespersons for the family and make decisions for the family. But always ask who the spokesperson will be.
- In many cultures, it is expected that family members will remain with the hospitalized patient. Try to be flexible regarding visiting rules.
- Involve the family in patient care when they so desire. Emphasize self-care only when it is desired by the patient or necessary for physical

recovery; do not impose the value of independence on those who do not share it.

- When appropriate, patient teaching should involve all members of the patient's family. They are the ones who will probably be caring for the patient at home.
- Show family members that you care about their loved one.
- Set up a schedule for updates on the patient's condition and stick to it. Explain any deviations from it.
- Ask your patients how much they know about their condition. Family members may try to protect them from a negative diagnosis/prognosis.
- When a patient gives you an inappropriate gift, try to refuse it graciously and offer an alternative. If possible, accept gifts and share them with the staff.

Chapter 7

Men and Women

Sex and gender are frequent sources of conflict and misunderstanding. Not every culture has been affected by the women's movement. Few share the American ideal of equality between the sexes.

Sex Roles

Since the advent of the women's movement in the 1970s, a concerted effort has been made to eliminate restrictive sex roles. Rather than having opportunities limited by one's sex, the emphasis is on treating each person as an individual and allowing free expression of their abilities. Admittedly, that is an idealized version of what is happening, but it reflects our cultural ideology and the direction in which we are trying to move. Not all cultures, however, share this notion of gender equality, as the following case illustrates.

Women as Caretakers

Amira Faroud was a three-year-old Middle Eastern patient, newly diagnosed with type 1 diabetes. Understanding the importance of involving the entire family in the patient's care, Lisa tried to get the patient's father, Mr. Faroud, to participate. She had seen other fathers reluctant to learn in the past, but eventually, they all were persuaded. But not Mr. Faroud. He would not even consider it. Eventually, Lisa changed the teaching plan to include Amira's grandmother rather than her father, and all went well.

In some cultures, there is a strict division of labor; men work outside the home and women are responsible for all duties within the home, including child care. This was the case in the Faroud household. While fathers should be encouraged to participate, if it is clear that they are not interested, involve other female members of the household instead. Remember to ask who is living in the home of the patient.

Men as Decision-Makers

Part of the ideology of gender equality extends to decision-making. The mainstream Anglo American ideal that husbands and wives should participate equally in the decision-making is not shared by all Americans and is often not the case for people from other cultures.

149 A twenty-six-year-old Mexican woman named Rosa Gutierrez brought her two-month-old son to the emergency department. She was concerned because he had diarrhea and had not been nursing. The staff discovered that he was also suffering from sepsis, dehydration, and high fever. The physician wanted to perform a routine spinal tap, but Mrs. Gutierrez refused to allow it. When asked why, she said she needed her husband's permission before anything could be done to the baby. The staff tried to convince her that this was a routine procedure, but she was adamant. Nothing could be done until her husband arrived.

Although legally she could have signed the consent, culturally she lacked the authority. In the traditional Mexican household, the man is the head of the family and makes all major decisions. Rosa was unwilling to violate that norm. Fortunately, her husband soon arrived and signed the consent.

A pediatrician working in an inner city clinic recently shared an observation that sheds further light on this case study. She said that it is often exceedingly difficult to get Hispanic parents' consent to a spinal tap. Their biggest concern is that the child will become paralyzed or mentally retarded as a result of the procedure. They must be convinced that the risk of meningitis is more deadly than that of a lumbar puncture. She also observed that when parents do consent, they often seem to hide the procedure from friends and family, for fear that their child will be labeled as having had the procedure, with all the implications to the child's future mental status. It's therefore not surprising that Rosa was adamant about obtaining her husband's permission for the procedure. The responsibility was too great to take on alone.

150 Another pediatrician who encountered a similar problem found a solution that proved effective. A female resident could not get a Hispanic mother to sign consent for a procedure for her child; she, too, insisted on waiting for her husband. In this case, however, it was urgent that the procedure be done as soon as possible. The resident asked an older male physician to speak to the mother. Apparently, the combination of his age and gender were enough to convince her to sign consent without speaking first to her husband.

151 Amiya Nidhi was a young woman in her twenties who had recently immigrated to the United States from India. She was in the hospital to give birth. Her support person was her sister, Marala. Marala kept telling

her to get an epidural, but Amiya said that even though she would like one, she could not get one; her husband would not allow it. Cindy, her nurse, overheard the conversation. Having learned that husbands are the authority figure in the traditional Indian household, she went to speak with Mr. Nidhi. She explained why an epidural would be advisable. She said that he seemed pleased that she came to him about it. He said he would think about it, and let her know. About thirty minutes later, he came to Cindy and told her that he would like his wife to have an epidural. Everyone was pleased. By using cultural competence, Cindy helped her patient get the care she wanted, while still respecting the authority structure within the family.

As a professional woman and wife who has always shared decision-making with my husband, I have to admit that it was hard for me to understand the position of women from other cultures who allow their husbands to make decisions. Although I understand it intellectually, it was something I never understood in my gut until one of my Filipina students shared her point of view. Rosaria was in her early twenties and had lived in the United States all her life. Her parents, however, were very traditional, and her father made all the important decisions. She had recently married a Filipino man who, she was a bit dismayed to learn, wanted her to share equally in decision-making. "It was so much easier having my father make all the decisions. There's so much responsibility involved in decision-making. I really hate it." That was something I *could* understand.

I should also point out that sex roles are changing as young women, growing up in the United States, become Americanized and educated. We were discussing this subject in one of my undergraduate anthropology classes that was populated largely by Mexican American students. The women told me that their grandmothers (living in Mexico) taught them that their husband was the boss and that their job was to make their husband's life easier. Their mothers (born in Mexico, but living in the United States) advised them to let their husbands *think* they're the boss, but to manipulate them to do what they wanted. The attitude of my students, born in the U.S. and planning to get jobs after college, was that there was no way they were going to let their husband be the boss; they would share that job equally. The Mexican male students were rather quiet on the topic, although a few expressed some regret over the changing norms.

Culture change is also occurring around the world, not just when people come to the United States. I was giving a talk to a group of nursing students visiting from Taiwan. Traditionally in Asian cultures, parents exert a great deal of authority over their children, even when they are young adults. Yet when I mentioned something to this effect to the students, they politely disagreed. They still respect their parents, but a number of the students insisted they did not feel they needed to obey them.

Men as Authority Figures

Male dominance is the norm in most cultures, a fact that can create problems for female health care providers, as in the following cases.

152   Anandi Kothari, a middle-aged Indian woman, was being discharged following an angioplasty. Her husband was at her bedside. Her physician wrote out discharge orders and left them at the nurse's station. The nurse, Athula, a female from Sri Lanka, entered Mrs. Kothari's room to remove her IV and give her discharge instructions. Unfortunately, Mr. Kothari refused to accept instructions from Athula. Zakia, a female nurse practitioner on the unit, got the same response. In the end, the male physician had to give the instructions to both Mr. and Mrs. Kothari. Mr. Kothari simply refused to take orders from a nurse, and a female one at that.

153   An Iranian mother and father admitted their thirteen-month-old child, Ali, to the pediatrics unit. After three days of rigorous testing and examination, it was discovered that Ali had Wilms' tumor, a type of childhood cancer. Fortunately, the survival rate is 70 to 80 percent with proper treatment.

Before meeting with the pediatric oncologist to discuss Ali's treatment, Mr. and Mrs. Mohar were concerned and frightened, yet cooperative. Afterward, however, they became completely uncooperative. They refused permission for even the most routine procedures. Mr. Mohar would not even talk with the physician or the nurses. Instead, he called other specialists to discuss Ali's case.

After several frustrating days, the oncologist decided to turn the case over to a colleague. He met with the Mohars and found them extremely cooperative. What caused their sudden reversal in behavior? The fact that the original oncologist was a woman.

Even though the Mohars had described themselves as "Americanized," the Iranian tradition of male authority was still strong. They could not accept a woman making life-and-death decisions for their son. Ali's treatment was too important to be decided by a woman.

Several weeks later, it became necessary to insert a permanent line into Ali to administer his medication. The nurse attempted to show Mrs. Mohar how to care for the intravenous line, but Mr. Mohar stopped her. "It is my responsibility only. You should never expect my wife to care for it." Throughout each encounter with the hospital staff, Mrs. Mohar remained silent and deferred to her husband.

Interestingly enough, the nurses had few problems with the Mohars. They were treated with respect because, as Mr. Mohar stated, they were functioning under the direction of the physician. Their only problem was in understanding why the Mohars initially refused treatment for Ali. They had assumed that because both parents were educated in American universities and had described themselves as Americanized, they would accept the American ideal of equality. The stress of their son's illness, however, had made them revert to traditional ways.

The dual role of father and male is evident in the following case study. 154 Magdi Bal was a twenty-seven-year-old woman from Saudi Arabia. Her father was at her bedside when Danielle was doing her preoperative assessment. The surgery Ms. Bal was about to undergo could result in sterilization. Danielle wanted to make sure that she understood before signing the consent. The problem was that her father refused to allow her to sign. Mr. Bal was insistent that she not have a hysterectomy under any circumstances.

The staff was outraged. If the surgeon found uterine cancer, as he expected, a hysterectomy might be the only thing that could save Ms. Bal's life. The physician, Dr. Allen, spoke with her. She said that she wanted to leave all decisions to her father. Dr. Allen spoke next with Mr. Bal. He was adamant—no hysterectomy, no matter what. The physician had no choice but to proceed without compromising her reproductive system.

Danielle spoke with Mr. Bal while Ms. Bal was in surgery. He explained that if she could not bear children, she could not get married. If she could not marry, her worth would be greatly diminished in the eyes of their culture.

Saudi culture is strongly male dominant. It was entirely consistent that an unmarried daughter, even a twenty-seven-year-old one, allowed her father to make all the decisions. Once she married, her husband would take over that job. Furthermore, it is common in Saudi Arabia for a woman to live with her husband's family after marriage. If Magdi Bal could not marry, she would be a burden to her family for the rest of her life.

The doctors and nurses involved in the case later met to discuss it. All were angry with the father for his apparent lack of concern regarding his daughter's health. The women were particularly angry with Magdi for not being more independent. They were further incensed when Danielle told them what Mr. Bal had said. "We are not baby-making machines and our ability to have a productive life is not dependent on having children!"

Once they had vented their anger, they realized that it was not their place to judge. The patient had maintained her rights—in this case, the right to choose someone else to make the decision. They recognized that their values were different from that of the patient's; in other words, they achieved a measure of cultural relativism.

Men as Spokespersons

155   A nineteen-year-old Saudi Arabian woman named Sheida Nazih had just given birth. Her husband, Abdul, had been away on business during most of their ten-month marriage but brought her to the United States to have their baby. He moved into the hospital room with Sheida immediately after she gave birth. He kept the door to their room shut and questioned everyone who entered, including the nurses. The nurses were not happy with this procedure but felt they had no choice except to comply.

Although Sheida could speak some English, the only time she would speak directly to the nurses was when Abdul was out of the room. Otherwise, he answered all questions addressed to her. He also decided when she would eat and bathe. As leader of the family, Abdul felt it was his role to act as intermediary between his wife and the world. This behavior is often interpreted as a sign of domestic violence, and can create additional confusion for Western health care providers (see case study #170 below).

156   Bella Abassian was an Armenian woman in her fifties who was always accompanied by a family member, either her son, her husband, or her daughter. When her physician, Dr. Chen asked her a question, she would allow her companion to answer for her. If a decision regarding her health needed to be made, she would defer to her son or her husband. Dr. Chen found this extremely irritating and frustrating. She considered herself to be a forward thinking, independent American woman, and she found this to be old fashioned and insulting. However, she reminded herself that this was typical in her patient's culture, and she developed what she felt was a successful approach. She learned to first address questions to Mrs. Abassian's husband and son, and then asked if she would like to add anything. She felt that in this way, she was respecting Armenian culture while at the same time, giving her patient a chance to speak.

Female Purity

Sexual Segregation

In the Muslim world, female purity is a major concern. This can have important repercussions in a health care setting.

Parey Assadian, a first-generation Iranian American, was admitted to   157
the hospital with heart problems. Her condition was serious; the moni-
tors showed her heart rate was greatly elevated. She needed to be seen
by a physician immediately, but her husband vehemently refused to
allow the doctor entrance to the room. Why? Simply because the physician was male. As a result, Mrs. Assadian's treatment was delayed and
her life endangered.

In a similar case, a twenty-eight-year-old Arab man named Abdul   158
Nazih refused to let a male lab technician enter his wife's room to draw
blood. She had just given birth. When the nurse finally convinced Abdul
of the need, he reluctantly allowed the technician in the room. He took
the precaution, however, of making sure Sheida was completely covered.
Only her arm stuck out from beneath the blankets. Abdul watched the
technician intently throughout the procedure.

Another time, the toilet in Sheida's room overflowed. Abdul flew into
a rage when three men from engineering and housekeeping were about
to enter the room after knocking. He refused to allow them in. The
toilet went unrepaired until the couple left the next day.

Both incidents stem from the fact that among Arabs and Muslims,
family honor is one of the highest values. Because family honor is tied
to female purity, extreme modesty and sexual segregation must be maintained at all times. According to Geraldine Brooks, author of *Nine Parts
of Desire* (1995), Mohammed, who did much to improve the condition
of women in the Arab world, began the segregation of women in order
to protect his wives from scandal. Others, wanting to emulate the great
prophet, followed suit. No matter what the origin, however, it is a tradition that has become firmly ensconced in the Muslim world. Hospitals
that do not have female physicians on staff should have a referral system
so one can be found when needed. Female housekeepers should clean
the rooms of Middle Eastern females. Male nurses definitely should not
be assigned to observant female Muslim patients. Same-sex staff should
be used whenever possible. For an example of a culturally competent
approach to treating observant Muslim women, see the next case study.

Leila Habib was a sixty-seven-year-old Lebanese women with a high-   *159*
risk mitral and tricuspid valve replacement. She was intubated and
sedated, and doing poorly. She required a great deal of inotropic support. Marion, the nurse caring for her, said that with patients requiring
as much care as Mrs. Habib did, cultural sensitivity and family support
tend to get ignored. When Marion was introduced to Mrs. Habib's son,
she noticed that he refused to shake her hand. She said that normally
she would have taken this as a sign of rudeness, but because she had
taken a cultural diversity course, she decided to investigate it instead.
She engaged the son in conversation, and learned that they had moved

to the United States fifteen years earlier. He wanted to make sure that his family did not lose their cultural roots, so he made sure his children learned both Arabic and English. He didn't want them to lose the ability to communicate with their relatives in Lebanon, where they visited often. Marion asked how she could support him and his mother in a culturally appropriate manner. He explained that it was inappropriate to touch members of the opposite sex (thus explaining his lack of handshake), and requested that she safeguard his mother's modesty as much as possible. Marion said that it was easy to comply, and told Mr. Habib that she would request female nurses when possible. As a result, Mr. Habib expressed great gratitude and Marion was able to build a trusting and rewarding relationship with the family.

Female Genital Cutting

One of the more controversial traditional practices is that of *female circumcision* (as it is seen from an emic perspective) or *female genital mutilation* (FGM in the human and women's rights literature). The origins of this tradition are ancient and largely unknown, but it is consistent with Islamic beliefs regarding sexual desire. As Brooks (1995) explains, it is believed that Allah (God) created sexual desire in ten parts; he gave nine to women and only one to men (hence the title of Brooks's book), which is why female sexuality must be kept under control. One way it is done is by keeping the woman covered, veiled, and segregated. Another method, used in some remote regions of Egypt, and particularly in other parts of Africa, is through FGM. It is believed that the practice reduces women's sexual desire, and that without it, women might be unable to control their exceptionally strong libido, and family honor might be lost. Although there has been a great deal of press coverage in the West of this tradition, nurses tell me that it is still extremely shocking to see.

160   In one instance, a twelve-year-old Somalian girl was admitted to the hospital with a temperature of 102 degrees. When the physician examined her, he discovered that her labia minora and labia majora had been sewn together so tightly that he could not insert a Foley catheter. He had to call in a urologist to place the Foley. The fever resulted from a severe urinary tract infection, likely caused by the infibulation.

The procedure is generally performed when a girl is seven or eight years old. Older women will come in the night, hold her down, and then start cutting. The most minor form involves cutting off the tip of the clitoris. The most severe, known as infibulation, is the removal of the entire clitoris, labia minora, and parts of the labia majora. The outer lips of the vagina are then held together with thorns, sutures, or a paste-like material. A small opening is left for urine and menstrual blood. The girl's legs are tied together for several weeks until she heals. As can be imagined, this practice often leads to myriad urinary, menstrual, and intrapartum problems, apart from the risk of infection and death at the time of the procedure.

In 1985, a world congress was held in Africa in an effort to reduce or eradicate the practice. Surprisingly, the greatest opposition to the elimination of the custom came not from men but from older women and young girls. The older women wanted to maintain tradition. The young girls were afraid that if they were not circumcised, they would be unable to find husbands. Circumcision is seen as the ultimate proof of purity; why would any man marry a woman without a guarantee of her virginity?

In the years since that world congress, little if any progress has been made toward eradication of the custom. In fact, newspaper and magazine reports indicate that it is spreading, as African women move out of Africa. Anthropologists recognize that it is difficult, if not impossible, to merely eliminate a traditional cultural ritual; efforts would be better aimed at trying to promote the *sunna* form, which involves cutting only the tip of the clitoris, over infibulation. Complicating the issue is that opposition to the practice has been associated with the Western world, and there is much anti-American feeling in parts of the world where FGM is practiced. For some, continuing the practice is an anti-American statement.

When the topic of female circumcision came up in one of my nursing classes, a student from Sierra Leone, where most (if not all) women are circumcised, shared something of the experience. She explained that they only cut off the clitoris there; they don't do the full infibulation. She felt the loss of the clitoris was no big deal. Her attitude was that sex is for procreation, not fun, and since African men generally do not perform oral sex on the woman, the clitoris was superfluous. She added that women there still have orgasms, since orgasms are more psychological than physiological. She had no negative feelings toward female circumcision, although she did not plan to have her daughter circumcised because it generally isn't done here. She said she would not hesitate to do it if they were living in Africa. To help us understand her perspective, she explained that there are a year's worth of festivities associated with the circumcision. It is a very big time in a girl's life. It is followed by an arranged marriage and "devirginization" (her term). This is the ceremony in which the girl is "deflowered" by her husband while all the relatives wait outside for the bloody sheet and listen for the appropriate moans of pain.

In another class, I happened to have two Nigerian students, both of whom were circumcised. But they were from different tribes, and had

161

162

very different experiences. The Igbo student had been circumcised as an infant and had no memory of it. She has had no problems resulting from it, and says if she had daughters and moved back to Nigeria, she would definitely have it done to them; it's their tradition. The Izon student had it is done when she was twelve. Her parents did *not* want to have her circumcised, but she was the daughter of a prince, and the first-born girl of his first wife (he had three wives), so they had no choice. She remembers being taken by women from the village, who held her down and performed the surgery with a sharp razor. No anesthesia was used, nothing to stop the pain. At the same time, because she was a princess, they also "tattooed" her stomach, creating a geometric pattern of keloid scars across her entire belly. This woman was completely traumatized by the circumcision and tattooing. She said that when she gave birth to her child here in the United States, the midwife delivering the baby didn't realize she was circumcised. When she saw her vagina, she reacted in horror. This led my student to believe that something was wrong with her baby and she was very distressed and embarrassed. Her son is autistic, and despite her training in biomedical nursing, she attributes his condition to her circumcision. She is adamantly opposed to circumcision and said she would never have it done to her daughter.

Doctors and nurses caring for circumcised women should be especially sensitive to their needs and feelings. Female providers should be used whenever possible, and the patient should be kept draped for privacy. Physicians need to know how to handle labor and delivery, because the episiotomy must be done at an earlier stage. Above all, do not express any ridicule or judgment. You might, however, gently discuss the relationship between their infibulation and any health problems they may have experienced, so that they can make an informed choice for their own daughters. It might also be appropriate to let them know that the practice raises issues of illegality and child abuse in the United States.

Female Virginity

163   The importance of female virginity and purity are unfortunately well illustrated in the following case. Fatima, an eighteen-year-old Bedouin girl from a remote, conservative village, was brought into an American air force hospital in Saudi Arabia after she received a gunshot wound to her pelvis. Her cousin Hamid had shot her. Her family had arranged for her to marry him, as was local custom, but she wanted nothing to do with him. She was in love with someone else. An argument ensued, and Hamid left. He returned several hours later, drunk, and shot Fatima, leaving her paralyzed from the waist down.

Fatima's parents cared for her for several weeks after the incident but finally brought her to the hospital, looking for a "magic" cure. The physician took a series of x-rays to determine the extent of Fatima's injuries. To his surprise, they revealed that she was pregnant. Sarah, the American nurse on duty, was asked to give her a pelvic exam. She confirmed the report on the x-rays. Fatima, however, had no idea that she was carrying a child. Bedouin girls are not given any sex education.

Three physicians were involved in the case: an American neurosurgeon who had worked in the region for two years; a European obstetrics and gynecology specialist who had lived in the Middle East for ten years; and a young American internist who had recently arrived. No Muslims were involved. The x-ray technician was sworn to secrecy. They all realized they had a potentially explosive situation on their hands. Tribal law punished out-of-wedlock pregnancies with death.

The obstetrician arranged to have Fatima flown to London for a secret abortion. He told the family that the bullet wound was complicated and required the technical skill available in a British hospital.

The only opposition came from the American internist. He felt the family should be told about the girl's condition. The other two physicians explained the seriousness of the situation to him. Girls in Fatima's condition were commonly stoned to death. An out-of-wedlock pregnancy is seen as a direct slur on the males of the family, particularly the father and brothers, who are charged with protecting her honor. Her misconduct implies that the males did not do their duty. The only way for the family to regain honor was to punish the girl by death.

Finally, the internist acquiesced and agreed to say nothing. At the last minute, however, he decided he could not live with his conscience. As Fatima was being wheeled to the waiting airplane, he told her father about her pregnancy.

The father did not say a word. He simply grabbed his daughter off the gurney, threw her into the car, and drove away. Two weeks later, the obstetrician saw one of Fatima's brothers. He asked him how Fatima was. The boy looked down at the ground and mumbled, "She died." Family honor had been restored. The ethnocentric internist had a nervous breakdown and had to be sent back to the United States.

Female Modesty

Female modesty is valued in many cultures. A Nigerian student shared that it may be difficult for a Nigerian woman to undress in front of a male health care provider, or to open her legs for a male gynecologist.

It would be best to assign female practitioners to such women. At the very least, they should be asked if they have a preference.

164　　While at an imaging center for a mammogram, I overheard Clara, the receptionist from El Salvador, closing the curtain where one of the patients was changing her clothes. The patient must have said something about it not being necessary, because I heard Clara say, "I don't want patients to have to expose themselves, even though we're all women here." I spoke to her about it afterward and she said that modesty is very important to her. Like her own mother, she will not wear low-cut dresses or short skirts. I was not at all surprised to find a Hispanic woman more concerned about the modesty of her Anglo patients than they were. A Guatemalan student once told me that her grandmother used to tell her that modesty is an asset, and not to let anyone other than her husband see her body. It shows that you have respect for yourself and gives you a sense of pride.

Southeast Asians consider the area between the waist and knees particularly private. Traditional Asian physicians did not touch a woman's body except to take her pulse. Instead, the woman pointed to the corresponding area of a doll to indicate the site of her problem. It was believed that only a woman's husband should see her genitals. Knowing this, Erin handled a potentially difficult situation with cultural competence.

165　　Erin was caring for Hoang Van Chau, a sixty-seven-year-old-Vietnamese patient with an irregular cardiac rhythm. As the nursing assistant began to do the EKG, she exposed the patient's chest. Erin noticed that Mrs. Hoang appeared embarrassed and tried to cover herself. The nursing assistant ignored her discomfort, and told her to keep her hands down. Erin moved to the head of the bed and pulled the covers over Mrs. Hoang, but kept them up so the nursing assistant could place the leads correctly. Mrs. Hoang relaxed a bit. When she completed her task, Erin let down the blanket and made sure her patient was completely covered. Erin removed the leads after the procedure and made sure the blanket stayed in place. Afterward, Mrs. Hoang took Erin's hand, bowed her head, and said "Thank you." The satisfaction Erin felt at making her patient more comfortable greatly outweighed the extra effort involved in keeping her covered.

166　　Sofia Toledo, a sixty-five-year-old upper-class Mexican woman, refused to be dialyzed when she learned that her usual dialysis station was unavailable. She said she would wait until her next treatment, when she could have her customary place. Unfortunately, this was not a viable alternative. Missing a treatment could result in serious complications or even death. When Julia, the nurse, asked her why the new station was unacceptable, Mrs. Toledo was very vague.

Julia finally called Mrs. Toledo's daughter, and together they solved the problem. Mrs. Toledo's usual station was unusual in that neither the nurses nor the patients at the other dialysis stations could see it very well. The rest of the stations were very open, designed for high visibility by the nurses. To be dialyzed, the patient had to remove her pants and don a patient gown. Her underwear was exposed during the process. Mrs. Toledo's sense of modesty, a quality very strong in Hispanic women, made the more open station intolerable.

Julia said that at the time she found Mrs. Toledo's behavior annoying. She and the other nurses saw it as a delay that would prevent them from leaving on time. They did not want to have the extra work of moving machinery or remixing the dialysate. She did not understand the importance of modesty in Hispanic culture, but she did realize that it was important to Mrs. Toledo, a normally "compliant" patient. In this case, a screen or curtain might have alleviated the problem.

Farishta Amanullah, a female Afghani patient with open reduction and internal fixation of her left hip, was labeled as "difficult," along with the rest of her family. When Harold, her nurse, went to change her dressing, Mrs. Amanullah's family refused to allow him to do the procedure. When it was time for her physical therapy, her relatives were reluctant to allow her to get out of bed. Tammy, the charge nurse, was taking a course in cultural diversity and decided to explore the situation. She realized that "difficult" patients are often patients with cultural issues. Tammy approached the family and asked if they had any concerns about Farishta's care. They told her that they preferred to have a female nurse care for her. They were also concerned about Farishta exposing her body in the open and revealing patient gown when she went to physical therapy. Tammy made sure to assign a female nurse to Mrs. Amanullah, and the director of the physical therapy department came to the room and told her that she would be given a second gown to cover her back and protect her modesty and dignity. Once these needs were addressed, Farishta and her family lost their status as "difficult" patients and in fact became quite cooperative. The beauty of cultural competence is not only that it makes medical care more pleasant for the patient, but that it also makes things much easier for the health care providers. All it takes is asking the right questions and making simple accommodations.

Aisha Nazir, a thirty-five-year-old Muslim woman, sat in her bed with a washcloth on her head. When Talia noticed it, she removed it, thinking that the last nurse had left it there by accident. Yet when she returned thirty minutes later, it was on her head again. It turned out that Mrs. Nazir's sister had placed it there, in an effort to maintain Aisha's modesty and symbolize her purity, since she didn't have a headscarf

167

168

with her. After Talia learned this, she told the family that they could certainly bring in a headscarf for Aisha, and she made sure it became part of the report from nurse to nurse. The staff made certain Aisha's headscarf was in place at all times.

I should point out that just as many Americans reading this might be surprised by the degree of modesty displayed by women from other cultures, many Europeans are surprised by the degree of modesty shown by American women.

169   Astrid, a thirty-six-year-old woman who grew up in Germany, made her first visit to the gynecologist in the U.S. When the nurse handed her the drapes and gown and left the room, she had no idea what to do with them. She told me, "In Germany, you go see the gynecologist, strip down, get on the table and spread your legs." She finds the modesty of American women rather amusing. It's all relative.

Domestic Violence

170   The next case both illustrates the value of modesty and raises the issue of domestic violence (also referred to as Intimate Partner Violence, or IPV). It began when Betty, an RN, looked over the chart given to her by the triage nurse. Betty's first reaction was irritation over the paucity of information. The chart noted only that the patient, an Iranian woman, had multiple injuries resulting from a fall. No description of the injuries was given, and only limited vital signs were noted. When Betty entered the room to meet the patient, she saw a woman completely covered in the dark, heavy cloth known as a *chador*, accompanied by her husband. The patient, Noor Esfahani, looked up at Betty for an instant, and then put her head down as her husband spoke. Mr. Esfahani explained that his wife was very clumsy and had fallen down the stairs in their apartment. Betty turned her attention to Mrs. Esfahani, asking simple, noninvasive questions. Before answering in halting English, Mrs. Esfahani would quickly look over to her husband for approval. When Betty asked her how she had sustained the injuries, Mr. Esfahani stopped her from responding with a quick shake of his head. He then repeated his original explanation.

Betty decided it was time to examine the patient, and asked her to put on a gown while she drew the curtain. Mr. Esfahani stepped outside the curtained area while she changed. Betty noticed that many of the bruises were on Mrs. Esfahani's stomach and inner thighs, locations inconsistent with the story of a fall down the stairs. At this point, Michael, the physician assistant on duty at the time, poked his head in the curtained area. Mr. Esfahani reacted to this intrusion by loudly yelling and pushing

Michael, while his wife grabbed sheets and blankets to cover herself. Betty tried to calm the situation, but Mrs. Esfahani quickly dressed and left with her enraged husband against all Betty's protests.

This case raises two issues. The first has to do with sexual segregation. The most obvious sign of cultural conflict occurred when the male physician assistant entered the room and saw Mrs. Esfahani without her *chador.* Although it was acceptable for Betty, a woman, to see Mrs. Esfahani undressed, it violated cultural norms for Michael, a man, to do so. The larger issue, however, has to do with domestic violence. Medical students are taught that one of the first signs of spouse abuse is when the husband speaks for the wife. In cultures in which males are dominant, including many of those in the Middle East, Asia, and Latin America, it is common for the husband to answer questions put to his wife. It is a way of "protecting" her from the outside world. Health care providers should not jump to unwarranted conclusions based on that evidence alone.

In this particular case, however, given the inconsistency of the location of the injuries with the explanation provided, spousal abuse was likely. What should have been done, aside from keeping male health care providers out of the room? Betty might have been more amenable to allowing Mr. Esfahani to answer her questions; this might have helped gain his trust. When she was ready to examine Mrs. Esfahani, however, she might have asked an assistant to get Mr. Esfahani something to eat or drink in another room, thus leaving her alone with the patient. She might then have said to Mrs. Esfahani something along the lines of, "Most couples fight at home and men sometimes lose their temper and hit their wives. Has that ever happened to you?" It is important that the health care provider make the patient/victim feel respected and supported, that she is being taken seriously, that she doesn't deserve the abuse, and that the health care provider is her ally.

Several nurses who work in an emergency room commented that they frequently see cases of domestic violence among Mexican immigrants. One said that she has had to testify against the husband for spousal abuse in two separate cases. One case involved a twenty-seven-year-old man who beat his fifteen-year-old wife badly enough that she suffered head injuries and required sutures to her face and mouth. She was holding their five-month-old son at the time. In the second case, the wife was not as badly injured, but the state pressed charges, even though the wife refused to do so. Another nurse reported that she has been asked on two separate occasions by Mexican employees *not* to report their husbands for abuse.

In one instance, Marta Villegas, a thirty-seven-year-old Mexican woman, had come into the emergency department after being beaten

171

172

by her husband. The attending physician, as required by law in his state, reported it to the police. Mrs. Villegas begged Rowena, her nursing supervisor, to tell the police that it was an accident; her husband didn't really mean to hurt her. Rowena told her that she could not do as she requested; she was concerned for her welfare. She offered some alternatives to returning home, but Mrs. Villega refused them. She knew that her husband would be even angrier now that the police were involved, and she feared reprisals.

Is spouse abuse a part of Mexican culture? No. However, aspects of Mexican culture and the living conditions of Mexicans in the United States may make it more likely. Traditional Mexican women are taught that a good wife should be submissive and take orders from her husband. She should not question him, but rather stand behind whatever he decides, even if she disagrees. She must also be tolerant of his behavior. The traditional male role emphasizes the concept of *machismo*. While a man with *machismo* is one who works hard, is a good provider, and lives up to his responsibilities, the term can also refer to a man who is a heavy drinker and can hold his alcohol, traits that are both socially acceptable and proof of manhood. There is a strong correlation between alcohol and spousal abuse. In addition, increased exposure of Mexican Americans to urban violence and poverty lead to feelings of alienation, powerlessness, and hopelessness—all conditions known to be associated with domestic violence. There is also a high degree of violence toward women in rural Mexico by husbands who migrate back and forth between the United States and Mexico. Many women feel that they must be subservient and obey their husbands, and accept violent treatment. "He works so hard for us. If he beats me when he's home, that's okay. It's only for a few weeks. It's a very small sacrifice for all he does for us."

It should be noted that as difficult as it is for physicians to get American women to admit to being victims of domestic violence, women from Middle Eastern, Asian, and Latin American cultures may be even more reluctant to discuss the issue. In these male-dominated cultures women may be both less likely to see domestic violence as a problem issue and less likely to report it. In addition, immigrant women from these cultures are generally dependent upon men for support, and there is greater stigma attached to divorce. A woman who leaves her husband may be completely without resources, and many of them realize this. They may seen the bad option of staying with their abusive husband as the *only* option. It will take an extraordinary amount of sensitivity on the part of the health care provider to get a woman to open up about her situation. It is important to explore options with the victim, especially resources within her own family. Social workers can often be very helpful in this regard.

Summary

What conclusions can be drawn from these cases? In general, same-sex physicians and nurses should be assigned if possible when dealing with non-Anglo ethnic groups. Try to keep patients' genitals covered whenever possible. Be alert for cases of domestic violence, but don't assume that simply because a man speaks for his wife he is abusing her. Recognize that sex roles and authority figures vary, though males generally hold the dominant position. Use that knowledge when dealing with patients or families from other ethnic groups. This advice may rankle many women, who may interpret it as reinforcing male domination. Perhaps it does, but if the goals are patient adherence, smooth working relationships, and the best possible patient care, this will be the most expedient way of achieving those goals.

Key Points

- In many cultures, males are the decision-makers. Respect family dynamics.
- If your patient comes from a culture which practices sexual segregation, do your best to assign female caregivers to female patients.
- Be especially sensitive to the needs and feelings of circumcised women.
- Try to maintain the modesty of women whenever possible.
- Inquire about the needs and concerns of your patients.
- Realize that domestic violence is an extremely complicated issue for women from many countries (even the United States).

Chapter 8

Staff Relations

Not only is the patient population culturally diverse, the staff population is as well. In addition to Anglo staff, hospitals frequently have large populations of doctors from Asia and the Middle East, nurses from the Philippines and Mexico, and orderlies from a variety of countries. This chapter addresses some of the problems and misunderstandings that can occur when hospital staff members from diverse cultural backgrounds interact, or as a result of differences in training.

Nurses and Doctors

Problems frequently stem from the differing status of both women and nurses in the United States and other countries. In many countries, particularly those of the Middle East and Asia, men have much higher status than women. In general, women are expected to obey men. Furthermore, physicians often have very high status. Even in the United States, doctors have always had higher status than nurses; they have many more years of education, and use their skills to "cure" patients; nurses merely "care" for patients. In recent years, however, nurses as a group have moved toward greater professionalism. Many are obtaining advanced degrees. In many hospitals physicians and nurses are taking more of a team approach, rather than the traditional hierarchical one. Most of today's nurses have grown up with the influence of the women's movement. More men are going into the profession. For these and other reasons many nurses are refusing to be subservient to physicians. This is not the case in many other societies, where traditional sex roles combined with the hierarchical nature of the health care profession create an even larger gap between nurses and doctors. This can lead to conflict between traditional foreign-born and American-trained health care providers.

The Role of the Nurse

The role of the nurse varies from country to country, as do expectations of appropriate behavior. In the United States, nurses are seen as an essential part of the health care team. They use critical thinking skills and the nursing process to assess, plan, and evaluate each and every aspect of patient care. They

- provide professional technical care;
- provide nonspecialized care (e.g., bathe patients, assist with bedpans, take vital signs);
- serve as patient advocates;
- provide psychosocial care;
- educate patients about self-care.

Critical thinking is an essential skill for nurses. It involves openness to questioning and the ability to reflect on the reasoning process. The goal is to ensure safe nursing practice and quality care. Nurses must be able to look at the entire situation—tasks, staffing, patient load, and acuity—in order to organize and prioritize their workload. RNs are expected to analyze the entire situation and think critically before delegating any tasks, especially to unlicensed staff such as nursing aides.

Managers at many hospitals say they have had numerous problems with nurses trained in other countries. Their technical skills are often excellent, but they often fall short in areas of patient advocacy and psychosocial care. They may not demonstrate the level of critical thinking skills required for the job. It's not that they are incapable of doing these aspects of the job; in many cases, they simply may not know that it's expected.

For example, a nurse trained in the Philippines said that when she came to the United States, she had trouble clarifying doctor's orders and decisions. Because physicians are in a position of authority, she didn't feel she could question them. In the Philippines, such behavior would be seen as "deviant and rude." Patient education was also difficult for her, because it was not emphasized in the Philippines; nor was psychosocial care. The family took care of any emotional needs.

A nurse working on a unit where many nurses were brought from India to work in the intensive care unit (ICU) and telemetry floor said they had a lot of problems getting the Indian nurses to advocate for patients, answer questions from patients and family members, and use critical thinking in anticipating patients' needs. She learned that in India a nurse is more of an assistant to the physician. The physician is always nearby, and is the one who talks with the patient. In India, nurses never discussed the disease or care plan with the patient or family members.

An American nurse working in Egypt reported that Egyptian nurses have little autonomy. They are essentially "handmaidens" (her term) to the doctors. The medical residents perform many of the more specialized tasks done by nurses in American hospitals while the nurses merely serve as aides to the physicians. Critical thinking is not part of the job requirement. The same is true in Nigeria, according to a nurse trained there. In addition, family members do a lot of the personal care for the patient. A nurse trained in Vietnam said that RNs there usually performed the duties done here by LVNs—monitoring blood pressure, changing dressings, and administering medication. They were not expected to do patient education, discuss the patient's condition, do personal care for the patient, or provide psychosocial support. They were trained to listen to physicians and *follow* their orders, not *question* them.

Duties of the Nurse

173   Vuong Hue disliked her job as a nurse when she first arrived in America from Vietnam. Before fleeing her native country for her life, she had been happy in her nursing position. However, she soon learned that nursing in America was far different from that in Vietnam. In Vietnam, she had but one function: to provide professional technical care. Nurses were responsible only for giving medications, taking vital signs, and changing dressings per doctors' orders. They were not required to attend to the patient's or family's emotional needs. Nor did they have to bathe, feed, or turn the patient, or make the patient's bed. Her coworkers thought she was stuck-up because she acted as if bathing patients and cleaning bedpans were beneath her dignity. It wasn't that, exactly; she just wasn't used to having to do it. As any American-trained nurse will admit, that is not the most pleasant part of the job! Psychosocial nursing was unnecessary as well; more than that, Hue viewed it as improper. The patient's family took care of personal issues; it was rude for her to pry into their personal lives. It took Hue several years, but she eventually became accustomed to the different roles that American nurses must take and her coworkers no longer saw her as stuck-up.

A nurse trained in China went into great detail regarding the differences between nursing in her home country and in the United States in the early part of this century. She felt that nurses in China lacked the professional autonomy and satisfaction enjoyed in the United States. She also described their job as largely that of "handmaiden" to physicians. They took vital signs, dispensed medication, and carried out doctors' orders. Family members were expected to feed and care for the patient, and often stayed in the patient's room, taking turns sitting at the bedside. She said that although nurses in China are trained in critical thinking, they don't get the opportunity to use these skills since physicians are available around the clock and are actively involved in patient care. Nurses do serve as the eyes of the physician, and alert them to any changes in the patient's condition. She contrasted this to nursing in the United States, where RNs perform in-depth physical assessments and gather data on the patient's physical and social history. She felt that American nurses are *encouraged* to use critical thinking skills and engage in the decision-making process. According to a 2008 study by Lu, While, and Barriball in *Journal of Clinical Nursing*, the role of nurses in China began to change in the first decade of the twenty-first century; however there is still much ambiguity regarding nursing and non-nursing roles.

Given the variation in the scope of nursing in different countries and the fact that roles are changing in some countries (so *when* a nurse was trained may have a significant effect on her experience and expectations), it might be helpful for American hospitals to have special in-service programs for foreign nurses to discuss explicitly the differences in nursing roles in various countries. It would go a long way toward avoiding misunderstanding.

Patient Advocacy

Before he left the hospital for the evening, Dr. Akram wrote orders for Mr. Harriman, a patient with emphysema, indicating not to use oxygen greater than one and a half liters, and not to do pulse oximeter checks or arterial blood gases. Tula, Mr. Harriman's foreign-born nurse, was concerned because too much oxygen can shut down the patient's respiratory drive, while not enough can provide less-than-optimal care to the patient. Without those diagnostic aids, there is no way to know how the patient is doing and what treatment would be most appropriate. Tula suspected that Dr. Akram didn't want these things done because he didn't want to be disturbed in the night with problematic values he would then be obliged to treat. Mr. Harriman was acutely ill, and complaining that he felt like he needed "more air." The problem, however, was that Tula didn't feel that she could question Dr. Akram's authority. Not only was he chief of internal medicine, but he was from Pakistan and had very traditional ideas regarding the authority of the physician and subservience of the nurse. Furthermore, Tula shared his notion of the authority of the physician, so she said nothing.

In fact, as a nurse working in the United States, it is Tula's *job* to question the physician's authority if she feels it is in the best interests of the patient. It is part of being a patient advocate. There are ways this can be

174

done, however, that minimize the potentially confrontational nature of advocacy. Tula might have said something along the lines of, "Dr. Akram, I feel like I need some direction. I know you've ordered no more than one and a half liters of oxygen, and I know it's important not to give COPD patients too much. However, Mr. Harriman is complaining that he feels like he needs more air, and I'm uncomfortable *not* doing an ABG to see what his oxygenation is like, and not monitoring him with a pulse oximeter. I can see you have a plan, but I'm worried about my inability to assess him properly. Would you be able to take a moment and help me understand what your plan is, and how you'd like me to respond to his needs?" After the physician clarifies his expectations, this often opens a chance for more dialogue. A last statement might be along the line of, "If he gets more symptomatic, what would you like me to do for him before I call you, so you can have the information you need?" This kind of approach maintains respect for the physician while still accomplishing the advocacy role of the nurse.

However, keep in mind that when American-trained nurses do their job as patient advocates, they can come into conflict with foreign-trained physicians who do not expect such assertive behavior from nurses, given physician-nurse relationships in their native country.

175   Annie, an American female nurse, had an unpleasant encounter with Dr. Rao, an East Indian male physician. He had ordered her to restrain a patient who she felt did not need restraining. When she confronted him with her opinion, he became angry and accused her of questioning his authority. When she asked him why he felt the patient needed to be restrained, his only response was, "Because I'm the doctor and I feel that the patient needs to be restrained." Annie was angry at this obvious non-answer. As a nurse, part of her job was to be a patient advocate, and she did not feel that the patient's needs were being met. As the argument continued, an East Indian nurse who had observed the encounter told the physician that this was America and the rules were different here. "This is not India where you can do whatever you want because you men are the only ones who have rights. You need to explain to her why you want the patient restrained, because the patient has rights and the nurse has the right to know why she's restraining the patient."

Upset by the support given Annie, Dr. Rao left the room. The East Indian nurse explained to Annie that his ego was hurt; in India, it is considered highly disrespectful for a nurse to question a doctor. Does this mean that nurses should never question Indian physicians? Obviously not. Perhaps the most effective solution would be to have all foreign health care personnel participate in an in-service seminar on the culture of the American health care system. However, until that happens, because such physicians are not as likely to change their behavior, nurses who want to communicate more effectively with such coworkers might use a less confrontational approach.

Dr. Fukushima, a Japanese physician, ordered Lisa to give a patient a certain dosage of a medication. Lisa refused on the grounds that the dosage might be harmful to the patient. Dr. Fukushima insisted, but she was adamant. The interesting twist to this situation is that when he reported Lisa to her supervisor, Dr. Fukushima suggested that she should have *agreed* to give the medication, but simply not have done it. The physician may not have realized that doing as he suggested is not legal in this country.

Asians generally believe it is important both to avoid conflict and to show respect for authority. Rather than refuse directly, it is more appropriate to agree to the supervisor's face and then not follow through. Americans, in contrast, feel it is important to be direct and honest. Disagreement is not avoided. Assertiveness is valued, as is an egalitarian ideal. Dr. Fukushima's major complaint was not that the nurse disobeyed him but that she disagreed to his face, thereby denying him proper respect.

It would be easy to suggest that nurses dealing with Asian physicians take that advice, but it is not that simple. Laws require nurses to follow through on orders they agree to. Nurses would be well advised, however, to remember that Asian men are very concerned about their dignity and self-esteem. And, once again, hospitals should consider offering foreign-born physicians training in clinical roles in American hospitals.

Jackie, a thirty-five-year-old Anglo American nurse, and Dr. Hussein, a sixty-seven-year-old Iraqi physician, got into a conflict over the timing of the discharge of a female cardiac patient. Dr. Hussein called in his order to discharge the patient. Jackie did not think the patient was ready to be discharged and refused, saying that she would not discharge her until Dr. Hussein examined her and read her chart. Jackie had noted several problems on the chart the previous day. Dr. Hussein was furious that she would not follow his orders, and insisted that she do so. Her response was to threaten to call the unit medical director, a threat she carried out. When Dr. Hussein came into the hospital, he became enraged over what he saw as her failure to "respect his word." He demanded to know why she was questioning his judgment. She replied, "Because your decision was not the right thing for the patient." They ended up taking the case to administration.

What went wrong? From the nurse's perspective, she was merely doing her job as patient advocate, since in her best clinical judgment the patient was not well enough to be discharged. From the physician's perspective, a subordinate and a female was questioning his authority and abilities. She was operating along American rules, he along Iraqi ones.

176

177

Jackie also felt that he valued the patient in question less than he did some of his other patients because she was a woman. She thought that he might have been prejudiced against the patient because he had made a notation in her chart that she had a reputation for promiscuity.

What could have been done to avoid the problem? This is a tricky situation. Most Americans, particularly but not exclusively women, would probably take the side of the nurse. However, if the goal is to achieve a smooth-running workplace, compromises must be made. When the physician first called, Jackie might have respectfully asked if she could review the events of the weekend with regard to the patient. For example, she could say, "I'd like your medical opinion on the events that have occurred since you last saw the patient. I think you'll understand why I'm worried about her." By showing respect for his opinion, he might have been more willing to listen to her. Instead, by demanding that he come in to see the patient before she would discharge her, she forced him into a position of having to defend his honor and clinical skills. Often, people feel compelled to maintain their position simply because someone has challenged it. Even if he had refused, she might have suggested that he choose another physician to review the patient's chart and status. This would protect the nurse from a legal standpoint, and the physician might have been more comfortable with the opinion of a professional equal. At the point when he asked why she was questioning his judgment, rather than acknowledge that she was doing so, she might have said that she was not questioning his judgment, but rather doing her job as patient advocate. Pleading that "the system" caused her to do this might have helped him save face. Because nurses are legally and ethically responsible for acting as patient advocates, he might see that by checking on the patient he would be helping her out. He could later have explained to her the importance of respect to him and that her lack of it made him feel defensive.

The comments of an American nurse who worked for several years in Egypt may shed some light on the attitudes of physicians from Middle Eastern countries. Nursing is a highly stigmatized occupation for women. Wages are very low and, as a result, nurses expect tips or *baksheesh* for patient care tasks, further contributing to the lack of professional status. Although male nurses generally treat only male patients, female nurses care for both men and women. In essence, this puts female nurses in the position of touching male strangers, something few women other than prostitutes will do.

Note that the suggestions for handling the situation put most of the burden on the nurse, despite the fact that her behavior was more in line with American cultural values. The truth is, however unfair, it is more realistic to expect the nurse than the physician to make accommodations. However, I would once again urge all hospitals to have an orientation for foreign-born staff on American cultural values in the workplace.

In case you're wondering how the incident was resolved: the patient remained in the hospital and had open-heart surgery the following week. The relationship between the doctor and nurse was permanently destroyed.

The following interaction between an authoritarian Asian physician *178* and an Anglo nurse illustrates how understanding culture can help improve working relationships. Kayla was a staff nurse on a medical-surgical floor when she first met Dr. Ling, an Asian physician. They got along well until Kayla transferred to the diabetes clinic. Clinic protocols allow nurses to order new medications, adjust medications, and order lab work as needed, as long as they get a physician to sign the order. When Kayla asked Dr. Ling for his signature, he would rudely question why she felt the medication was necessary, and on a few occasions refused to sign, stating that he disagreed with the medication she had ordered. After learning more about Asian culture in a cultural competence course, she realized he probably perceived her approach as showing a lack of respect, despite the fact that she was following clinic protocols. She then changed her approach. Rather than just asking him to sign the medication order, she would go to him, explain the situation with the patient, tell him what she was considering, and ask him what he would like done. Kayla reported that Dr. Ling was much more receptive to this approach, probably because it allowed him to feel respected and in control. Taking the extra time to do this repaired the lines of communication between them. Although it could be argued that Dr. Ling is the one who should have changed his behavior, that is probably less realistic than having Kayla apply her cultural knowledge to achieve the results that she wanted.

Patient advocacy also involves asking questions, something foreign-born nurses may have a problem doing.

Dr. Kim, a Korean physician, ordered Isra Srisai, a Thai nurse, to give *179* Digoxin to a patient. Isra, however, thought he had said Dilantin. When she repeated the order to Rowena, the charge nurse, Rowena corrected her. She had been in the room at the time Dr. Kim gave the order. Rowena told Isra that she would have to clarify the order with Dr. Kim. Isra, however, clearly did not want to do that. Rowena, concerned with the safety of the patient, went ahead and clarified the order with Dr. Kim and presented the information to Isra. Fortunately, nothing bad happened in this situation.

However, nurse managers often report that Asian-trained nurses are hesitant to question physicians, either when they disagree with their orders or when they don't understand an order. Asian respect for authority and concern with self-esteem often conflict with the patient advocate aspect of the nurse's job in the United States. If the physician is male and the nurse female, respect plays an even bigger role. It is important that foreign-trained nurses be taught that patient advocacy is an important aspect of their job and that it is okay to challenge a physician if they think it is in the best interests of the patient. Suggestions for how to do that in a diplomatic manner can be found in some of the previous cases.

Many Asian-trained nurses also find it challenging to ask questions when they don't understand something, for fear of seeming incompetent. Again, hospital orientation for foreign-trained nurses should emphasize that it is expected they will ask questions.

Critical Thinking

180   Susan, an Anglo American nurse, asked Marietta, a nurse trained in the Philippines, to cover for her while she took a lunch break. Susan told her that one of her patients, Mrs. Smith, would probably want her pain medication while she was at lunch, since it would be exactly four hours since her last dose. Mrs. Smith had severe chronic back pain and was in for some tests. As predicted, Mrs. Smith called for the nurse while Susan was on her lunch break. Marietta brought her the pain medication. Mrs. Smith told Marietta that her pain was much worse and that she now also had a terrible headache. Marietta told her to see if the medication also helped her headache, and to tell Susan if it didn't. When Susan returned, Marietta reported to her that she had given Mrs. Smith the pain medication. When Susan made rounds after returning from her break an hour later, she ended in Mrs. Smith's room. Susan didn't start with her because she was (supposedly) recently assessed by Marietta. She found Mrs. Smith slumped over and slurring her words; she was having a stroke. Her physician ordered procedures and medications to treat and manage the severity of the stroke, but unfortunately, it was too late to prevent lasting affects. Mrs. Smith could no longer speak and was paralyzed on her dominant side. Marietta asked Susan whether Mrs. Smith had told her about her headache. She hadn't, because she was having a stroke when Susan first saw her.

This tragedy occurred because the role of the nurse is different in different countries. *In many other countries, nurses are primarily seen as aides to the physician. They are not expected to think on their own.* They are expected to carry out physicians' orders, but not to analyze and assess patients on their own. Nurses trained in such diverse countries as Nigeria and Iran report the same thing. Nursing in the United States has a much broader

scope. Nurses are expected to apply critical thinking skills in the performance of their job. In this case, Marietta should have done several
things beyond simply giving Mrs. Smith her pain medication. She should
have also:

- assessed Mrs. Smith and found out that the headache was a new
  symptom, and assessed for pain level;
- documented the complaint of headache and pain level;
- checked the chart for other diagnoses that would trigger a need to
  call the doctor (such as severe headache in a patient with
  hypertension);
- checked on Mrs. Smith or assigned an aide to sit with her;
- reported the headache to Susan when she first returned.

Whatever happens to the patients during Susan's break is Marietta's
responsibility. Just because the only thing Susan told Marietta about this
patient is that she would need pain medication doesn't mean that that
is all Marietta had to do for her or Susan's other patients. As an RN in
this country, Marietta is expected to assess any situation she walks into
and handle it appropriately. The sudden severe headache was a signal a
stroke was occurring. This was essentially ignored by Marietta, an RN
who had been trained to assess symptoms. It was her duty to report any
significant change in the patient's condition to the physician. Unfortunately, Marietta didn't do her job, and the patient suffered permanent
damage because of it.

In the United States, nurses are accountable for everything they do or
don't do. RNs are responsible for people's lives in the same way physicians are. Marietta was too task oriented and took her "assignment" too
literally. She merely gave out the pain medication as requested, and
neglected the more important aspect of her job—to use critical thinking
skills to assess and care for *all* the patients she sees. It is essential that
hospitals realize that the scope of nursing is different in different countries, and that they provide orientation and training on the specific
expectations for nurses working in the United States.

Psychosocial Care

I often hear the same complaint from Anglo Americans who have been
hospitalized. They criticize what they perceive as the "coldness" of many
Filipino nurses. I brought this up in one of my classes that was populated
largely by Filipino nurses. I was curious as to how they would respond to
the charge. They explained to me that what is perceived as "coldness"
is intended to be a display of "professionalism." It is a sign of respect to
show distance. Further adding to the Anglo perspective is the fact that

Filipinos are raised not to be physically affectionate in public, so they may not touch as much as other nurses. Another contributing factor is the lack of training in psychosocial care. In the Philippines, as in many parts of the world, family members remain with the patient day and night. They take care of any psychosocial needs the patient might have. In fact, it would be considered rude for a stranger to involve herself in the personal life of a patient. In the United States, the situation is different. Family members often live in different cities, or even in different states. Thus, they may not be available to take care of the patient's psychosocial needs. Nurses are expected to take on that function. While, of course, there will be much individual variation, it is important for all foreign-born health care professionals to receive training in American culture, so that they understand that distance is perceived not as professionalism but rather as a lack of warmth and caring and that psychosocial care is not only appropriate, but expected.

Cultural Influences on Nursing

In addition to differences in role expectations, cultural differences also affect the relationships between nurses on the job and lead to misunderstandings and conflicts between nurses of different cultures.

Gender Role Conflict

181 Traditional dominant and subordinate roles can be a source of friction among hospital staff. For example, Ikem Nwoye, a Nigerian male nurse assistant, would have what one nurse described as a temper tantrum whenever a female registered nurse asked him to do something. At other times he would sulk and simply leave the room. What he would not do was take instructions from a woman. In Nigeria, men are considered superior to women. Men tell women what to do, not the reverse.

Nursing is a hierarchical profession in which orders are followed according to rank, not sex. The nurses thus expected the nurse assistant to do what they told him. As a Nigerian male, Ikem felt he should not have to take directions from females, despite his lower professional rank. Unless someone with this cultural disposition can be placed under the supervision of another man, it will be difficult to maintain a viable working relationship on the floor.

A Team Approach

182 Josepha, a Filipina nurse, did not get along well with her coworkers. The nursing staff on her unit was composed of two Anglo Americans, two

Nigerians, and Josepha. She felt her coworkers were taking advantage of her, because they would ask for assistance whenever they saw her. Josepha was angry over what she perceived as obvious discrimination. She cheered herself by reminding herself that she was a better nurse than the others; she could do her work without their help. In addition, she was not lazy like they were. She took care of her patients; the other nurses insisted that their patients take care of themselves.

One day, Rena, one of the Anglo nurses, was unusually friendly, so Josepha opened up to her. As they got to know each other better, Josepha shared her feelings of being taken advantage of. Rena explained that it was common procedure for the nurses to help each other with their work. Rena confided that the others thought Josepha was being snobbish and proud because she never asked for help. They saw what Josepha had interpreted as laziness on the part of the others as being team players. Rena also explained that American health care providers believe that independence is important and encourage self-care among their patients.

Josepha was stunned by Rena's revelations. Rena offered to help bridge the communication gap between Josepha and her coworkers. She explained to the others that Josepha was trying to save face by never asking for help; she didn't want them to think she couldn't do her job. Josepha began to teach her patients self-care and to ask her coworkers for assistance. Over time, the cross-cultural misunderstandings were resolved, and Josepha's coworkers became her best friends.

Leadership

Problems also arise from the traditionally passive female roles valued in most Asian cultures. Myung Soon Park, a Korean charge nurse in intensive coronary care, was an excellent worker. She was quiet, industrious, and knowledgeable. She gave the patients good care and was proficient in using the specialized equipment in the unit. In her role as charge nurse, however, Myung Soon was perceived as incompetent. She was unable to lead. She did not offer strong guidance to her staff. She did not counsel or reprimand them. She was indecisive and became apologetic when anyone made a mistake. 183

Although Myung Soon's personality was partly to blame, her submissiveness was consistent with the traditional role of Korean women. Korean culture is hierarchical, and the ideal woman is passive and subservient. She is taught to avoid conflict and maintain harmony. These values made it difficult for Myung Soon to perform the functions of a good charge nurse. Her coworkers liked her personally but were frustrated by her professional performance.

Myung Soon was aware of the problems she was having. Counseling helped her to realize she could not handle her job. She resigned as charge nurse but continued on as a staff nurse.

Passive Versus Assertive Behavior

A few examples have been given of the passive, submissive behavior of Filipino and other Asian nurses. Many other nurses, however, report the complete opposite. They say that Filipino nurses, for example, can be very assertive, to the point of aggressiveness. What accounts for this discrepancy?

As in any culture, people are born with personality traits that fall along a continuum. Different cultures, however, value and reinforce different aspects of the continuum. If a child is by nature passive and the culture reinforces passivity, socialization will be easy. If the child is by nature assertive, socialization will be difficult but possible. When that child grows up, if he or she moves to a country where assertiveness is valued, years of socialization to be passive may be suddenly undone, as the individual's true nature comes through. The assertiveness may even be exaggerated as a result of years of repression.

Thus, passive Filipino nurses are the ones who were by nature passive even before being socialized in that direction. It will be very difficult to train them to be assertive. The aggressive ones are most likely those who were socialized to be passive against their inherent nature and who now find in America cultural permission to be assertive. At the same time, it can also reflect generational differences and location of training.

184   Lily was a new nurse, born in the Philippines but trained in the United States. She was working at a teaching hospital. One day she told the intern about the condition of one of their patients. He gave her instructions on what to do for the patient, but they didn't sound appropriate to Lily, so she told him she would page his resident and speak to him about the situation with the patient and what should be done. Sarah, an older Filipina nurse trained in the Philippines, overheard their exchange. After the intern left, she scolded Lily for what she had done, saying "He is the doctor and he knows what to do and you need to follow his orders." She added that it was inappropriate to call physicians by their first name; she should address them as Dr. so-and-so. Lily observed that many of the older nurses trained in the Philippines showed a lot of respect for physicians and accepted whatever they say. But she was trained to think critically, act as her patient's advocate and see physicians as members of a team.

Hierarchical Cultures and the Meaning of Criticism

Lourdes Balmonte was a sixty-year-old Filipina patient with pulmonary   185
tuberculosis. Her physician had ordered strict home isolation, but she
was not complying with the order, so the county health department
issued an order that if she did not remain in her home, she would be
confined in a treatment facility or jail, according to the California Code
of Regulations. Josephine, a middle-aged Filipina nurse with the county
health department, was asked to act as interpreter when Rebecca, an
Anglo American county health supervisor, served Mrs. Balmonte the
medical order. Josephine agreed, both out of respect for her supervisor,
and because she was still on probation at the job and wanted the chance
to impress Rebecca with her interpreter skills. Unfortunately, it didn't
work out that way.

Several times during the session, Rebecca stopped to criticize Josephine. First, she criticized her for smiling and talking in too friendly a
manner to Mrs. Balmonte. "This is a legal matter and must be taken
seriously," she informed Josephine. She also disapproved of the way
Josephine was doing the interpreting. Josephine's translations were
often much longer than Rebecca's statements. Each time this happened,
Rebecca would pause and give Josephine a look of annoyance.

After the session, Rebecca pulled Josephine aside. She thanked her
for helping out and said she had done a good job, but then pointed
out some things that Josephine should remember next time. First, she
explained, "Smiling and making friendly gestures will make the patient
take the matter lightly." Then she said that she should translate only the
exact words and not embellish on the speaker's statements. Josephine
was devastated by Rebecca's criticism, and two months after the incident
was still worried that it would affect her probationary status.

What went wrong? What Rebecca didn't realize was that the dynamics
of the situation put Josephine in a very awkward position. Filipino culture is hierarchical, and the elderly are accorded great respect. Even
though Josephine was only interpreting for Rebecca, she felt extremely
awkward having to scold Mrs. Balmonte for disregarding the doctor's
orders. Smiling and making friendly gestures was her way of conveying
respect. She felt she had to go beyond merely translating Rebecca's
words, for many English words lack an exact counterpart in Tagalog.
Josephine felt that the only way she could translate Rebecca's meaning
was by citing examples. In addition, she had to use both Tagalog and
the Ilocano dialect from the region Mrs. Balmonte was from.

Did Josephine explain all this to Rebecca? No. Rather than defend
her actions, Josephine merely listened quietly to Rebecca's criticisms. It
would have been against Filipino cultural norms to "talk back" to her

supervisor. Instead, Josephine was afraid the incident would result in her not getting the permanent position once her probationary period was over. She felt caught between her values and her job, and feared that honoring her values would cause her to lose her job. In all likelihood, Rebecca forgot the incident, or, if she remembered it, assigned little or no importance to it. Because of the hierarchical nature of Filipino culture, criticism from a supervisor carries much more impact than it does in our more egalitarian culture. Rebecca probably saw her comments as helpful; Josephine saw them as questioning her ability to do her job.

This situation underscores the need for cultural competence training. Rebecca needed to understand some of the difficulties in translating from one language to another, as well as the awkwardness of putting Josephine in a position where she had to "scold" an elder. Had an older or male Filipino been available to act as interpreter, it would have been a better choice. Josephine needed to understand that criticism has a different connotation in American culture and that it is acceptable to offer an explanation for one's actions without appearing to show a lack of respect. Practice in cross-cultural communication skills is essential.

Hierarchical Cultures and Offering Help

186   Another incident based on status differences involved an Anglo nurse who was in the habit of helping out nurses' aides when her own work was done. All the aides but one accepted Sylvia's assistance gratefully. When Sylvia offered to help Celina, a Filipina aide, with the difficult care of her quadriplegic and stroke patients, she declined. Rather than feel grateful for the offer of assistance, Celina was insulted, because in the hierarchical culture in which she had been raised, a supervisor would offer to help only if she felt the worker could not do her job properly. Sylvia then responded, "Don't be silly! It's crazy to do this alone. You could get a bad back." Celina took the word "crazy" literally, that it meant Sylvia thought she was mentally ill, a condition that is highly stigmatized in Filipino culture. No wonder she was insulted. Celina also interpreted the original offer of help to mean that Sylvia thought she was slow and incompetent. Her *amor propio* (self-esteem) had been wounded.

Sylvia learned of Celina's reaction from another Filipina aide. Celina had not said anything directly to Sylvia because she wanted to avoid conflict and show respect for authority—important values in Filipino culture. Although Sylvia at first perceived this as "going behind her back," she later learned that the use of a third party go-between is common in many Asian cultures. The next time Sylvia saw Celina, she apologized, saying that she had not understood how Celina felt. Celina explained that she had been raised with certain ideas and was having trouble adjusting to American ways. For example, Filipino nurses feel they have failed if they do not complete all their work on an eight-hour shift. American nurses will simply tell those on the next shift that they were very busy and could not finish everything. By the end of their discussion, Celina and Sylvia came to an understanding and never had any further problems. It is important to realize that words and actions can carry greater significance than we might intend.

Terry eventually came to a similar understanding, but not before experiencing great frustration. She was acting as a preceptor in her unit to two new hires—Sally, an Anglo American nurse and Hue, a Vietnamese nurse. All went well with Sally; they maintained good eye contact, and she felt there was trust. When Sally didn't understand something, she let Terry know. The situation was quite different with Hue. Hue avoided eye contact with Terry and never asked questions. When Terry asked if she understood something, Hue would nod affirmatively, but later it often became clear that she had not. Terry was extremely frustrated and felt Hue was unhappy being assigned to her. Since Hue was a new grad, she was going to be working with her for 12 weeks. Terry was ready to withdraw from the role. She finally asked her manager to get feedback from Hue about how she was doing and whether she wanted Terry to continue as her preceptor. To Terry's great surprise, her manager told her that Hue *did* want to continue with Terry as her preceptor and furthermore, thought she was the best nurse she had ever worked with.

At the time this was happening, Terry was enrolled in a class on cultural diversity. About five weeks into the preceptorship, Terry realized that the problems she was having with Hue might be due to cultural differences. At that point, she decided to adopt a different approach. Rather than giving Hue instructions and asking if she understood, she would ask her to repeat and demonstrate the instructions. She also had a heart to heart talk with Hue, and told her some of the frustrations she was feeling. Hue was a bit embarrassed; she hadn't realized that something as simple as eye contact could mean something so different in the United States. She had been avoiding eye contact to show respect. She also had not asked questions of Terry because she felt it would be rude to question her preceptor. The very behaviors that led Terry to think she was doing a poor job with Hue were Hue's way of showing respect for Terry's higher position. After their discussion, things got much better. They both learned about each other's culture. Terry felt that it helped her become a better preceptor because it made her realize that not only did individuals have different learning styles, but that cultural differences could also play a role. In the end, Terry and Hue developed

187

a very good relationship. Often, being aware of cultural differences and bringing them out in the open for discussion can make a huge difference.

Medicine

The Role of the Doctor

A cross-cultural misunderstanding between a Middle Eastern male physician and an Anglo American female patient sheds interesting light both on the roles of men and women in Middle Eastern culture and on the roles of doctors and patients.

188   Roberta Hansen had been admitted for pneumonia. Abbas Mehraban had been called in to consult when her own physician found some lab results he could not explain. Dr. Mehraban questioned her about her symptoms, and then told her how he was going to treat her condition. He neither explained his rationale nor included her in the decision-making process. When Ms. Hansen tried to question him about her treatment, he gave her only vague responses. She became increasingly angry and yelled at him, using profanity. Her behavior angered the physician so much that he resigned from the case.

Most Americans can probably understand why Ms. Hansen was angry, but what about Dr. Mehraban? In the Middle East, doctors are seen as authority figures and their decisions are not to be questioned. Ms. Hansen breached proper Middle Eastern etiquette regarding patient and physician roles. Dr. Mehraban needed some teaching on the relationship between American patients and their physicians, including the patient's "right to know."

Although by American standards Dr. Mehraban would not be considered a "good" doctor—he certainly did not practice patient-centered care—there are other cultures in which he would. In many Native American and Asian cultures, a "good" doctor does not need to ask the patient a lot of questions. The doctor should be able to diagnose the patient by reading the proper signs. This is in direct conflict with the American approach, which values physicians who *ask* their patients a lot of questions and *listen* to the responses. "Good" American doctors may thus unwittingly lose the respect of some their patients. Recall case study #10, in which the Vietnamese patient felt she couldn't trust a doctor who had to ask *her* what was wrong. In such situation, physicians might judiciously choose to have a nurse interview the patient before they begin their examination.

The American legal and medical systems recognize the patient's right to know all the details of his or her condition. The high incidence of medical malpractice suits also dictates that physicians share all possible complications of any surgical procedure or medication. Such openness and honesty can sometimes have a negative effect, especially when dealing with patients from other ethnic groups.

In China and Japan, where doctors are seen as authority figures in a hierarchical and patriarchal society, patients are told little about their condition. Lawsuits are extremely rare. The physician is expected to know best and to use good judgment. If the patient has cancer, the family might be told, but the patient is rarely given the diagnosis. Asians have a tremendous fear of cancer, perceiving it as a death sentence, even though many forms can be successfully treated. Patients told they have cancer often mistakenly assume the situation is hopeless and give up. Loss of will to live can lead to premature death.

Imagine the situation of a Chinese or Japanese patient new to the United States who is told he or she has cancer. The physician may believe it is easily treatable through a combination of surgery, radiation, and chemotherapy. The patient, knowing that doctors never reveal a diagnosis of cancer to a patient, assumes the worst—he or she is going to die immediately. The psychological ramifications can be devastating. In such a case, it might be advisable to use a technical medical term other than cancer (lesion, growth, etc.) and begin by emphasizing the success of treatment. This topic is discussed in more detail in Chapter 10.

Language and Communication Problems

Speaking in the Native Language in the Workplace

One of the most common problems mentioned in my workshops is that of nurses speaking their native languages in the hospital. This is a very interesting issue, with legitimate explanations and concerns on both sides.

The most important reason for nurses not to converse in a language not spoken by the patient is that the patient may think they are talking about him or her.

Harry Davisson, a Vietnam veteran, was in the recovery room follow-   189
ing surgery. Two nurses in the room were speaking to each other in Tagalog about their weekend plans. Mr. Davisson was disoriented due to the anesthesia. He thought he was in a prison in a foreign country. When he later told his family about this, they were quite upset and went to speak to the charge nurse. They felt that the two nurses had added unnecessarily to their father's anxiety. A staff meeting resulted. Such incidents can be easily avoided by strictly following the rule of only English around patients.

It is less critical, but still hurtful, when nurses speak in their native tongues around other employees. American nurses frequently report feeling left out when they walk into a room and several Filipinos continue to converse in Tagalog. They see it as extremely rude.

When this issue comes up in groups, I usually ask the Filipinos to explain why they speak in Tagalog at work, even though they can speak English. Some of their answers are to be expected; others are surprising. Among the expected answers: away from their native land, it brings them a sense of home and belonging. One Filipino stated, "Speaking our own language reassures Filipinos that even though we are here in the United States, we still have something that bonds us together, something that we have in common that gives us a sense of belonging." In an emergency situation, they feel they can communicate more quickly in their native tongue. Some things, like jokes, do not hold up in translation. Or they may be embarrassed by their thick accent in English.

I've heard two other explanations that were less predictable. One is that in Filipino culture it is important to show respect to your superiors in the hierarchy—for example, anyone older than you. Tagalog has different words that do this; English does not. It could therefore be seen as rude for a Filipino to talk to an elder in English. Another explanation has to do with the fact that, in the Philippines, speaking English is associated with higher social status. If you are Filipino and speak to another Filipino in English, you will be seen as conceited, as acting as though you are better than the other person.

In discussions of the topic at hospital workshops, Filipinos often seem surprised that the other nurses don't just ask them to switch to English and join in. Anglo Americans say they could never do that; it would be rude. They want to be invited. Sarah Lanier, author of *Foreign to Familiar* (2000), contrasts hot-climate "inclusion" cultures with cold-climate "privacy" cultures. In inclusion cultures, individuals know they are automatically included in conversations, meals, and any other activities of the group; it is rude to hold a private conversation. In privacy cultures, private conversations are acceptable and people are expected to ask permission to interrupt a conversation. It's clear that such a distinction may be in operation when an Anglo nurse enters a break room and finds a group of Filipinas in conversation. They may assume she knows she's included, while she may feel she cannot join in without an express invitation.

It is important for native English speakers to realize that Filipinos are not intending to be rude when they speak in Tagalog in the presence of others. But Filipinos must also realize that it can be very distressing to patients and can make non-Filipino coworkers feel excluded. Open discussion of all perspectives is usually quite effective. The most equitable solution is to allow hospital employees to speak in their native tongues when on break, as long as no one else is around. When nonspeakers enter the room, they should immediately switch to English. Under no circumstances should they converse in anything other than English around patients (unless, of course, the patient is fluent in that language).

One of my students reported an interesting solution that her hospital implemented. They did an experiment in which they formed groups in which everyone spoke a language other than English. One group spoke Spanish, another German, another Italian, and another Tagalog. They put a single Filipino in the Spanish group, a single German in the Italian group, and so forth. They continued to rotate individuals until they had all been in a group where they were the only one not speaking the language. At the end of the day, they all got together to express their feelings. The experiment was successful, and from that point on nurses were much more careful about using their native language around the hospital, coworkers, and patients. No one likes to feel like an outsider.

Another student shared a "game" they use at her hospital. Every time someone uses a word in Tagalog, they have to put money in a jar. The money they collect goes toward a staff party. Everyone gets a good laugh when someone has to pay. This is a lighthearted way of drawing attention to the problem.

Open Communication

The next example underscores the importance of open communication. Making assumptions is dangerous, while asking questions can lead to greater harmony.

Natasha, an Eastern Orthodox Christian nurse from Russia, was the only non-Filipino staff member on the unit. The Filipino nurses organized a potluck dinner one night, and kept inviting her to have some of the Filipino delicacies they had brought. The problem was that it was in the 40-day period before Easter, when Eastern Orthodox Christians do not eat meat. Many of the Filipino delicacies have meat in them. Rather than tell them the truth, she would simply refuse, saying, "Thanks, I'll have some later on my break." Finally, they just made up a plate for her with her name on it. This created conflict for her, since she felt it was disrespectful not to eat food that is given to you, but eating it would go against her religious beliefs. She finally decided the only thing to do was tell them the truth. When she did, they burst out laughing. They had perceived her refusal as some sort of discrimination—as if she was "too white" to touch their food. They also thought it might be because she was anorexic; she was very thin. It never occurred to them that it could

190

be a religious issue. This incident broke the ice and now their communication is much more open and filled with questions about each other's religion and culture.

191   The next case involves me in the culturally inappropriate position. I was giving a talk at a conference. Although I would have liked to attend the entire conference, I arrived just prior to my talk and had to leave right afterward. My husband had had knee replacement surgery earlier in the week, and I needed to get home to take care of him. I made the comment at the end of my talk that I couldn't stay for the rest of the conference; I had to leave to "play nurse." I used the term "play" because I'm not a nurse. As in "I'm not a real doctor, I just play one on TV." After my talk, I was in the lobby area, talking to conference attendees. A woman, a nurse, came up to me to tell me that she really enjoyed my presentation, but that I said something that rankled her a little. I asked her what. She said it was when I said I had to go home to "play nurse." She interpreted it as a way of demeaning nurses. She felt that society in general did not appreciate nurses and was always stereotyping them as sexpots, etc. I really appreciated her saying something, and she did it in the nicest possible way. I hadn't given any particular thought to the comment; it was off the top of my head. I taught in a nursing program for thirty years, and have nothing but respect for the work nurses do in an important and often underappreciated job. Her comment was a revelation to me. She said I should have said, "I have to go home to care for my husband." I explained to her what I had meant and apologized for offending her. It was not awkward. She understood, I understood. But if we were in a health provider/patient or colleague relationship, if we had not talked about it, the comment might have damaged any rapport we had or could have had. It was an important reminder of how easily things can get off-track, and how simple it can be to repair a relationship, as long as lines of communication are kept open.

Demeanor

192   Eva, a Chinese nurse, was caring for a young girl. Eva had been directed by the intern to keep the girl under close observation because she was becoming diaphoretic and pale. After two hours, these conditions continued to worsen, and she was breathing abnormally. Eva was alarmed, but tried to stay calm and composed when she called the patient's doctor. The physician was unavailable, so she spoke to his associate. She said, "The patient is looking dusky. Can someone come to look at this patient?"

Three minutes passed, and the patient's condition had worsened, yet none of the doctors had arrived. Eva eventually had to call a "code" over the phone, which summoned every doctor at once.

Afterward, Eva was chided by her nurse manager for not indicating the seriousness of the patient's condition when she called the doctor. She should have used the word "now" emphatically, and conveyed a sense of emergency by her tone of voice.

Eva was offended at first, but then realized it was a cultural problem. As a Chinese woman, she had been raised to control her emotions and to remain calm in an emergency. Since that incident, she has learned to employ more "American" communication skills and call for help more assertively when necessary.

Tone of Voice

As in the last case and case study #29 with the "rude" cafeteria workers, tone of voice can be a major source of misunderstanding.

Kiyoko was a Japanese nurse with a problem. She had taken several   193
years off work to raise her children. When she returned to work, many of her new co-workers were Nigerian. She was disturbed by the fact that some of them spoke really loudly, even on the night shift when the patients were sleeping. It sounded to her as if they were yelling at the patients and their family members. When they spoke to her, she felt they were being rude and trying to overpower her. In response, she tended to keep her distance from them and limited her socializing with them. At least, until she took a cultural diversity course and one of her classmates was from Nigeria. She came to understand from her classmate that a loud tone of voice was the norm in her culture, and was not intended to project any of the meanings Kiyoko had associated with it. As a result, Kiyoko began to talk with her Nigerian coworkers more often and became more accustomed to their tone. She realized that they were not rude, but in fact were very caring and attentive to their patients. She no longer expects them to lower their tone of voice, but now respects it as part of the diversity among them.

When "Yes, I Understand" Means "No, I Don't"

Marsha, an Anglo nurse, attempted to assess the knowledge and techni-   194
cal skills of the critical care nurses in her hospital. Most were from China, Laos, Korea, Vietnam, and the Philippines. The first phase of testing involved a written exam focusing on general principles. Confusion reigned, and the scores were low. Thinking the problem lay in the language of the test, Marsha rewrote the exam. In the new version, the

nurses had only to answer yes or no to questions about their knowledge of a specific procedure (e.g., "I understand the principles of hemodynamic monitoring"). Over 90 percent of the questions received a "yes" response. Disturbed by the contradictory results of the two tests, Marsha interviewed several of the test takers, asking open-ended questions that required them to demonstrate their knowledge. Although their English was proficient, many were unable to answer correctly. Why had they said they understood procedures and principles they clearly did not?

Recall the discussion in Chapter 2, "When 'Yes' May Mean 'No.'" The Asian nurses were probably too embarrassed to admit they did not know something. Education is highly valued, and a lack of knowledge indicates a lack of education. The result is a loss of self-esteem. The lesson here is the same as earlier—try to avoid asking yes or no questions. Ask that people *demonstrate* their knowledge instead.

195   Speaking of exams, Celine was involved in an incident with Malea, an older Filipina nurse who was taking a CEU class to renew her nursing license. As Celine passed the nursing station, she saw Malea asking two younger Filipina nurses the answers to some of the questions. They answered several questions for her before making excuses about having to get back to work. Celine noticed them rolling their eyes when Malea wasn't looking. When Malea later asked Celine for help, she refused. For Celine, it was a matter of integrity. She saw Malea as "cheating." She felt the younger Filipina nurses helped Malea out of respect for elders and avoidance of conflict. It's likely that for Melea, it wasn't a matter of cheating, but the kind of sharing that is expected in a culture that values *inter*dependence. A friend who taught English as a Second Language told me that she often had problems giving exams to assess the level of her students because students from some countries would all "share" answers. In their culture, they were expected to help each other out. This made it rather difficult to assess their skill level!

"Please" and "Thank You"

196   Patty, an Anglo nurse, had been working with Maria, a Korean nurse, for two years. Their relationship had been rather hostile. Patty felt that Maria was a very bossy person, never saying "please" or "thank you." Maria was also perceived as rather cold and standoffish, as evidenced by the fact that she would rarely call her coworkers by their first names, especially the older ones, even after being asked to do so. Patty decided to interview Maria for a class assignment in order to understand her better.

When discussing her values, Maria explained the importance of respect in Korean culture. People will call each other by their last names, and use special terms when addressing people older than themselves. However the hierarchy works two ways. When asking something of someone younger than yourself, it is unnecessary to say things like, "please," and "thank you," since you are in the higher position and can act more informally. The respect is understood. Thus, because Maria was older than many of the other nurses, she rarely said "please" or "thank you," assuming it was understood. It wasn't; the others thought she was rude. According to a Korean medical student, the gratitude and apology for asking a favor that are implied in "please" and "thank you" are conveyed in the tone used and incorporated in the conjugation of the verb. Furthermore, the Korean word for "please" (*jae bal*) is reserved for very serious requests, and is often used when begging or desperate. Thus, in Korean, "please" wouldn't be appropriate when making an ordinary request of a colleague.

After the interview, Patty realized that her impression of Maria had been totally wrong, and they soon became friends. It is important to recognize that what is polite in one culture may be seen as rude in another. Open discussion of cultural differences, however, can help alleviate such problems, as it did in the case of Patty and Maria.

Leslie reported that her hospital had recently hired five new Korean *197* nurses. Unfortunately, they did not get along well with the rest of the nursing staff. They rarely said "please" or "thank you" and were generally perceived as rude. Leslie was reading an earlier edition of this book and suddenly realized that the Korean nurses were older than the other nurses on the unit and probably felt that "please" and "thank you" were implicit. Leslie then showed the other staff nurses the section on "Please" and "Thank You." She reported that morale on the unit is much improved. Sometimes, all it takes is a little understanding.

"With Your Permission"

An American physician and professor, consulting in Japan, was about to   198 address a group of university physicians; it was fully understood by all that he would give his talk in English. He nevertheless prepared a brief introduction in Japanese, concluding with the statement, "My Japanese is limited, so with your permission, I will continue in English." When he asked his Japanese secretary if his statement was grammatically correct, she seemed uncomfortable. On further questioning she reluctantly admitted that, grammar aside, it was not appropriate for someone of his stature to ask the audience for permission, and that this would diminish the audience's ability to respect anything else he said. Instead, she suggested, he should merely announce that he would continue in English. In this context "asking permission" was entirely pro forma in American culture; it would be seen as a polite gesture. In Japan, however, it was considered inappropriate from someone in a position of authority, and would likely result in a loss of respect for the person doing the asking. It is easy to see how in the United States, a Japanese physician who believes that asking permission is inappropriate, even simply as a matter of courtesy, would likely be perceived as rude and could inadvertently cause major conflicts with other staff.

Religious Conflicts

Medical personnel also face conflicts between their duty to patients and their own religious beliefs.

199   Elisa, a nurse of the Jehovah's Witness faith, was temporarily transferred to the intensive care unit, where she admitted a patient with gastrointestinal bleeding. He required several units of blood. Elisa refused to hang the blood. It was against her religious beliefs even to participate in a blood transfusion. Reluctantly, she did agree to watch it infuse after someone else started it.

200   Carmen, a Filipina nurse, was informed that she was to be the circulating nurse on a therapeutic abortion. She immediately began to cry and told her supervisor that she would leave work unless her assignment was changed. Carmen was a devout Catholic and refused to participate in an abortion. Joyce, her supervisor, was upset. Other Catholic nurses had worked on abortions before. Besides, she was short of personnel and cases were already running over schedule. Joyce agreed to find someone else to circulate, but she asked Carmen to gather the equipment and supplies for the case. Even this was a problem. "If I set down the room, it's just the same as if I were doing the case," she explained. "I have assisted or aided in taking a life." Joyce finally changed her assignment, but not without some resentment.

A number of the medical students I've taught said they would have problems performing abortions. In order to best serve the needs of their patients, they should be able to discuss, without prejudice, the various options available to the pregnant woman, and be prepared to refer their patients to someone who is not uncomfortable with the procedure.

201   David, an RN from the step-down unit, applied for and received a position as an ICU/CCU staff nurse. When he received his new schedule, he went to the unit director to ask to have his schedule changed. He was scheduled to work on Saturdays. As an Orthodox Jew, he needed Saturdays off to observe the Sabbath. The unit director refused his request, saying that it would cause them to be understaffed on Saturdays. Rather than compromise his religious practices, David decided to

go back to the step-down unit. The unit director could have handled this situation better by asking if any of the other nurses would be willing to trade days off with David. When some of the other ICU/CCU nurses who had Saturdays off found out what happened, they said they would have traded with David. Unfortunately, the unit director didn't think to ask.

It is often very difficult for people to understand others' religious practices, especially when they cause inconvenience. But it is best, whenever possible, to avoid giving assignments that conflict with individuals' religious convictions. Jehovah's Witness nurses, for example, can be assigned to coronary care or well-baby units, where there is rarely a need to hang blood. Days off can be traded. Nurses assigned occasional duties that conflict with their religious beliefs can arrange to switch tasks with a coworker. If their beliefs get in the way of their job too often, however, they should be advised to look for a new job.

Summary

Given the vast cultural diversity of the health care staff in American hospitals, it is sometimes surprising that more conflicts do not occur. The major problems seem to stem from the different roles doctors and nurses are assigned in different cultures. These are often accentuated by gender role differences. Thus, male physicians from male-dominated countries tend to be even more authoritarian than American male doctors, and female nurses from such countries tend to be more submissive than American nurses. Rules of polite behavior vary cross-culturally, and are often a source of misunderstanding.

Because rules of behavior are rarely made as explicit as rules of grammar or rules of the road, conflicts and misunderstanding abound. In most cases, such problems can be avoided or resolved through cultural education. Doctors and nurses from foreign countries could be required to participate in an in-service on the culture of the American hospital system. In addition, workshops in which staff are led to discuss the way things are done in their culture, and in which participants can feel free to ask questions and share their feelings, are often successful in alleviating conflicts and misunderstandings.

Key Points

- One source of staff conflict is the fact that in many cultures men have much higher status than women, as do physicians compared with nurses. This can create conflict between American-born nurses and foreign-born physicians.

- The scope of nursing in the United States is much broader than that in other countries, in that it includes both patient advocacy and psychosocial care. It also requires critical thinking skills.
- Foreign-trained clinicians need to be trained in the "culture" of American medicine and nursing.
- American nursing is based on a team approach, while Asian nursing is based on a hierarchical one. This is the source of much conflict and misunderstanding between American- and Asian-trained nurses, particularly with regard to the meaning of offering help.
- American patients often expect to be a partner in the decision-making process. In other countries, physicians often take on a more paternal role.
- When foreign-born nurses speak in their native tongue at work, they do so for many reasons; they don't realize that nurses who speak only English feel excluded.
- Many problems between staff could be resolved through more open communication.
- Avoid asking yes or no questions whenever possible; when checking competence skills, look for a demonstration of skills.
- Words like "please" and "thank you" are often thought to be understood, and thus unnecessary to say, in hierarchical cultures.
- Try to avoid giving assignments that conflict with individuals' religious convictions.

Chapter 9

Birth

Increasingly, people enter the world in a hospital. Birth is an emotional and generally painful occasion imbued with cultural ritual and thus, once again, we find the potential for misunderstanding and conflict, as well as opportunities for cultural sensitivity.

Antepartum

Pregnancy Taboos

A classic anthropological theory, formulated by Bronislaw Malinowski, states that under conditions of chance or uncertainty, when things cannot be controlled by knowledge, people will turn to magic. Pregnancy certainly fits that condition, and thus it is not surprising that there are numerous beliefs regarding what one should and should not do during pregnancy. One of the most common taboos involves reaching your arms over your head. Doing so is thought to result in the cord being wrapped around the baby's neck. This belief is found among African Americans, Anglo Americans, Asians, and Hispanics.

An Anglo student once told me that when she was pregnant she was warned against raising her arms. As a nurse, she knew there was no medical connection between the activity and the presumed result, so she ignored the warnings. Her son was born with the cord wrapped around his neck. Fortunately, the hospital staff were able to save him. She said that the next time she became pregnant, she was careful not to lift her arms above her head, even though she knew there was no medical basis for it. Why take a chance?

This case illustrates the probable origin of many of the pregnancy taboos found around the world. Throughout human history, childbirth has been a dangerous enterprise. There is much that can go wrong during pregnancy, much that we have little or no control over. After carrying a child for nine months, learning that the child is dead at birth must be devastating for the mother. The first question that must come to her is "Why?" If she can figure out why the baby died, she can prevent it from happening again. Looking back over all the incidents that occurred during pregnancy, you find one that makes some sense to be connected to the baby's death. You then avoid that behavior the next time you are pregnant, and warn other women as well. If the next child is born healthy, that is seen as proof that the connection was valid. And thus, a taboo is born. Pregnancy taboos include such things as avoiding lunar eclipses to prevent the baby from being born with a deformity (Mexican), postponing a baby shower until after the birth to prevent the baby being stillborn (Sephardic Jewish), and avoiding tying knots or braids, which can result in a difficult labor (Navajo).

Miscarriage

203   Bella took care of Anna Boswell, a Roma (Gypsy) woman in her mid-twenties who had come in for a procedure following a miscarriage. Her physician had written orders for her to be discharged. Bella noticed that female relatives surrounded the patient. They asked Bella numerous questions about how much bleeding would occur, and argued against her being sent home. Bella explained that bleeding was normal, and that if any complications arose, Mrs. Boswell could call her physician. Yet she begged to be allowed to remain in the hospital, offering cash to stay.

Why were they all so concerned about normal bleeding, and so adamant about remaining in the hospital? It reflects the Roma concept of *marime*, or impurity. The Roma believe that a woman is "impure" for six weeks after giving birth. (Note that six weeks is the length of the traditional lying-in period, and the time biomedicine says it takes the woman's uterus to return to normal after childbirth.) As long as Mrs. Boswell was bleeding post-miscarriage, she was considered "polluted." It also explains why no males were in the room. Men are to avoid women while they are *marime* so they do not become contaminated. Culturally, it would be much easier for her if she were to stay in the hospital until the bleeding stopped and she was once again *wuzho* (pure).

Dietary Prescriptions and Food Cravings

As described in Chapter 5 in the section on diet, many Asian and Hispanic cultures practice a system of hot/cold body balance. Pregnancy is generally thought to be a "hot" condition, and thus foods that are considered "hot" are restricted so as not to exacerbate an already out-of-balance body. Unfortunately, many foods that are high in protein are considered "hot" foods. It is important for physicians to carefully assess the pregnant woman's diet to make sure she is getting enough protein. Many Hispanic women also avoid iron supplements and prenatal vitamins, which are considered "hot." A culturally competent physician will recommend that she take them with a neutralizing "cold" beverage, such as fruit juice.

Food cravings are a common feature of pregnancy. I've been told that many African American women believe that unsatisfied food cravings can cause birthmarks on the baby.

Estelle Lincoln, a pregnant thirty-two-year-old African American woman, was getting ready for bed when she discovered she was hungry. She went to the kitchen, but nothing looked appetizing. What she wanted, she realized, was fried chicken. In fact, she *had* to have fried chicken; nothing else would do. She begged her husband to go to the local KFC, but he was tired and refused. Five months later, their son was born—with a birthmark in the shape of a drumstick. When Estelle saw it, she looked accusingly at her husband; she *knew* what caused that birthmark!

Some women crave and eat nonfood items, a condition known as pica. Mexican American women often crave magnesium carbonate or the ice that forms in non-frost-free freezers. Unsatisfied cravings (*antojos*) are thought to cause injuries or birth defects in the infant. Physicians should be aware of the prevalence of pica, and question pregnant patients about it in a nonjudgmental manner.

Prenatal Care

A common complaint of health care providers is that many women do not seek prenatal care. Although this can sometimes result in problems, the primary difficulty is a conflict in perception. Americans are raised to see pregnancy and birth as medical conditions; therefore, births usually occur in hospitals under the supervision of doctors. Medical culture also values education (thus, childbirth classes) and a future time orientation (preparation for the coming birth). Prenatal care is an essential part of this package.

One nurse reported that in the small California town in which she lives, Hispanic women often do not come in for a prenatal visit until they are well into their second trimester. This is the case even though the health care staff repeatedly try to "educate" the women, using interpreters. The nurse who shared this wondered if it was due to stubbornness on the women's part, or because interpreters did not adequately relay the information during their previous pregnancy. Neither is the most likely explanation. Pregnancy is generally seen as a "normal" condition rather than an illness and thus not necessarily requiring the assistance of a physician. Elder women provide the support and information needed. Time orientation is focused on the present rather than the future; hence a frequent lack of prenatal care. Although health care professionals should strive not to impose their values on their patients, if a woman who has just given birth can be predicted to have high-risk pregnancies in the future, health care providers should take the time to explain why prenatal care will be important next time.

A Vietnamese nurse said that Vietnamese women believe pregnancy is a natural process and, like many Hispanic women, therefore do not seek prenatal care. They also may avoid prenatal vitamins, thinking they are too "hot" (in the yin/yang sense) for the fetus. Instead, they will eat more "cold" (yin) foods during the last trimester. These foods include eggs, steamed rice, and pork. Physicians should thus carefully explain why prenatal vitamins are need, or ensure that women get the proper nutrients from their diet.

Labor and Delivery

Labor Pains

Individuals respond differently to pain, although cultural norms often dictate how it is expressed. This holds true for the pains of labor.

205   Miguela Coronel, a Filipina woman, was delivering her baby. Her contractions were very strong and closely spaced. The baby was positioned a little too high, and there was some discussion of a possible caesarean section. Despite her difficulties, she cooperated with the doctor's instructions and labored in silence. The only signs of pain or discomfort were her look of concentration and her white knuckles.

206   Doris Davis, an African American woman, lay in the delivery room across the hall, moaning and groaning. Although the delivery was progressing normally, her cries increased in intensity. Finally, her blood-curdling yells resounded through the halls. The hospital personnel compared the behavior of the two women and naturally rated Mrs. Davis's unfavorably. Why was she acting like such a baby? Why couldn't she control herself as Mrs. Coronel did?

Cultural differences account for the behavioral differences. Miguela Coronel's culture values stoicism; Doris Davis's culture does not. Filipinos believe that a woman must experience pain and discomfort as a part of childbirth. To express these feelings, however, brings shame upon her. This is true in most Asian cultures. One of my students from mainland China once explained to me that any woman, "even a queen" (who presumably can do whatever she wants), would be ashamed to cry out in childbirth. A nurse who works frequently with Hmong patients noted that it is imperative to monitor their facial expressions very closely to determine if they've entered Stage 2 (pushing) because they are very stoic, rarely uttering a word during the process. As Anne Fadiman describes in *The Spirit Catches You and You Fall Down* (1997), moaning or screaming is thought to thwart the birth.

The culture of African Americans does not place such restrictions on its women. Varied emotional expression has always been a part of African American culture. Mrs. Davis was culturally appropriate in expressing her pain. Another African American woman might have suffered in silence and still have been culturally normal.

Maricela still remembers the time she assisted Galilahi Hayes, a Cherokee patient, while doing a rotation at a birthing center. Although it was her first baby and she was already four centimeters dilated when she came in, Mrs. Hayes was in complete control. Her grandmother, a Cherokee healer, was attending her, along with her mother and sister. Despite not using any pain medication, Mrs. Hayes barely made a sound during the ten-hour labor. When the time came to deliver the baby, her grandmother helped her into a squatting position while the midwife sat on a stool at the side of the bed. After twenty minutes of pushing, the baby was born into the grandmother's hands. Maricela said it was the most amazing birth she had ever witnessed.

In contrast, Mexican women are notorious for loud behavior during labor and delivery. It is often possible to identify a Mexican woman in labor simply from the *aye yie yies* emanating from her room. Although this chant can be annoying to nurses and patients alike, it can be seen as a form of "folk Lamaze." To repeat *aye yie yie* several times in succession requires long, slow, deep breaths. *Aye yie yie* is not just an expression of pain; it is a culturally appropriate method of *relieving* pain. However, it is important, as always, not to stereotype. As a third-year medical student doing her obstetrics rotation noted, although the two Hispanic women she observed giving birth to their first child were loudly yelling, another Hispanic woman having her fourth child was completely silent during labor and delivery. It is important to remember that there are always individual differences; some cultures simply allow free expression while others discourage it.

Women from some cultures may profit greatly from emphasizing their pain during childbirth. A labor and delivery nurse reported that the most difficult patient she ever attended was Robabeh Farag, an Iranian woman, who yelled and screamed for the entire duration of her labor. After she delivered their child, her husband presented her with a three-karat diamond ring. When her nurse commented on the expensive gift,

207

208

she responded dramatically, "Of course. He made me suffer so much!" Iranian custom is to compensate a woman for her suffering during childbirth by giving her gifts. The greater the suffering, the more expensive the gifts she will receive, especially if she delivers a boy. Her cries indicate how much she is suffering. A young Iranian doctor recently told me that when his wife has a baby, he will present her with a diamond ring or a Rolex watch.

As a side note, an article in the December 6, 2007, *New York Times* described the new "tradition" among Anglo Americans of the "push present"—a gift, usually jewelry, given to the new mother for having pushed out the new baby. A study of 30,000 new mothers found that 38 percent received a gift from their mate for birthing their child; 55 percent of pregnant women wanted one.

American nurses value cooperation; a cooperative patient is one who is stoic and follows directions. "Uncooperative" patients like Robabeh Farag are often avoided. How can hospital personnel deal with the variety of expressions of women's pain during labor and delivery? As one nurse put it, there are techniques for controlling pain that are more effective than yelling, but the delivery table is hardly the place to educate women in coping skills. If nurses understand why patients behave the way they do, however, they can be more supportive.

As for the patients themselves, it might be very disconcerting for an Asian woman accustomed to controlling her emotions, to labor next to a highly expressive Mexican or Middle Eastern woman. Ideally, women might be placed in rooms with women from cultures similar to theirs. Unfortunately, this is not always possible. Sometimes, a brief explanation of cultural differences in the expression of pain might help, particularly for a first-time mother who is laboring next to a woman from a more expressive culture.

Labor Attendants

It is currently standard American practice for a woman's husband to assist her in labor and in the delivery of their child. Husbands are expected to be helpful and to attend to their wives' needs. Unfortunately, things do not always work out this way.

209   Naomi Freedman, an Orthodox Jewish woman, was in labor with her third child. She had severe pains, which were alleviated only by back rubs between contractions. Her husband asked Marge, a nurse, to remain in the room to rub his wife's back. Because she had two other patients to care for, Marge began to instruct him on how to massage his wife. To Marge's surprise, he immediately interrupted her, explaining

that he could not touch his wife because she was unclean. Marge, assuming he meant she was sweaty from labor, suggested that he massage her through the sheets. In an annoyed tone, he again explained that he could not touch his wife because she was unclean. He then left the room.

Marge later learned from Mrs. Freedman that "unclean" referred to a spiritual, rather than a physical, condition. According to Orthodox Jewish tradition, the blood of both menstruation and birth render a woman unclean and her husband is forbidden to touch her during those times.

Labor and delivery nurses must do everything for the Orthodox Jewish patient whose husband will not participate. This often generates resentment toward both the patient and her husband. Nurses sometimes try to avoid being assigned to Orthodox patients or assign a Jewish nurse to attend to them. As always, a good solution is education. If nurses understand why an Orthodox husband cannot get involved in his wife's labor, they may be more accepting. If any female relatives accompany the patient, they might prove to be more willing aids.

An Arab husband can be similarly unhelpful during his wife's labor   210
and delivery. After his wife Azar was admitted to the unit, Ahmed Ramzy told the nurse that he would wait outside. Realizing that her patient did not speak English, she asked him to stay and act as interpreter. (This incident occurred before CLAS standards were instituted, and interpreters were less accessible.) At first, he refused, insisting that it was a woman's place to help in birthing, not a man's. Since there were no Arab women available to interpret, however, he reluctantly agreed to stay.

During her entire labor, Ahmed ignored Azar except to interpret as requested. She was obviously having a difficult time, expressing her pain quite loudly, but he did nothing to comfort her. The staff grew angry with him. It was in fact inadvisable to insist that he stay with his wife during childbirth. Because it was inappropriate for him to be there, he felt extremely uncomfortable and did little to help her situation.

Some nurses have reported that Middle Eastern men often do accompany their wife or sister in the delivery room, but not to assist her. Rather, they are there to "protect" her virtue.

A similar case involved a young Mexican couple. Judging from her *aye*   211
yie yies, Juanita Guerrero was in a great deal of pain. When the nurse insisted that her husband, Carlos, attend to her, he very reluctantly entered the room. Rather than help soothe her by holding her hand, speaking gently to her, or wiping her brow, he stood in the corner. He looked up, down, everywhere but at her. The nurse became very angry. She felt that because he had gotten her into this position in the first place, he should be willing to comfort her.

212   In another instance, Julio Gomez, a fifty-one-year-old father-to-be for the sixth time, became so upset when the staff nurse insisted he join his mother-in-law and sister-in-law in attending his wife in the delivery room that security had to be called. Fortunately, the security guard was an older Mexican man who understood why Mr. Gomez preferred to be in the waiting room with his brothers, uncle, and sons. He explained to the staff nurse that the husband's responsibility was to be strong for his wife—*outside* the delivery room.

213   In Mexico, it is inappropriate for a husband to attend his wife during delivery. It is a woman's job—ideally the job of her mother. This may be related to the extreme modesty of Mexican women. American nurses who have difficulty believing that the modesty of a traditional Mexican woman can extend to her own husband should be told of the eighty-five-year-old Mexican woman with a tattoo of a small cross on her upper thigh. No one in her family—including her husband and daughters—had ever seen it. It is likely that during all the years of her marriage she undressed in another room and made love in the dark. She told the nurse who was caring for her that she had gotten the tattoo in her "wild and crazy youth."

Whatever the reason, a number of cultural traditions dictate that a husband not see his wife or child until the delivery is over and both have been cleaned and dressed. For those who find these cultural practices hard to understand, consider suddenly being forced to watch your parents have sex. How would you feel? Would you stand there and coach them? Wipe their sweaty brows? Or would you stand in a corner, looking up, down, everywhere but at them? Sexual relations occur in the presence of children in some parts of the world but are taboo in American culture, just as it is taboo for a traditional Mexican man to watch his wife give birth, though it is a common practice for American men. Younger, more Americanized Mexican couples may want to participate in the delivery process together, but it should not be assumed that the husband is the proper person to coach his wife in this situation.

In general, traditional Latina women often prefer that their mothers attend them in labor. This is also true of Asian women, although sometimes the mother-in-law is considered more appropriate. A Korean nurse shared this information in class one day, to the general shock and horror of the rest of the class. As she explained, traditionally, when a Korean woman marries, she goes to live with her husband's parents and spends much of her married life taking care of the needs of her in-laws. This is reversed during childbirth. A mother-in-law must attend to the needs of her daughter-in-law, both during delivery and throughout the month-long lying-in period.

Caesarean Section

Chue Hong, a Hmong refugee woman, was pregnant with twins. Early   214
in labor, it was discovered that the second twin was lying across the
uterus rather than head down. The attending physician recommended
a caesarean section. The woman's husband and mother refused, stating
their fear that she would die during surgery. Although the doctors and
nurses continued to try to persuade the patient and her family that she
should consent to the surgical delivery, they remained adamantly
against it. As a result, although the first twin was delivered without problem, the second twin died. The next morning, the husband returned
and requested the placentas, explaining that they had to be separated
in order to protect the live infant from death.

Why was the family so opposed to a caesarean section? Perhaps
because, like many non-Christian rural Southeast Asians, they believed
that souls are attached to different parts of the body. During surgery,
they can leave the body, causing illness or death. In such a situation,
there is little the health care team can do except respect the wishes of
the patient and family. This case resulted from a conflict in beliefs, and,
in the United States, the patient has the right to refuse medical care.

One day I received an email from a social worker who had attended   215
one of my workshops. The small Midwestern hospital in which she
worked was faced with a dilemma that she hoped I could resolve. She
said that her hospital had a significant population of Somali women who
had had caesarean sections in the past, which had made them a high
risk for vaginal births later. However, even though their physicians had
tried to educate them as to the risks, they were still refusing to have a
caesarean. The physicians generally referred these women to their closest affiliated larger hospital that was better equipped, but the women
usually refused. The hospital had had one woman who did successfully
deliver a child vaginally after having had a caesarean section (despite
the warnings of her obstetrician), and now another woman wanted to
do the same thing. The medical staff were concerned for the health and
safety of the patient and unborn baby. They were planning on hosting
an ethics forum discussion, and wanted my input.

I did some research and learned that in Somalia, caesarean deliveries
generally take place under very dire circumstances, and there are high
rates of maternal mortality. It is generally believed that women who have
a caesarean section will suffer later on. However, in Somalia, the caesarean incision is usually done vertically, whereas in the United States, it is
done horizontally, and is less risky.

I consulted a well-known obstetrician, and she described it as a "major
risk management issue." If the second baby is larger, there is a $1/200$

chance that the old uterine scar will rupture, often leading to the death of the mother and infant.

What I found most interesting—and curious—was that they agreed to the first caesarean section, but not to a following one. I suggested that rather than focus on trying to "educate patients" per se, they instead try to understand their patients' specific concerns with a caesarean section (recall the 4 C's), and then address those.

The hospital did have the ethics meeting. The concerns were, of course, both ethical and legal. Unfortunately, the OB/GYNs who had raised the issue did not attend the meeting, but a labor and delivery nurse was able to provide insight into the staff's thoughts and concerns. In the end, the committee concluded that it was a situation of "our culture vs. their culture." They decided to start education at the first office prenatal visit, and to create a "waiver of treatment" form to offer patients.

Postpartum

Burying the Placenta

216   Farhana Setrak, a young Muslim Arab woman, was giving birth in a rural hospital. Two older women accompanied her. She was very expressive in her pain. During the long labor, several staff members heard the women talking about a burial. Although they didn't quite understand what she was referring to, the news quickly spread throughout the unit. There was much speculation on the part of the staff, especially since the women grew quiet right afterward. Were they fearful that they had been overheard? The women also wanted to know how soon after delivery the new mother and baby would be released. The staff grew concerned. Why was the family so secretive? Why were they so eager to leave the hospital?

Mrs. Setrak gave birth to a baby girl. Speculation continued, especially since some staff members knew that Arab culture often prefers sons to daughters. Was the family planning on killing the baby girl? Was that the "burial" they referred to?

Fortunately, no. It was the burial of the placenta that concerned the family, a fact known to the physician but one he had failed to communicate to the rest of the staff. Once the staff understood the situation, mother, baby, and placenta were quickly discharged so they could perform the ritual burial.

Many cultures have a tradition of burying the placenta. In her book *The Spirit Catches You and You Fall Down* (1997), Anne Fadiman describes how the Hmong word for placenta also translates to "jacket." It is this "jacket" that the soul must don at death in order to make the dangerous journey to the place where it will be reunited with its ancestors and await rebirth. Without the placental jacket, the soul is doomed to wander, alone and naked, for eternity. That is why the placenta must be safely buried. A traditional Arab belief holds that the future fertility of a woman is connected to the disposition of the placenta. Should something happen to it, the woman might be rendered sterile. This belief does not appear to be currently widespread among Arabs, and it is not known why Jasmine and her family wanted to bury the placenta, but health care personnel should not be surprised if a patient requests to take the placenta home. At least one hospital has worked with the health department and its own infection control department to allow the placentas of African women to be stored in a container for them to take home for burial.

Umbilical Cord

In some cultures, parents may want to keep part of the umbilical cord. A Vietnamese student shared that in Vietnam the umbilical cord is dried and kept for good luck. Her mother still has her dried umbilical cord in a small box. Others put it in wine to drink. A Japanese student said there is a similar custom in Japan. Traditionally, the cord is dried and placed in a small box that the mother keeps for a lifetime; it is usually buried with her as proof that she gave birth to children and brought spirit to the future. The student said that when she herself gave birth in the United States, she would have liked to do the same, but was ashamed to ask. She thought it would be nice if nurses would remember to ask.

Breastfeeding

It is well known that the colostrum that fills a new mother's breasts before her milk comes in is rich in antibodies that fight infections to which newborns might be subject. Western doctors and nurses emphasize the importance of feeding infants colostrum. Women from many ethnic groups, however, refuse to do so.

Sofia Salgado, a young Mexican woman, gave birth to a son. The nurse wheeled the baby into her room and handed him to her to be nursed. Instead, Mrs. Salgado pointed to her breasts and said, "*No leche, no leche*" (No milk, no milk). Pedro, her husband, explained to the nurse that she would bottle-feed now and breastfeed when she returned home.

According to the nurse who related this example, most Mexican women who gave birth in a hospital near the Mexican border followed the same

217

pattern—early bottle-feeding, later breastfeeding. Because colostrum is so important, this practice worries health care professionals.

Many Mexican women believe they have no milk until their breasts enlarge and they can actually see it. Some perceive colostrum as "bad milk" or "spoiled" and thus not good for a baby. Many do not realize that nursing stimulates milk production. Still others are very modest and are embarrassed to expose their breasts while nursing in the hospital.

The best way to deal with this situation is through education. Explain the importance of colostrum to the baby's health. If the mother's concern is to provide "real" milk for the baby, tell her that nursing on the colostrum will help it to come more quickly. The new mother should also be given privacy while nursing her infant.

Similar advice could be given to the Vietnamese mother who refused to breastfeed in the hospital, explaining that she would do so when she returned home. The Vietnamese also believe that colostrum is dirty and often delay nursing until after their milk comes in.

Postpartum Lying In

218   Angela Wong, a Chinese American woman, had had a caesarean section the day before. She was covered with eight blankets and sweating profusely; her patient gown was drenched. When Celia, the nurse's aide, tried to remove the blankets and offered her a sponge bath, she refused both. Lourdes, one of the other nurses on the unit, explained to Celia that Mrs. Wong was practicing the traditional postpartum lying-in period. Lourdes then spoke to her about the importance of movement to recovery and in preventing pneumonia and deep vein thrombosis. In an example of cultural compromise, they came to the agreement that Mrs. Wong would take a short walk once a day, and that every couple of hours she would move in bed and practice deep breathing. Lourdes showed cultural sensitivity in respecting traditional practices, while at the same time promoting the kind of care she felt was necessary.

219   Maria Salazar was a thirty-two-year-old recent immigrant from Mexico with an infected incision from a caesarean section. She asked Tonya, her nurse, for some water. When Tonya grabbed the bedside pitcher to refill it, she discovered it was full. When Tonya pointed this out to her, she answered in Spanish, "Yes, but I have a fever and a cough. If I drink that cold water I will get even more sick." Tonya, who spoke some Spanish, was taking a course in cultural diversity at the time and was elated to see hot/cold beliefs in action. She then emptied the ice water and refilled it with warm water. Curious, Tonya asked her if there were any changes she would like to see in her treatment. Mrs. Salazar nodded her head. She said she didn't understand why the nurses kept insisting she do

things that would make her ill—things like taking a shower. Didn't they understand she had a fever and had just delivered a baby? And why did they want her to spend so much time walking, when she knew she should stay in bed and rest as much as possible?

Angela Wong and Maria Salazar were both practicing versions of the traditional lying-in period observed throughout much of Asia and Latin America. For a period of time after a woman gives birth, her body is thought to be weak and especially susceptible to outside forces. The new mother is encouraged to avoid both exercise and bathing. These traditional practices come into direct conflict with Western health care, which promotes exercise and bathing for new mothers as soon as possible following childbirth.

The traditional practice in China is called *zuo yuezi*, or "doing the month." It is important to keep the room warm, lest cold or wind enter the new mother's joints. Bathing is considered dangerous for similar reasons. No matter how hot the weather, a traditional Chinese woman will want the windows closed and the air conditioning off.

In Asia, health is believed to depend on keeping the body in a state of balance. As stated earlier, pregnancy is generally thought to be a "hot" condition. Giving birth causes the sudden loss of yang, or heat, which must be restored. The most effective way to do this is to eat yang foods, such as chicken. Cold liquids should be avoided lest the system receive too great a shock.

Traditional Asian thought has it that the price for not "doing the month" is aches, pains, arthritis, and other ailments when one is old. Although practical circumstances may prevent a woman from observing the entire month, many want to practice at least a shortened version of it. This explains why the patients in the cases described above refused ice water in preference for warm and rejected bathing or exercise, insisting on keeping extremely warm. For Chinese new mothers in the heavily Asian immigrant neighborhoods of Queens, New York, there are postpartum confinement centers catering to middle-class immigrant women who are living far from their families in China. They provide the warmth, food, and rest believed to be necessary for new mothers. In Los Angeles, there are Chinese food delivery services for women who observe the custom of *zuo yuezi*.

As noted above, in Mexico the lying-in period lasts for six weeks, the time believed necessary for the womb to return to normal. The customs involved are essentially identical to those of the Asian practice: the woman is to rest, stay very warm, and avoid bathing and exercise. Special foods designed to restore warmth to the body are prescribed. Disregarding these practices is believed to lead to aches and pains in later life.

There are three additional points to be made about the postpartum lying-in period. First, it is designed to give a woman a period of rest between childbirth and returning to work. The women who practice this custom are usually Asian and Latin American. In these cultures women traditionally did not return to office work, but went back to physical labor in the fields. Because they usually had large families, it might be the only time they had to rest.

Second, avoidance of bathing may have practical origins. In many countries the water is impure and filled with harmful bacteria. Bathing could introduce these organisms into the body and cause illness. Although conditions in the United States are different, the custom continues.

A third point involves the ways different generations adhere to customs. Sometimes, in order to avoid her mother's nagging, the daughter may comply with cultural traditions when the mother is present. When the patient is alone, she may be more receptive when a nurse suggests bathing, exercise, and so forth.

Compromises can be made. Although it is important for a patient to drink fluids after childbirth, hot tea and hot water with lemon deliver the same amount of liquid as ice water without violating custom. Using boiled water (cooled down) may make a sponge bath more acceptable. (This was done in China to remove impurities.) The patient should be kept covered and given socks or slippers to walk in. It is important to explain the reason for bathing and exercise and not to assume that the patient will follow orders that violate the traditions and wisdom of her own culture.

Admittedly, this is less of a problem today than it was a few decades ago, given the limited amount of time most insurance companies pay for women to remain in the hospital after giving birth.

Bonding

Maternal-infant bonding has become a major concern of Western health care professionals in the last several decades. Poor bonding has been associated with failure to thrive, child abuse, and psychological problems. It is therefore not surprising that doctors and nurses become concerned when they observe cultural beliefs and practices that appear to reflect poor bonding. However, these observations are often misleading and do *not* indicate poor bonding.

220   An example is the case of Ngo Lien, a Vietnamese woman who came to the hospital to deliver her fifth child. After giving birth to a son, she refused to cuddle him, although she willingly provided minimal care such as feeding and changing his diaper. The nursery nurse, feeling

sorry for the "neglected" baby, picked him up, cuddled him, and stroked the top of his head. Seeing this, Mrs. Ngo and her husband became visibly upset. The baby, who had jaundice, had to remain in the hospital for several days after Mrs. Vo went home. She did not visit her baby even once during the time he remained in the hospital.

In the past, nurses who worked in areas with a large Vietnamese population often referred these mothers to social services. Eventually, however, they came to understand that the apparently neglectful behavior did not reflect poor bonding, but indicated cultural beliefs and traditions. Many people in the more rural areas of Vietnam believe in spirits. Because spirits are particularly attracted to infants and likely to "steal" them (by inducing death), it is important that parents do everything possible to avoid attracting attention to their newborn. For this reason, infants are not verbally fussed over. They are sometimes even dressed in old clothes to "fool" the spirits. The apparent lack of interest new parents demonstrate reflects an intense love and concern for the child, rather than the opposite.

A Vietnamese nurse also pointed out to me that Vietnamese women are socialized not to show emotion in public, and thus may not be displaying the emotional attachment they feel while health care providers are in the room. That doesn't mean they don't play with the infant when they are alone.

Mrs. Ngo and her husband were probably distressed over the nurse's attention to their baby for two reasons. First, they may have feared having attention drawn to their baby. Second, Southeast Asians view the head as private and personal. It is also seen as the seat of the soul and is not to be touched. Not only did the nurse risk attracting the attention of dangerous spirits, but she stroked the child in a forbidden area.

Why did Mrs. Ngo not come to visit her son in the hospital after she was discharged? She was probably practicing lying-in and was at home resting while her internal organs resumed their normal position in her body.

Nurses can best deal with Vietnamese mothers by following their lead. If the parents do not fuss over the child, nurses should not either. In any event, they should avoid touching the infant's head. And as long as a mother can feed and hold her baby properly, they should not be concerned about an apparent lack of interest; it is merely an illusion.

Nurses were similarly disturbed when a woman from India refused to hold her babies except to feed them. Shankari Prabhu, a young Indian woman, gave birth prematurely to twin girls. Although the father was out of town on business, numerous other relatives were there, including the mother-in-law, aunts and uncles, nieces and nephews, and cousins.

221

Shortly after the delivery, Indira, the father's sister, came to speak to Edith, the nurse, explaining that Mrs. Prabhu was too tired to speak with her, but did plan to breastfeed the babies. Edith explained the importance of breastfeeding to the sister-in-law, and emphasized the importance of the mother spending time with the babies.

The next day Indira spoke to Edith again, giving her the names of the babies to put on the crib card. Although Edith knew enough about East Indian culture to realize that Mrs. Prabhu was practicing the lying-in period and had designated her sister-in-law to care for the infants, she reiterated the importance of having her spend time with the babies. She also explained that it was not enough for Indira to tell her the babies' names; that information had to come from the parents. Realizing the cultural importance of Indira's role as caregiver, she encouraged her to change the babies' linens and diapers, and hold the girls. But she was adamant in insisting that Mrs. Prabhu visit the babies because she was concerned about bonding.

Mrs. Prabhu finally came to visit her babies the next evening. She held them only briefly, and then passed them on to one of the many family members who were there with her. When Edith questioned her, she remained passive and allowed family members to respond for her. Fortunately, Edith had enough cultural competence to put aside her ethnocentric expectations that the mother should take full control in caring for her infants. This is not an expectation or common practice in Indian culture. It is traditional to have a female companion who does everything for the woman—feeding her, taking care of her hair, pouring beverages, and all infant care. The only care many Indian new mothers provide for their infants is to nurse them. A family member takes over its other care. In a variant of the lying-in period common in Asia and Latin America, the new mother is encouraged to rest in bed and eat a special diet including large amounts of milk, cooked butter, ghee (clarified butter), and high-protein foods.

Edith was able to adjust her expectations, thus creating a more pleasant situation for the patient and her family, as well as a less stressful situation for herself.

Baby Naming

222   When the subject of baby naming came up in class, Leila, a Hindu nurse from India, shared her own experience. She said that when she and her husband had their first son, they wanted to name him in the traditional Hindu manner, which meant waiting until he was seven days old. Before choosing a name, they would have to consult an astrologer who would give them a list of auspicious letters, based on the baby's time and date

of birth. These letters would be given to her husband's sisters, who would then choose a name beginning with one of the letters on the list.

What they had not counted on was the response of the hospital. Despite the fact that Leila was a nurse, she did not realize the importance placed on filling out the birth forms. When she refused to fill in the baby's name, the nurse reported her to the head nurse. This resulted in visits from the hospital administrative nurse, the chaplain, and the social worker. They all seemed concerned about Leila's plans for the baby once they got home. When she asked the social worker why everyone seemed so disturbed, the social worker admitted that they were worried that she wasn't bonding properly with the baby—why else would she not have named him?

Leila and her husband were both shocked and embarrassed that anyone would think they did not want their child. She quickly explained the Hindu tradition to the social worker, who noted the information for the nursing staff. Leila also recommended that, in the future, a patient who refuses to fill out the child's name should be asked *why* before any misunderstandings result.

Leila was told to call the hospital as soon as they named the baby, but apparently the hospital could not wait. On the morning of the seventh day, Leila received a call from the social worker, wanting to know the child's name so the forms could be completed.

When Leila asked her mother and grandmother why they were to wait until the seventh day to name the child, they told her that it is the day the stump of the umbilical cord falls off, and is thus the baby's first day of life. It is also the first time that the baby really opens his eyes and looks around. Although they did not mention it, it is probably related to high infant mortality rates. If the baby survives the first week, she or he is more likely to make it.

This custom of delaying the naming of the baby is found in many Asian cultures. Traditional Chinese will often give the baby an unattractive nickname at birth, such as "Little Doggie," or "Ugly Pig," to make the child seem less attractive to any spirits who might want to steal the infant.

Suk Luu, a Chinese man from Vietnam, had a daughter who grew up to be healthy, talented, and intelligent. His mother is convinced it was because Suk and his wife took the precaution of calling her by an "ugly" name; her "real" name was used only on her birth certificate. As Mrs. Luu explained, her granddaughter's ugly name ensured that no devils paid attention to her; who would be jealous of an "ugly name girl"? Mrs. Luu had learned the importance of names the hard way. Years earlier, she had ignored her own parents' warnings and given Suk's older brother a name that meant "intelligent" or "bright and clear." Mrs.

223

Luu is convinced that the reason he suffered serious illnesses for many years and died as a military prisoner in South Vietnam when only thirty was due to the devils' jealousy over his name.

Rejection

224   Occasionally parents will reject a newborn. Such was the case with a Middle Eastern couple after the wife, Salomi, gave birth to a baby girl. At the moment of delivery, while the doctor and nurses were oohing and aahing over the infant, her father turned and abruptly left the delivery room. The mother herself would not hold or even look at her child. When a nurse approached the lobby where many of the woman's relatives had earlier been anxiously awaiting the birth, she found that they had all left. Later, she held her child, but she refused to lavish any loving attention on her.

The nurse who reported this incident could not understand why parents would respond so negatively to such a joyous event. A Middle Eastern acquaintance later told her the reason. The couple had two daughters but no sons. Males are extremely important in Middle Eastern culture because they carry on the family name and all wealth is passed on through them. Many groups trace descent through the male line only, unlike our own system, which recognizes both the mother's and father's sides of the family. Even in groups that have adopted more Western patterns of inheritance, the traditional importance of the male may remain. A third daughter was a great disappointment.

There is little that the staff can do in such a situation, other than refer the parents to social services—and that may not be entirely welcome. Parents will rarely change ideas that have years of cultural tradition behind them. The important thing for clinicians to do is to watch for signs of neglect.

Infant Care

225   Kelsi was working in the NICU taking care of Ashur Algafari, a Syrian newborn. His father came to visit him while his mother was recuperating after a caesarean section. He seemed somewhat reluctant to hold or feed his baby. Kelsi assumed he was uncomfortable since this was his first child and he didn't know what to do. However, when Kelsi tried to show Mr. Algafari how to change Ashur's diaper, he declined, saying that he wasn't interested. Kelsi playfully responded that he should practice, so when the baby went home he would know what to do, but he still refused. At this point, Jesse, a nurse taking a cultural diversity class, pulled Kelsi aside and explained that in some cultures the father does

not participate in child care. Although economic and other factors may intervene, there is generally a very strict delineation of sex roles in the Middle East. Childrearing is a woman's responsibility. A man deals with his children later in their lives. In such situations, if the husband clearly does not want to get involved, it's best not to push it. Recall case study #148 in which a Middle Eastern father refused to be involved in the care of his young daughter, newly diagnosed with type 1 diabetes. The culturally sensitive nurse instead brought in the girl's grandmother to help care for her.

Belly Buttons

American medical professionals fear germs. For this reason, they are almost obsessively concerned with cleanliness. A custom practiced by Mexicans and other groups designed to create an attractive belly button is thus likely to disturb them. A coin is applied to an infant's navel and the area is wrapped tightly with a cloth to keep the coin in place. Sometimes the job of keeping the navel flat is left entirely to the bellyband. In any case, a protruding belly button is considered unsightly. Loving mothers will do what they can to ensure that their babies are attractive.

Health care professionals are concerned about the possibility of infection from a dirty cloth or coin. To respect their tradition and address health concerns, mothers who practice this custom should be taught the importance of using clean cloths and wiping the coin with alcohol before putting it on the baby's body. Most mothers are willing to make the minor adjustments necessary to ensure the health of their children.

Birth Control

A chapter on birth must also acknowledge efforts to prevent the event. Limiting the number of children is an extremely complicated issue in many cultures. Often, women and men take different positions on the issue, particularly in cultures where women have the primary responsibility for raising the children and men's major access to status and prestige is through the number of children they sire. Although a woman's status in such cultures may also derive from her role as a mother, women generally take the more practical stance.

Summary

Different cultures have different traditions regarding the process of birth. Some cultures dictate that a woman suffer the pains of labor in silence; others encourage her to express or even exaggerate her pain. The husband, mother, or mother-in-law may attend the birth. Some cultures have postpartum rituals a new mother must observe that contradict the recommendations of Western medical science. Some bathe and exercise as soon as possible, while others are taught to lie in bed and avoid showering and physical activity. Some have customs that may appear to reflect a lack of bonding but, in fact, do not. Although doctors now encourage immediate breastfeeding, women in some cultures believe it is necessary to wait several days lest the "dirty" antibody-rich colostrum harm their child. Finally, many cultures do not share our advocacy of birth control, in part because children are a major source of self-esteem for those who would otherwise have no access to status.

Some of these differences affect the health of the mother or child but others do not. Health care professionals must learn to recognize the difference. Detailed explanations and compromise are necessary when good health is the issue; cultural relativism must be exercised when it is not.

Key Points

- Most pregnancy taboos originated in the desire to control the outcome of pregnancy.
- Pregnancy is considered a "hot" condition in cultures that practice a system of hot/cold body balance (many Asian and Hispanic cultures). Because foods that are high in protein may be perceived as "hot" and thus avoided, physicians should carefully assess the pregnant woman's diet to make sure she is getting enough protein. The same is true for prenatal vitamins. If they are too "hot," taking them with a "cold" beverage can often neutralize them.
- Prenatal care may be avoided because many women see pregnancy as a "normal" condition and thus not requiring the assistance of a physician.
- Some cultures dictate stoicism during labor; others allow free expression of pain.
- In many cultures, female relatives are the preferred labor partner. If the husband seems unwilling to be in the room with his wife, do not force him to be.
- In some Southeast Asian cultures, surgery may be avoided due to the beliefs of the patient.
- In some cultures, patients may want to keep the placenta or the umbilical cord.

- Some women may want to postpone breastfeeding, believing that colostrum is bad for the baby. Patient teaching may be necessary.
- Many Asian, South Asian, and Hispanic women may practice a post-partum lying-in period in which they are to rest, stay warm, and avoid bathing and exercise. Compromise when possible.
- Do not be concerned if Southeast Asian women do not appear to be bonding with their infant, as long as they hold and feed the baby properly. If they are not fussing over the infant, follow their lead.
- In many traditional Asian and South Asian cultures, baby naming may be delayed for up to a month.

Chapter 10

End of Life

In the past most people died at home, cared for by their families. Today, however, people are dying more frequently in hospitals, cared for by professionals. Thanks to improved medical technology, people are also taking longer to die. The end of life is often fraught with difficulties for patients and their families. In addition, there are complications that can occur because cultural traditions vary significantly on a variety of issues, including whether or not to reveal the diagnosis to the patient, attitudes toward removing life support, expression of grief at the time of death, attitudes toward organ donations and autopsies, and beliefs and customs surrounding the moment of death.

Dying

Revealing/Withholding a Negative Diagnosis/Prognosis

One of the first cultural issues that arise with regard to the end of life is whether or not to reveal a terminal diagnosis to the patient. From the perspective of traditional American culture, which values individualism and autonomy, this is not even a question. *Of course* the patient is told if she or he has a terminal condition; it is one of the basic patient rights to know. However, the situation becomes complicated when the patient is from a culture that values the family over the individual. Studies have found that 52 percent of Mexican Americans feel that dying patients should not be told their prognosis, and 65 percent of Korean Americans believe such information should be withheld (see Kagawa-Singer and Blackhall 2001). In many Asian countries, including China and Japan, it is customary for the physician to reveal a cancer diagnosis only to the patient's family, and leave it up to the family whether to tell the patient. A nurse in Boston, Massachusetts shared that a Chinese physician friend told her that giving a patient the diagnosis without first consulting the family could cause a physician to be barred from practice in China. She was rather surprised to hear this, and checked with two more Chinese physicians, one a pathologist and the other an oncologist. Both confirmed what the original physician had said.

In some cultures, it may be seen as insensitive to tell a patient he or she is dying. It may be thought to create a sense of hopelessness and hasten the dying process. A Mexican American woman explained that the stress of knowing your condition would only cause you to get worse. The very devout may believe that only God knows when someone will die. Among the Hmong, to tell someone they are dying is thought to curse them. How could you know they will die unless you plan to kill them yourself?

For the health care staff, however, honoring the patient's culture may mean ignoring the American values of autonomy and individualism as well as creating potential legal complications. One solution is for the physician to discuss with the patient—ideally, before the need arises—to whom the patient wants information about his or her condition to be given. Does the patient want the physician to speak directly to a family member, or to him or her? How much does the patient want to know about his or her condition? Whom does the patient want the physician to speak to for decisions regarding treatment? It is important that any conversations regarding how much the patient wants to know be held in private, in order to ascertain the patient's true feelings.

In the state of Washington, there is a law that allows patients to waive personal consent authority for making their own medical treatment or nontreatment choices. They may sign a document that says they waive their consent authority freely and voluntarily, and do not wish to be informed of the nature and character of the proposed treatment/procedure; the anticipated results of the proposed treatment/procedure; the recognized alternative forms of treatment/procedure; or the recognized serious possible risks and complications of the treatment/procedure and of the recognized alternative forms of treatment/procedure, including nontreatment. They may also assign authority for decision-making to a third party. Recognizing the patient's "right *not* to know" is an important step in cultural sensitivity. Keep in mind that people from *any* culture—including middle-class Anglo Americans—may choose *not* to know.

Suken Hashimoto, a seventy-eight-year-old Japanese woman, was scheduled to receive chemotherapy for cancer. Normally, her nurse would explain to a patient why she was receiving chemotherapy, but Mrs. Hashimoto did not know she had cancer. Her physician had carefully discussed Mrs. Hashimoto's plan of care with her son; he had told

226

the physician and the nursing staff not to let his mother know her diagnosis. The staff had a hard time understanding this wish, and felt they needed to call in the ethics committee. Before this, however, they asked Mrs. Hashimoto if she wanted to know her diagnosis and why she was receiving (chemotherapy) medication. To their surprise, her answer was "no." She said, "Tell my son. He will make all of the decisions." The situation was resolved by having her sign a durable power of attorney for her son to make all her health care decisions. This is something hospitals can routinely do at the beginning of a hospital stay. Some patients will choose to be informed; others may prefer to defer that right.

227   Felix Andrada, a seventy-nine-year-old man living in the Philippines, was dying of lung cancer, but he didn't know it. He knew he had cancer, but he didn't know that it was stage four and that he only had perhaps six months to live. The physician gave the prognosis to his wife, who chose not to tell him. Mrs. Andrada refused hospice care, telling her daughter Celia, a nurse in the U.S., that hospice was "a death sentence." Celia did her best to explain that people outlived hospice all the time and that it provided excellent palliative care, but her mother's mind was made up. The physician felt that chemotherapy was not an option due to his age, nearly eighty, but he was able to complete a cycle of radiation therapy. At that time, the radiologist told him that he was now "cancer free." Mr. Andrada called his daughter to share the happy news. He did well for a short while after that, and was able to enjoy a huge eightieth birthday party. He died four months later. Celia recalls being upset with the radiologist for telling him that he was "cancer free," for clearly he wasn't. But reflecting back two years later, she was grateful to the radiologist because her father was able to live the last six months of his life to the fullest, unburdened by the loss of hope that would have accompanied an honest prognosis. She came to see that her mother and the physicians were right to withhold the prognosis from her father. As she says, it was for the best. Although prognostication is always a tricky and often dangerous business, the point is that people will respond differently to a negative prognosis. Some will find it a burden that leaves them feeling hopeless; others will use the knowledge to take care of business and complete their "bucket list."

Sometimes it's more complicated than whether or not the patient wants to know, as in the following case.

228   Raul Santiago was a Hispanic male in his seventies who had been in the hospital for seven months. He had been admitted for abdominal pain, but it soon became apparent that he had advanced stage pancreatic cancer. Mr. Santiago had 12 children, who all conspired to avoid using the word "cancer" in front of their father or to even acknowledge

his fatal prognosis. Instead, they referred to his condition as "abdominal pain." During the time he was in the hospital, Mr. Santiago became close to the nursing staff. One day while Tiffany was administering his pain medication, he looked directly at her and said with resignation, "I'm going to die, aren't I?" Without waiting for her to respond, he continued. He explained to Tiffany that he didn't want his children to suffer because of his illness, and he knew that if *they* knew that *he* knew he had cancer, it would cause them great distress. He told her that he was ready to be with his wife who had died two years earlier. He was content to pretend to be ignorant of his disease if it eased his family's suffering. Whether it would have caused his children to suffer or would have been a relief if they knew he knew is unknown. But the nurses honored his decision.

In Chapter 2 we addressed why it's best to avoid using family members as interpreters. The following case is another example that illustrates how the family's agenda can interfere with hospital care, as well as the lengths to which family members will go to protect patients from a negative diagnosis.

Pepe Nunez, a sixty-four-year-old Latino male with a poor prognosis, had family members at his bedside around the clock despite strict visiting rules. Whenever the nurses asked them to leave, they would argue and insist on staying. When one of the nurses finally asked about their concerns, the patient's daughter explained they were afraid that one of the staff might tell their father he was dying. The family felt that being told death was imminent would cause him to lose his will to live, a will that would provide him strength to fight the disease. 229

The problem was solved by documenting their request in the nursing process notes and verbally passing on the information during shift change. They also informed the physician and nurse practitioner of the family's wishes. The patient was told that his condition was critical, but that they were taking it one day at a time and hoping for the best. When the patient died, the family expressed their gratitude to the staff and physicians for going along with their concerns and wishes. The staff did well by respecting the family's wishes, but it would have been better to ascertain the desires of the patient by finding out from him how much *he* wanted to know.

It is also important to remember that not all members of the same culture will make the same choices.

Freya Castro and Eunice Mercado were two Filipino students who had both recently lost a grandparent. Freya's family followed the more traditional pattern of withholding that information from the patient. Afterward, they were pleased with their choice, feeling that their loved one was able to live out her days without the added burden of knowing she 230 was dying. Eunice's family decided to tell the patient. They, too, were content with their choice, knowing that the patient was able to make her final arrangements and say goodbye to everyone. Two Filipino families, two different choices, both leaving the family feeling satisfied. In these two instances, it's unclear whether the patients were given the opportunity to choose, but the cases underscore the importance of both not imposing American values on others, and not stereotyping. The culturally competent health care provider will neither assume that the patient does *not* want to know, nor impose American ways and tell the patient everything. Instead, she or he will come to the situation knowing the cultural possibilities and ascertain what the individual patient wants. Acting in such a culturally competent manner can help physicians avoid potential problems, as described in the following cases.

231   A nursing student told me about a physician who strongly feels it is his moral and legal responsibility to tell patients their diagnosis. This attitude has created problems with several families who did not want their family member to know. Some of these patients frequently missed appointments; others never returned. It is likely their family members refused to bring them to this physician to "protect" them from hearing their diagnosis.

I want to emphasize the importance of finding out from patients how much they want to know about their condition and prognosis. I've had several well-meaning students who in their role as nurses felt they were being culturally competent by respecting the family's wishes and not telling the patient about her prognosis. What if the patient truly *does* want to know? Making assumptions in either direction can be dangerous. At the same time, be aware that even when the patient *does* want to know, there can still be problems with the family.

232   Rachelle was caring for Lidia Medina, a sixty-one-year-old Hispanic woman with stomach cancer. She had always been the strong person in her family; her husband and children depended on her. When she first became ill, her family kept reassuring her that she would get better and encouraged her to fight twice as hard. Her physician gave the family a lot of hope—false hope, in Rachelle's opinion. Her family avoided any mention of the word cancer and informed the staff they were not to say anything negative to Mrs. Medina. They insisted she continue treatment. She was assigned to both a hospitalist and an oncologist. At one point, Mrs. Medina was alone in the room with Rachelle when the hospitalist, Dr. Cherry, came to assess her. Dr. Cherry asked her what she knew about her condition and how she felt about the treatment. Mrs. Medina responded that she knew very little; her family refused to discuss her condition with her. Nor would they allow her to research her disease or ask the staff any questions about it. Since a family member was nearly

always in the room with Mrs. Medina, they were able to enforce it. Dr. Cherry spent a fair amount of time with Mrs. Medina, sitting at her bedside and answering all her questions. She felt good about what she thought—and what was objectively—excellent patient-doctor communication.

After Dr. Cherry left, Mr. Medina returned and learned what she had done. He was irate and called the oncologist to see his wife right away. After speaking with the family the oncologist called Dr. Cherry and began what Rachelle described as "ranting and raving and chewing her a new one." He told her that she had no right to tell *his* patients that they are going to die or that they should consider hospice care. He said she needed to "grow up and have some compassion." Without having observed the situation myself, it sounds as if Dr. Cherry was the one who acted appropriately by responding to the needs expressed by the patient, and that the oncologist was misguided in serving the needs of the family over the patient.

After this incident, the family told Mrs. Medina that Dr. Cherry was wrong and that she wasn't going to die. This was of course very confusing for Mrs. Medina, who then asked Rachelle if she were going to die. Rachelle had a long, honest, heart to heart conversation with her about her cancer and prognosis and support resources. Mrs. Medina never told her family about their conversation.

Hospice and Palliative Care

A growing trend in care of the dying is hospice. Unlike Western medicine, which is dedicated to preserving life as long as possible, hospice emphasizes palliative care—comfort rather than cure. Hospice, however, tends to be used largely by Anglo Americans, which is rather ironic, given that it more closely approximates the conditions of dying in more traditional cultures. Part of the problem is that many people have misconceptions about the nature of hospice care. Many mistakenly believe that hospice care is provided only at special facilities and they don't want to "abandon" their loved one to such a facility since they feel it is the duty of the family to take care of its own members. This duty is particularly important in Asian cultures where filial piety is highly valued. Calling in hospice may be perceived as not fulfilling one's responsibility. The reality is that most hospice care is provided at home, where family members can continue to care for their loved one with the aid of a visiting hospice nurse who can provide palliative pain medication. It should be emphasized that hospice is meant to *assist* rather than *replace* the family. Teaching them what they can do to help their loved one feel more comfortable during their last days should be encouraged.

For Spanish-speaking patients, the concerns may be exacerbated by the fact that "hospice" in Spanish translates to "hospicio," which can also mean a place of poverty and asylum, or orphanage. Who would feel right about that? Specifically addressing these concerns and explaining how involving home hospice can be the most loving and kind way to care for a loved one may help overcome the reluctance to utilize hospice.

For some religious patients, there may be some concern that it shows a lack of faith in God since the patient is acknowledging that he or she has a terminal condition. This is an attitude held by many Muslims. If you have no faith in Allah, why would Allah save you? Plus it is complicated by the fact that many want to withhold a terminal diagnosis from the patient, as discussed in the previous section.

When talking to a patient or family about hospice, one approach would be to discuss how treatment will shift to palliative care, providing comfort and pain relief. It's important to emphasize that if the patient develops a treatable condition—pneumonia, for example—it *will* be treated. And it is always possible to leave hospice. It is not an irrevocable death sentence. Sometimes people receiving only palliative care live *longer* with the same condition than do those who receive chemotherapy. Chemotherapy can take a huge toll on the body and result in a heart attack or death from a newly acquired infection.

Fear of addiction to the pain-killing drugs used in hospice care may be another factor leading to a lack of acceptance of hospice care. Recall the Filipino nurse (case study #78) who halved the doctor's prescribed dosage when administering pain medication to her dying mother. It is essential that health care personnel discuss with the family the nature of addiction and why it generally is not a concern in the case of dying patients. The need for pain medication during terminal illness is different from the need for pain medication during addiction and does not involve drug-seeking behavior, which is often the major source of concern in drug addiction.

Use of traditional remedies and healers should be opened as a topic of discussion. Although remedies that conflict with hospice medications will need to be avoided, anything else should be investigated and, if it poses no harm, allowed and respected. The next case, although it did not occur in the context of hospice, is a good example of how integrating a traditional healer into the care of a dying patient can be beneficial for all concerned.

233   Matilda Salazar, an extremely ill Hispanic patient, was dying as a result of sepsis, acute respiratory distress syndrome (ARDS), and multiple organ failure. Her family asked that a *curandera*, a traditional healer, be allowed to come pray with her and massage her with oil. Dr. Edgar, a culturally sensitive physician, not only agreed to this but requested he

be called to the bedside when the healer arrived. Using an interpreter, Dr. Edgar spoke with the *curandera* about the rituals that would take place. He stayed to watch from the corner of the room as the *curandera* chanted, prayed, and massaged oils into Mrs. Salazar's body. Although the ceremony did nothing to affect the patient's prognosis, the family and patient seemed more at peace afterward, and the experience improved the family's rapport with the physician. When the time came for Dr. Edgar to tell the family there was nothing else they could do for Mrs. Salazar, they accepted it calmly and began saying their goodbyes. After she died, the family remained grateful to the doctor and staff for respecting their traditions. This case is important because it shows how respect for a patient's cultural traditions can have a positive effect on the relationship between the staff and the patient (and family). It also underscores the fact that the point of medicine doesn't always have to be to cure, but to *care* for the patient.

One final thought on hospice and its under-utilization by non-Anglo Americans. Perhaps because hospice allows patients greater control over their own death, it is a better fit with the worldview of the dominant American culture, which views nature as something that can be controlled. For many other ethnic groups, including those in the Middle East and Latin America, life and death are up to the will of God. *Qué será será.*

Advance Directives and Removing Life Support

A culture's worldview will also have a strong influence on the willingness of an individual or family to learn about or consent to "Do Not Resuscitate" (DNR) orders, or to Advance Directives.

Advance Directives are the written directions a patient gives to family members and health professionals to guide decision-making about end of life care, including the use, or not, of extraordinary measures to prolong life. A relatively new phenomenon (the Federal Patient Self-Determination Act was enacted in 1990), Advance Directives are legally binding in some states. Nurses, in their role of patient advocate, as well as physicians have the responsibility to ascertain the wishes of the patient regarding the use of and adherence to Advance Directives. Depending on cultural beliefs about health care practices and treatments, as well as the meaning of life and death, patients may accept or reject the option of Advance Directives.

Although it is difficult for anyone to actively allow a loved one to die, cultural and religious influences play an important role in determining whether or not a family member is willing to remove life support. Jill Klessig (1992) studied the effect of values and culture on life-support decisions and found that members of several cultural and religious groups were reluctant to withdraw life support, for a variety of reasons. These groups included Muslim Iranians, Orthodox Jews, Korean Americans, African Americans, Mexican Americans, and Filipino Americans.

Muslim Iranians were generally opposed to removing life support, not only because is it seen as an obligation to seek medical attention, but also because only Allah can decide when someone will die. Note that although *starting* life support is using the "gift" of technology that has been given to man, it is not seen as interfering with God's will the way *removing* life support is. Even if a patient is suffering, this is not a reason to remove life support because suffering is an opportunity to show courage and faith in Allah.

234   An example can be seen in the case of Noor Gatrad, an elderly Iranian woman. Mrs. Gatrad was slowly dying. The staff felt that nothing could be done to improve her condition, and that her son's refusal to sign a DNR order and his insistence on doing everything possible to prolong her life was causing her to endure needless suffering. Her son steadfastly held to his decision, despite the assistance and recommendations of the ethics committee. Her nurse shared this case with me during a course I was teaching on cultural competence. She said that at the time, she felt only frustration and could not understand Mrs. Gatrad's son's behavior. After learning about Iranian attitudes toward the removal of life support, she suddenly understood. Such knowledge might have enabled the staff to feel less stress while caring for Mrs. Gatrad.

Orthodox Jews also generally want to prolong life support. Because there is no belief in an afterlife, and life itself is considered sacred, it should be preserved whenever possible. However, because suffering is not thought to bring redemption, it is acceptable to remove life support if the patient will die within seventy-two hours.

Klessig found that Korean Americans were generally opposed to removing life support because stopping it (although not starting it) is seen as interfering with God's will. In addition, stopping life support, even if that is the wish of a parent, may be thought to dishonor family members in the eyes of relatives or community, due to the importance of filial piety.

She found that African American families were more likely than Anglo Americans to want life support continued. Some distrusted the largely white medical community, and feared that life support would be withdrawn early for racist reasons. Others were very religious and believed that God could provide a miracle cure, as in the following case.

235   A fifty-two-year-old African American man named William Jefferson was admitted to the critical care unit with a diagnosis of pneumonia. On

admission, he was offered an Advance Directive, which he refused, saying that God would help him with his illness. His lung cancer had gone into remission after radiation treatment; he believed that God had helped him through that illness, and would help him through the current one. He thought that signing a Do Not Resuscitate form or Advance Directive would be a sign of giving up or losing faith in God. Unfortunately, he died ten days later, after enduring a great deal of suffering.

Klessig also found that Filipino Americans and Mexican Americans were often opposed to withdrawing life support. Catholicism strongly influenced their attitudes. It is seen as morally wrong to encourage death with any action or omission ("suicide"), and if the illness is punishment by God, one should not interfere with the opportunity to redeem one's sins through suffering. It is important to note that traditional respect and courtesy toward physicians may lead patient or family to agree with a doctor who suggests removing life support, even when they are opposed to it.

Klessig found a dual attitude among Chinese Americans: it is acceptable both to stop life support *and* to do everything possible to extend a patient's life. Because the family is valued over the individual, if life support is an economic or emotional burden on the family, the patient who forgoes it is seen as performing an act of compassion, which is highly valued. In contrast, among Buddhist Chinese, there is a precept that prohibits killing and a concern that stopping life support will interfere with a person's karma. Issues of filial piety may also be involved.

Other, more unusual, circumstances can contribute to a refusal to remove life support, as the following case illustrates. Ngoc Ly, a twenty-five-year-old Vietnamese man, was hit by a car while riding his bicycle to work. Paramedics were able to resuscitate him, but the physician at the local trauma center determined that Mr. Ly was clinically brain dead. He placed him on life support until the family could be notified.

An interpreter explained Mr. Ly's condition to his wife and parents. They nodded in understanding and quietly left the hospital. Normally, the staff neurosurgeon would then have pronounced Mr. Ly dead and removed him from the ventilator, but he was suddenly called to surgery.

Later that afternoon, Mr. Ly's family met with Dr. Isaacs, the physician they had spoken to earlier. Dr. Isaacs intended to tell them of the plan to pronounce Mr. Ly dead and discontinue the ventilator, but the Lys had other plans. They informed him that they had consulted a specialist who said this was not the right time for him to die. Dr. Isaacs was confused. What kind of specialist would make such a recommendation? An astrologer who had read Ngoc Ly's lunar chart advised that his death be postponed until a more auspicious date.

236

The physician had never encountered a situation like the one now facing him. Fearing legal repercussions if he did not abide by the family's request, he agreed to keep Mr. Ly on life support until further notice. A little less than a week later, the Lys called to tell him that Ngoc could now die.

Most members of the staff were stunned by this incident. Mr. Ly's body was starting to decompose and smell. People looked up books on astrology and questioned Vietnamese coworkers. They learned that many Asians take astrology seriously. When an important decision is to be made, they will often consult a *bomoh* or *dukun* to interpret the astrological charts.

Although most people cannot predict or control the date of their death, they believe that simply knowing when someone has died can be helpful in terms of knowing what fate has in store for the deceased's descendants. If a person dies at the "proper" time, his or her children will be rewarded with good health and goodwill. If the time is inauspicious, the children will suffer financial losses, unhappy marriages, or similar negative fates. A *bomoh* can tell people what the future holds for them so they can be prepared.

The Ly family had an opportunity denied to most people. By delaying removal of Ngoc Ly's life support, they could influence the fate of his descendants for generations. How could they not do everything possible to bring good luck to his fatherless children?

Death

What Constitutes Death

The biomedical definition of death focuses on the cessation of brain function, but not all cultures view it that way. In many cultures, it is the absence of warmth, pulse, breath, and heartbeat that serves as the criteria for death. Machines that perform these functions can give the appearance of life. Many believe that the person declared brain dead is actually in a coma, and they may have the idea that a miraculous recovery is possible.

237   Nizam Koury was a twelve-year-old Middle Eastern boy who tragically suffered a ruptured brain aneurism and was pronounced brain dead. The staff made the decision to leave the ventilator on until relatives arrived from overseas later in the day. Prior to this point, the staff had held numerous conferences with the family to explain the meaning of brain death, and how taking the patient off the ventilator was not actually "removing life support" since there was no longer a life to support.

The family always indicated that they understood. Although the staff knew that legally they did not need the family's permission to turn off the ventilator, they were trying to be sensitive to the family's needs and to give them a reasonable amount of time to grieve. When the members of the extended family arrived at the hospital, the Kourys asked the physician to hold another conference to explain the situation to them. After several lengthy conversations, it was determined that the time had come to take the next step, but the extended family had trouble with the idea of turning off the ventilator. They kept saying that the parents would have to live with this decision for the rest of their lives. In their view, Nizam was not "dead," and by removing life support (turning off the ventilator), they were taking the decision for his death out of Allah's hands and into their own. The physicians decided that the most sensitive way to handle the situation would be to gradually wean Nizam off the vasopressors that were keeping his heart beating, so that when his heart stopped, he would appear to have died "naturally," rather than unnaturally from turning off the ventilator. It was a creative solution to a tricky problem.

My own brother, a thirty-seven-year-old Sephardic man, died in the 238 ICU in 1993, after a week on life support. The night he died, he appeared to be still breathing, since a machine was doing the work for him. A nurse told us that his brain activity had ceased and that he was dead. It was a Sunday evening in a small hospital, and the few physicians there were busy in the emergency department. That meant no one could officially pronounce him dead and remove life support for more than an hour. Although intellectually I understood that my brother was dead, watching his chest rise and fall with each breath made it very difficult to believe. It is much easier to accept what we can see and feel—like a heart that is no longer beating. Brain activity is invisible from the outside. I truly understand why many cultures don't share the same understanding as that of biomedicine.

The Moment of Death

The moment an individual makes the transition between life and death is significant in numerous cultures. Many Americans feel it is important to be with their loved one at that instant, so that they do not feel alone. However, the opposite is the case in the Sephardic (Spanish Jewish) tradition.

When Leon Levy, a forty-eight-year-old Sephardic man, lay dying, his 239 family made a point of leaving his room for five minutes every hour. Like many Sephardics, they believed it is too hard for the dying to let go of life in the presence of loved ones. Leaving the room regularly gives the dying patient the opportunity to pass on, unencumbered by the emotional ties created by family members. Mr. Levy made the transition when his family was out of the room.

Other customs are followed by the Roma (Gypsies), as illustrated in the following cases.

240   Philip Maturo, a Roma (Gypsy) king in his late seventies, was brought to the hospital and diagnosed with pneumonia. The severity of his illness necessitated an oxygen tent. Clan members caused pandemonium; they crowded into Mr. Maturo's room, blocked the doorways, and filled the cafeteria with their coffee cups and cigarette smoke. This behavior, however, was merely a nuisance. The greatest problem was that they insisted on keeping a candle on the shelf at the head of Mr. Maturo's bed. The nurses lived in fear that it would be lit while the oxygen was turned on and cause an explosion. Many animated discussions were held on this point, but the Roma were adamant. If their king died, the candle would be lit at the moment of death to guide his spirit to heaven. Fortunately, Mr. Maturo recovered and the hospital survived.

241   Another hospital witnessed a different Roma custom regarding death. When the end was imminent, the clan received the hospital's permission to move the king outside, bed and all. They felt this would help free the soul of their dying leader, now unencumbered by walls and ceilings.

Concern for the ability of the spirit to soar to freedom is common in many cultures. One nurse who worked at a hospital close to the Hoopa Valley Indian reservation in northern California told of how, when someone died, the nurses would open the windows to allow spirits to leave. The importance of this custom to the Native Americans made it difficult for her when she moved to a hospital where none of the windows opened.

242   In an example of how cultural sensitivity can be advantageous for both the patient and the clinician, Christina said that the most memorable death she ever participated in as a nurse was that of Mr. Shi, a practicing Buddhist. When the time came to remove the ventilator, she helped the family dress him in a suit that had had its buttons removed, to enable his soul to slip out easily. She was given a bag of coins to place in his left hand and a bag of food to place in his right hand, sustenance for the journey. Finally, she was told to place a coin in his mouth. After Mr. Shi was extubated, his entire family came and took many photos of him after his final breath. Christina was asked to return the bag of money, but the deceased kept the food, coin, and suit.

243   Reina also had a positive experience helping the family of Cadeo Kieu, an elderly male Vietnamese patient who died from a chronic illness. It was Thanksgiving, and when she saw that he was about to die, she called her husband at home and had him read to her from her

course textbook about Vietnamese culture with regard to death. She was amazed to see that the words in the text so accurately described the scene that was unfolding before her. The eldest son made all the decisions and arrangements. He requested that Reina bathe and dress his father in his own clothes. Reina said the other nurse looked at her as if she were crazy for doing this. Steeped in the importance of culture from the class she was taking, she said she was keenly aware of why she was doing it, and how important it was to the family. She watched as his son placed a small gold medallion in Mr. Kieu's mouth. His family asked her to place several items in his pockets, including a handful of play money and simulated food items.

Later, several of her coworkers told her that if they had been in her shoes, they would have told her to tell the family to do it themselves. Although she said her first instinct was to chastise her coworkers for their callousness, she instead used it as an opportunity to explain the cultural significance of her actions. Acting in such a compassionate—and culturally competent—manner not only helped the patient's family, but made Reina feel good.

Expression of Grief

Individuals express grief over the death of a loved one in a variety of ways. Furthermore, culture may influence whether it is more appropriate to cry and wail without restraint or to present a stoic face to the world. Anglo American culture tends to value emotional stoicism. Older readers may recall how Jacqueline Kennedy was praised for the way she maintained her composure in public after her husband, President John F. Kennedy, was assassinated. Hospital culture reflects the dominant culture and tends to find stoicism more admirable as well as easier to cope with, which can present problems when people from more expressive cultures die.

Mustafa Mourad, a Muslim Arab, was admitted to the oncology floor. *244* A few weeks earlier he had been diagnosed with extensive colon cancer. His family kept him at home until he went into a coma. On admittance, it was determined that he was a "no code," but little else had been discussed. There had been no time to develop rapport. Six to ten family members were at his bedside throughout the night.

At 2 A.M., the daughter ran to get the nurse—he had stopped breathing. When the nurse confirmed that he had no pulse, several family members began to cry and wail loudly. The nurses tried to comfort them, but Mr. Mourad's son pulled them away. Soon the entire family joined in the wailing. The son asked the staff not to interfere, stating that the loud display was part of the grieving process. He added that it was necessary in order for his father's soul to be released.

The problem was that it was 2 A.M., and the wailing and crying were disturbing all the other *non*comatose patients, who were pushing their call buttons. They were angry, concerned, and frightened, and wanted to know what was going on. When the nurse asked the patient's son to have them please soften the noise, he became angry and accused her of being disrespectful.

The nurse had called Mr. Mourad's physician earlier to report the death. He instructed her to call the emergency department physician to pronounce the man dead. They were still waiting for him. Meanwhile, the nurse called the nursing supervisor. She also, unsuccessfully, tried to speak with the family about lowering the noise.

The doctor from the emergency department arrived nearly an hour later. When he requested they stop their wailing, they complied. He arranged to have the body moved to the chapel where they could continue mourning without disturbing the other patients. The physician also instructed the nursing staff not to call the mortuary until told to do so by the family, which they did at 10 o'clock the next morning.

There are a number of cultural elements displayed in the Moustafa case. No plans had been made with the mortuary regarding the impending death because to do so would interfere with the will of Allah. The most disturbing element of the case for the staff was the loud crying. Wailing is an important cultural ritual. The nursing staff, unaware of this, was totally unprepared.

Another cultural aspect was the fact that the family ignored the requests of the nurses but complied with those of the physician. Arabs have a great deal of respect for authority—of physicians, not nurses. This was accentuated by the greater respect the culture has for men.

In this situation, the physician demonstrated an important understanding of cultural diversity and suggested a solution (moving to the chapel) that allowed the family to continue their ritual without compromising other patients. It is generally more productive to work within the culture rather than impose solutions from without.

Postmortem Organ Donations and Autopsies

Most religions have rules regarding what can be done to the body after death. Although there will be variations according to how devout the family is, there are some practices that health care professionals can anticipate. Orthodox Jewish and Muslim patients may be opposed to organ donations and autopsies (unless required by law). According to Jewish belief, the body must be whole for resurrection when the messiah comes. For that reason, Jewish families may request that the deceased be buried with amputated limbs and bloody clothing, for example, if they died in an accident (see case study #87). Furthermore, many Jews believe that the body belongs to God, and that we do not have the right to disfigure it without a good reason. There are mixed feelings regarding organ donation among Muslims. Those who are opposed say the body can still feel pain, and that life is a "trust," so you cannot donate part of your body to anyone else. It should be returned to Allah in the same shape in which it was given, and that was not with body parts missing. Those Muslims in favor of it say that because it can save a life, it falls under the Islamic doctrine that "necessity allows the prohibited." Hmong families are also likely to refuse autopsies and organ donations because they believe that whatever is cut will be missing when they are reincarnated.

Burial and Funeral Practices

Humans have disposed of the dead for at least the last 90,000 years. The earliest records we have of burials are associated with the Neanderthals of western Europe, whose skeletons have been found with the remains of wild flowers, animal bones (food for the journey to the afterlife?), and stone tools. Disposal of the corpse is important both as a public health measure and as a mirror of religious and cultural beliefs. The means of disposal, like most cultural traditions, often reflect both practical circumstances and ideology. The two most popular means of disposing of a dead body in the United States are burial and cremation. Generally, Muslims and Jews will be opposed to cremation, while Buddhists and Hindus may prefer it. The views of the Catholic Church have shifted on this issue. Cremation used to be forbidden due to the belief that the body must be whole for resurrection. However, in recent years, probably due to the practical influence of overcrowding and lack of burial space, it has been thought that as long as there is even a chunk of bone left, resurrection can occur. This is an excellent example of how cultures adapt to changing circumstances.

We can see how traditions regarding disposal of the body relate to both environmental conditions and beliefs regarding the afterlife. For example, among Orthodox Jews, cremation is forbidden. This reflects the Jewish belief that when the messiah comes, we will be resurrected, and so we need our bodies to be whole. It also reflects the ecological circumstance of the Middle East. There is not a lot of wood for burning bodies in the desert, but there is plenty of room for burial. This helps explain why there are so many similarities in Jewish and Muslim funeral traditions. Orthodox Jews are buried in a plain white shroud. The belief is that we are all equal in the eyes of God, and should thus appear that way. Judaism itself is a very egalitarian religion, compared with, for example, Roman Catholicism, which is very hierarchical. All members of the Jewish community are to assist in the actual burial by shoveling dirt onto the coffin. This reflects the strong value of community and the fact that Jews have always been outsiders and have had to rely on their own people.

Cremation is part of both Buddhist and Hindu traditions. From an adaptive perspective this makes sense. Japan, a traditionally Buddhist culture, is a small but highly populated island. There is little room for burial, but there are plenty of trees to provide wood for burning bodies. Although India is a large country, there is tremendous overcrowding in the major cities. Cremation makes sense as both a public health measure and a way of disposing of corpses easily. I have one vivid memory from my seventh grade science class. The teacher had been to India that summer. On the first day of class, he described how in the morning, the street sweepers would sweep up the bodies of the dead, along with the garbage. I've never forgotten that image, and for me it underscores the practicality of cremation. At the same time, both Buddhism and Hinduism believe in reincarnation. Given the ideological belief that we are born into new bodies in our next life, there is no need to maintain the integrity of our current bodies. Again, the practical and ideological merge to create a tradition.

Numbers and Death

Most Americans would be uncomfortable if they were assigned to room 13, because the number 13 is considered by many to be "unlucky." Many buildings do not have a 13th floor, at least, not one labeled as such. In Japan, while most high-rises do have a 13th floor, they lack a 4th floor, due to the association of the number four with death.

245   A young Japanese woman named Kieko Ozawa was being wheeled into operating room 4 when she noticed the number over the door. She began to cry softly. The nurse became concerned and asked what was wrong. Kieko was embarrassed but explained that the Japanese character for the number 4 is pronounced the same as the character for the word "death." Already concerned about her health, Kieko was disturbed to be wheeled into a room labeled "death."

Although she said it was just a silly superstition, Kieko was unable to let go of her fear. The surgery went well despite the room number, but the patient suffered needless anxiety. Had the hospital personnel mentioned to Kieko that she was being scheduled for room 4, her feelings might have become known in time to reschedule her into a different operating room. Room 3, for example, would have been appropriate because 3 in Japanese characters also means "life."

The same is true for Chinese and for Koreans. In fact, the administration at a hospital in a largely Chinese neighborhood realized that they needed an in-service workshop on cultural diversity when a Chinese man on their board of directors became quite upset during his hospitalization. He had been put in room 444.

246

Whenever possible, avoid putting Chinese, Japanese, and Korean patients in rooms with the number 4. As a side note, 4 is not the only number with special significance for the Chinese. They regard numbers 8 and 9 as lucky. The character for 8 signifies wealth and the character for 9 means long life. (For the Japanese, however, 9 may represent "suffering.") In Hong Kong, most of the expensive luxury cars owned by Chinese include the number 8 on the license plate. The Chinese pay extra money and wait in long lines to get a plate with that number. An expensive car without an 8 on the license plate is generally owned by a foreigner.

Although the number 4 has negative connotations for the Chinese and Japanese, the opposite is the case for the Navajo, who see much of the world in terms of four. Phrases are repeated four times in their ritual chants, pollen is thrown to the four directions in many of their ceremonies, and they revere four sacred mountains. A Navajo might find it easier to remember to take medicine four times a day than three or five times.

Summary

Although this chapter has only touched on some of the issues caregivers face when working with dying patients, it demonstrates the importance of culture in shaping people's attitudes and behavior in the face of death. At the same time, remember that culture does not explain everything; people's responses at this momentous life transition are often purely personal.

Key Points

- Because it is common in some cultures to withhold a negative diagnosis/prognosis from the patient, it is important to discuss with the patient—in private, and ideally, before the need arises—to whom the patient wants information about his or her condition to be given. Does the patient want the physician to speak directly to a family member, or to him or her? How much does the patient want to know about his or her condition? To whom does the patient want the physician to speak for decisions regarding treatment?

- When raising the subject of hospice care with families, make sure they understand that care can be provided in the patient's home. This will allow family members to continue to care for their loved one.

- Cultural and religious influences play an important role in determining whether or not a family member is willing to remove life support. These influences can include the belief that only God can make that decision, the belief that suffering is an opportunity to show courage and faith in God, the need to show filial piety, and distrust of the white medical establishment.

- There is cultural variation in how death is defined. For some, it is when the heart stops beating. In biomedicine, it is the cessation of brain activity.

- Many cultures have beliefs regarding the moment of death, including whether or not someone should remain at the bedside and what needs to be done to free the individual's soul.

- Many cultures have specific practices regarding how the body should be prepared after death. Health care providers can play an important role in assisting families at this time.

- There are cultural variations in the expression of grief, as well as attitudes toward organ donations and autopsies (see Appendix 2).

- Traditions regarding disposal of the body relate to both environmental conditions and beliefs regarding the afterlife.

- Numbers can have significance for people; 13 may be seen as unlucky by many Americans; 4 is associated with death by many Asians.

Chapter 11

Mental Health

The mental health profession is paying increasing attention to the effect of culture on individual psychology. Many graduate programs in clinical psychology now offer courses on treating clients from culturally diverse backgrounds. Knowledge of the range of what is considered "normal" is essential to effectively treating both private practice clients and hospital patients. Unfortunately, psychiatric diagnoses of foreign patients can be inaccurate, due to health care workers' ignorance of cultural patterns. This chapter will address some issues that relate to the mental health of patients.

Mental Illness

Defining Mental Illness: Deviation from the Norm

One definition of mental illness is behavior that deviates significantly from the norm. Because each culture values different behavior in its members, what is considered normal in one culture may be perceived as deviant in another. In a culture that values emotional control, expressiveness can be seen as a sign of instability. In a culture that values independence, the desire to live with one's family after adolescence may be seen as something that needs to be worked on in therapy. When diagnosing patients it is essential to distinguish mental illness from culturally supported behaviors and personality traits. In fact, the 2013 edition of the Diagnostic Statistical Manual (DSM-5) has added for at least one condition (Dissociative Identity Disorder) the following criterion: *The disturbance is not a normal part of a broadly accepted cultural or religious practice.*

The following case took place in 1974. Current laws and cultural change make it unlikely that it could happen today, but the role of culture makes it an extremely relevant case example.

247   Chio Yamamoto, a forty-six-year-old Japanese immigrant woman, was committed to a state mental institution by her husband on the basis of what he termed a major personality change and uncharacteristic behavior. The problems began after her three children went to college. Mrs. Yamamoto decided she wanted to attend college as well, something that was rare among Japanese women at the time. When her husband learned of her intentions, he had her committed. Her primary diagnosis was "chronic undifferentiated schizophrenia" with an acute psychotic episode and a secondary diagnosis of "hypochondria with multiple somatic complaints." Clearly, she did not belong in an institution simply because she wanted to attend college. Then why was she diagnosed with psychiatric problems once in the mental hospital? Probably it was due to her behavior, which, though consistent with Japanese culture, was misinterpreted as psychotic.

The staff at the institution documented her "noncompliant" behavior. She was "sullen," quiet, and would not participate in group therapy. Furthermore, she would not make eye contact with anyone. She also had multiple somatic complaints with no medical basis. These included vague abdominal pains, extremely poor appetite, and general weakness.

What were the cultural bases for these "symptoms"? At that time in Japan, women were raised to show respect for authority and to be submissive. It would have been culturally inappropriate for Chio to have questioned the therapists who were treating her. Eye contact was to be avoided in order to show respect. It was not surprising that she was extremely withdrawn in therapy; to call attention to yourself and talk about your feelings was completely antithetical to the Japanese notions of inconspicuousness (consider the Japanese saying, "the nail that sticks out gets hammered down") and emotional control. In addition, mental illness carries a tremendous stigma in Asian cultures. Chio must have certainly been burdened with the shame of her diagnosis, causing her to withdraw even farther.

Rather than express her feelings, Chio somaticized them. Psychosomatic complaints are common among the Japanese, who are allowed few acceptable outlets for their anger. Stomach pains are commonly associated with emotional distress. It is difficult to eat when your stomach hurts, and if you don't eat, you become weak. Thus, the chain of her "symptoms."

Chio was falsely institutionalized for eight months. Though it is now much more difficult to commit someone against his or her will, the error was compounded by a lack of understanding of Japanese culture on the part of the psychiatric hospital staff.

248   Culture can add a layer of complexity to psychiatric diagnoses. Miya Fukui, a Japanese woman who had been living in the United States for more than thirty years, was admitted to an inpatient psychiatric hospital. She had been referred by the emergency department for attempting to commit suicide "for no reason" by overdosing on Tylenol. The physicians at the psychiatric hospital assumed her attempted suicide was due to depression.

Sonya, her nurse, had a long discussion with Mrs. Fukui and asked her many questions about her life. Mrs. Fukui said that she had been unhappy in her marriage but stayed with her husband for the sake of her three children, who were now grown. Just recently one of her daughters was arrested for drug trafficking. The shame Mrs. Fukui felt over the arrest was so intense that she chose to kill herself rather than live with it.

Sonya explored with her patient the concepts of honor and shame in Japanese culture. Although Mrs. Fukui still felt suicidal, and her shame was intensified by her failure to die on her first attempt, she developed a strong enough bond with Sonya to contract with her for safety. Why did she trust Sonya to that degree? Because Sonya was the only clinician to try to comprehend her perspective. Mrs. Fukui thanked Sonya for "understanding" her.

Sonya then spoke to the psychiatrist and treatment team and shared Mrs. Fukui's perspective. Together, they were able to address all Mrs. Fukui's issues with her family and help them understand her situation as well. Sonya's cultural competence in asking the right questions may have saved Mrs. Fukui's life.

Consider another case, this time involving a Hispanic woman. Rosa Valdez was a forty-seven-year-old woman who, though born in the United States, considered herself Puerto Rican, because that is where her family was from. Spanish was her primary language. She was a long-term patient in a state psychiatric hospital, diagnosed with "schizoaffective disorder-depressed type" along with borderline, histrionic, and dependent personality traits. Although she clearly suffered from mental problems, hers was a case in which a lack of understanding of cultural traits may have affected her personality disorder diagnosis.

Puerto Ricans often tend to be vocal, expressive, and dramatic. When seen through the perspective of a culture that values rational, controlled behavior with a minimum of emotional expressiveness, such behavior could be interpreted as dramatic and attention seeking; in other words, *histrionic traits.* Puerto Rican females were traditionally taught to be modest, submissive to males, and demonstrate a strong sense of closeness to the family; such traits could well be interpreted as *dependent* in a culture that values independence and individuality.

One of her psychiatric "symptoms" was that she would not make eye contact when speaking with the psychiatric nurse. In fact, Puerto Rican

249

women of her generation were taught to lower their eyes and avoid eye contact. It should not have been interpreted as a lack of ability to relate to others.

Ms. Valdez often complained of physical symptoms; she claimed she felt "feverish," or that her eyes "felt funny," or that she suffered from a stomachache or headache. It is common in Puerto Rican culture to convert emotional feelings to physical symptoms. As Rosa explained, in her culture you are not expected to talk about feelings. She referred to her psychiatric illness and depression by saying, "My heart is hurting me."

When she spoke of her family, it was of the large, Latino extended family, which includes aunts, uncles, grandparents, and cousins. Although she would have liked to return to them, her prognosis made it unlikely. Each time she progressed to a point where she could be discharged to a personal care boarding home, she regressed quickly and was returned to the hospital. It is likely that the hospital had taken on the role of her family—the traditional, hierarchical family structure in which her needs are all taken care of, but where her illness frees her from any obligations or expectations.

Again, it is not that the patient had been misdiagnosed as mentally ill on the basis of culturally normal behavior. Rather, some of the traits she displayed were not necessarily symptomatic of psychiatric illness but part of her cultural upbringing. Her culture confused her diagnosis.

250   In the next case, behavior that is seen as normal in one culture is perceived as abnormal in another. Esperlita, a Filipina nurse, began acting strangely. Her aunt and uncle had died in a fatal car crash on their way to Reno. A week after the funeral, Esperlita began to see visions of them. She would hear someone calling her name, smell the scent of her uncle's hair dressing, and feel a cold breeze on her face. The experience disturbed her so much that she began having trouble sleeping and was losing her appetite.

Esperlita shared her experience with Jackie, an Anglo American nurse, who strongly advised her to get psychiatric help. Jackie believed that the stress of her relatives' death was leading Esperlita to a nervous breakdown.

Esperlita related the same story to Araceli, a Filipina coworker. Araceli had a completely different interpretation. She thought that Esperlita's dead relatives, having died in a foreign country and lacking the proper burial ritual, were having trouble making their journey to the next world. Or perhaps they simply wanted to say goodbye. Whatever the explanation, Araceli saw the experience as normal, not as a sign of impending psychosis.

Convinced of Araceli's interpretation, Esperlita and her family offered masses for her departed aunt and uncle over the next two weeks. They also lit candles on their graves each night. At the end of two weeks, the voices, visions, and scents disappeared, Esperlita could sleep undisturbed, and her appetite returned.

What is interesting about this case is the difference in the interpretation of the same behavior by an Anglo American and by a Filipina. The former's culture does not allow for the existence of spirits; the latter's does. Seeing spirits is not interpreted as a sign of mental illness in cultures where people believe spirits exist.

Diagnosing and Treating Mental Illness

As mentioned in the first two case studies above, diagnosing mental illness can be complicated by the fact that in many cultures, including Puerto Rican and Asian groups, emotional stresses are converted to physical symptoms. Consider the following case.

Canh Cao was a thirty-four-year-old Vietnamese woman who was treated by a medical student at a public health clinic. She had made several visits for various physical complaints—abdominal pain, backache, headaches. She was diagnosed with somatoform pain disorder—preoccupation with pain in absence of physical findings.   251

Several months later, Cao attempted suicide. She was sent for evaluation to a psychiatrist, who at that point diagnosed her with depression. She had been depressed all along, but the medical student was both inexperienced and unaware of cultural issues, so he missed it.

It is often difficult to diagnose depression in Vietnamese American patients because they tend to focus on physical complaints rather than underlying emotional problems. As I've mentioned, mental illness carries a great stigma in Asian cultures, and thus individuals will tend to somaticize their problems and report only the physical symptoms. Clinicians need to be aware of this.

Also remember that when dealing with refugees from any country, you must consider numerous other conditions that can affect their mental health, including homesickness, concern for the future, loss of family members, adjustment to a new culture, language problems, and job dissatisfaction. These factors can all lead to depression and suicide attempts.

The Stigma of Mental Illness

Maria Kim was a twenty-four-year-old Korean woman, admitted after   252
overdosing on Valium and Xanax. She was also diagnosed with

decreased blood pressure. Celia, the admitting nurse, was Filipino; Roberta, the charge nurse, was Anglo American. Celia called Roberta to request a room assignment. Roberta reminded Celia that Ms. Kim would have to be admitted to the intensive care unit for constant observation, as per procedure with all overdoses, because such patients are considered a threat to themselves. Celia explained that the patient's physician, a Korean named Dr. Chee, had insisted that the overdose was accidental. Roberta would have questioned Dr. Chee's pronouncement, but Celia's Filipino background would not allow her to insult his authority in that way. Roberta compromised by assigning Maria Kim a room in front of the nurses' station, where she could be observed.

The patient was extremely withdrawn and would not speak. She crawled under the bed covers, while her brother stood watch all day. At 5:00 P.M., Dr. Chee arrived, noted that her blood pressure was now stabilized, and discharged her. When Roberta suggested to him that Maria have a psychiatric evaluation, he simply replied that it was an accident and that the family wanted to take her home.

Although Maria Kim's behavior seems to indicate that she was extremely depressed and probably suicidal, the fact that her physician was also Korean influenced the way the case was handled. Because of the stigma associated with mental illness in Asian cultures, people with such problems are generally taken care of by the family. Dr. Chee recognized this, and did not stigmatize her with the label "depressed" or "suicidal." Her problem was handled by her family, who watched over her and took her home with them.

Roberta, the Anglo nurse, was uncomfortable with merely letting Ms. Kim go without evaluation, so she referred her to Social Services for follow-up. The results are unknown.

Why is mental illness so highly stigmatized in Asia? As a Korean student explained to me, mental illness is thought to be inherited. If it were known that someone in the family was mentally ill, no one would want to marry into that family. When I've mentioned this in class, students from other Asian countries nod in agreement. This is consistent with the fact that in Asian cultures the family, not the individual, is the primary unit. It is not just individuals who marry, but families.

When I was teaching a class of nurses from mainland China in the 1980s, they were quite astounded to learn that many Americans sought psychotherapy for minor problems. They believed that you were either sane or hopelessly mentally ill. There was no middle ground, no category of "neurotic," only that of "psychotic." I once met a Chinese psychiatrist in Los Angeles. When I mentioned that it was surprising to me to hear the combination of "Chinese" and "psychiatrist," he nodded understandingly and said that his parents were ashamed that he was a psychiatrist due to his association with the mentally ill. To hide their shame, they told their friends only that he was a "doctor." Sometimes it can be helpful for practitioners to discuss such diagnoses as depression as a "chemical imbalance" in order to get them to accept medications to treat it.

Although mental illness is highly stigmatized in Asian countries, family members often take care of mentally ill family members. In contrast, a student from Cameroon, Africa, shared that in her town, schizophrenics were regarded as outcasts, and treated "like scum." They often became homeless because no one wanted to take care of them or be associated with them. Family members would usually disown them.

Stress and Mental Health

Culturally Induced Stress and Depression

In December 2012, the secretary of state at the Ministry of Public Health in Cameroon called for citizens to curb depression, as it is one of the leading causes of mental disorder. My student from Cameroon explained that in her culture, women experience depression more commonly than men, and she related that to the social structure of society. Because many African men are polygamous, many mothers are left with the task of bringing up about five children on their own, without support from family members. This puts tremendous stress on women, leading to depression. The Cameroon government is hoping that the campaign will draw attention to the need for patients to get help for depression.

Discussing Emotional Problems

Although mental illness carries a stigma for most Americans, a distinction is made between psychosis and the stresses of everyday life. Seeking counseling to deal with such stresses does not carry the same burden of shame for most of us, at least in the major urban centers. However, talking about personal problems to strangers is not something that is comfortable for everyone. Few African Americans will turn to therapists, because most therapists tend to be white, and they may distrust white institutions in general. Furthermore, it is difficult for a white person to fully understand the stresses of being Black in America. Often, African Americans will turn to the church instead. As mentioned earlier, many Puerto Ricans and Asians will somaticize their feelings and seek treatment for physical symptoms instead.

One might think that having a counselor of the same ethnic background as the patient/client would make it easier to talk, because the counselor would have a better understanding of the cultural stresses, but, surprisingly, this is not always the case. Ethnic communities tend to be very tightly knit, and the (unfounded) fear that the therapist will talk within the community may keep the client from opening up in therapy.

253   Many Italians and Hispanics will turn to their families, rather than discuss their personal problems with strangers. A fifty-five-year-old Mexican American woman named Maria Ibañez was admitted to the coronary care unit with chest pain. She appeared withdrawn and was crying. When asked what was wrong, she shook her head and replied, "Nothing." She gave brief answers to Dr. Mandel, the physician who took her family history, but offered no additional information. Her crying continued even after her chest pain ceased, so Dr. Mandel asked why she was depressed. Still she did not answer.

Eventually Mrs. Ibañez's thirty-five-year-old daughter Cecilia arrived and explained that her mother had been in a state of emotional upset since her father had left home two weeks before. At this Mrs. Ibañez cried out, "No, no! You must not say anything. It is private." Her daughter quietly replied that she could not stand to see her mother suffer so and that she was frightened by her chest pains. Dr. Mandel then suggested that Mrs. Ibañez might want to talk with the staff psychiatrist. In response Mrs. Ibañez exclaimed, "No! No other people should know about this!" Dr. Mandel drew Mrs. Ibañez closer to him, held her hand, and gently said, "Okay. But we need to talk about this." Cecilia, who was visibly disturbed, pleaded with her mother, "Please, Mama."

Why was Mrs. Ibañez so reluctant to discuss the problem that was most likely causing her chest pains? A Mexican nurse on staff later explained that Mexicans feel personal matters should be handled only within the family. They should not be discussed with strangers. Furthermore, a traditional Mexican woman's status is in large part derived from her role as a wife. If her husband leaves, she is nothing. Mrs. Ibañez's pride and embarrassment probably prevented her from talking about the situation. Her daughter, a second-generation Mexican American, was more Westernized and thus more open with outsiders about personal matters.

As it turned out, Mrs. Ibañez did not have a heart attack and was transferred to the postcoronary care unit the next day. The nurse attending her case stopped by her room several times before she left. Although she still did not want to discuss her husband, she had stopped crying and was feeling somewhat better emotionally. What she needed most from the staff was nonintrusive warmth and support. In this case, the underlying emotional nature of the problem was discovered due to the intervention of the more Westernized daughter and the sensitivity of the physician. At the same time, potential medical problems should not be assumed to be somaticized emotional problems.

It is important for health care providers to remember the strong connection between the mind and the body. People often somaticize their emotional stress. The potential for this is further increased when culture dictates a withholding of feelings. It may take a great deal of sensitivity and luck to get patients to discuss their feelings with health care providers. Whenever possible, try to involve culturally appropriate individuals, such as clergy members, traditional healers, or more acculturated family members.

Psychotherapy is not common in most cultures. In traditional, non-Western societies, mind and body are not seen as separate. The same healer—be it shaman or *curandero*—will treat the problem, without distinguishing between emotional and physical ailments.

Acculturation and Mental Health

Depression and anxiety are very common in immigrant populations. Individuals are often alone, without their extended family. They are frequently busy trying to make a living, with little time to talk to one another. Although there are medications to treat depression and anxiety, patients often don't want to take them because of the stigma associated with any kind of mental illness. This is particularly true in Asian populations. A Korean physician has found that when she tells Korean patients that it sounds as if they're suffering from depression, they often break down and cry. Although counseling would generally be appropriate in such a situation, she said she rarely refers them, because they won't go due to the stigma of "mental illness." She finds she has more success if she herself does supportive counseling. Patients will often spend some time talking with her. She typically assures them that anxiety and depression are very common; they won't be on medications forever, but the medications will help them get through the difficult time. She says it may take a few visits to convince patients to take medication, but eventually, they usually do. She also encourages them to look for support in their church or community. Traditional healers can be helpful as well.

While Myra was doing a psych rotation, she cared for Zulema Herrera, *254* a Mexican patient who had been diagnosed with major depression. Mrs. Herrera was also experiencing delusions and her husband had her hospitalized because he was afraid she might harm their young daughter. Mrs. Herrera had moved to the United States two years earlier. She was not responding to medication, and the psychiatrists were considering electroconvulsive therapy. Mr. Hererra disagreed with their diagnosis and plan; he believed his wife was suffering from *susto* and needed treatment from a *curandero*. (*See Chapter 12 for more on* susto.)

A team of psychiatrists, nurses, and social workers met to discuss her situation. The nurses and social workers felt that Mrs. Herrera's illness was related to the stress of being in a new country and far from her family in Mexico. They thought she would benefit from seeing a *curandero*. They physicians reluctantly agreed but insisted they meet first with her husband and the *curandero* to discuss what would take place. They decided to allow the *curandero* to treat Mrs. Herrera with prayer, massage, and herbal teas. After the *curandero* performed his healing ritual, Mrs. Herrera was noticeably less depressed and was more responsive to the therapy prescribed by the psychiatrists. The fact that when physicians work *with* traditional healers, patients usually benefit is a common theme throughout this book.

With the increasing numbers of immigrants in this country comes the growing problem of children who are raised at home with one set of cultural values and are exposed to another set at school and with friends. This can create stress for first-generation Americans.

255   Tammy Tang was born in China, but her family moved to the United States when she was in elementary school. Her parents were very traditional. Although she was now in college, she still lived at home. In fact, she attended the specific college she did because her parents would not let her enroll in any university that was too far from home for her to commute. She was not allowed to date and had a very early curfew. If she were living in China, these restrictions would not have been a problem; however, she was living in the United States. Most of her friends could date and stay out as late as they wanted. Many lived in the dorms or had their own apartments. Tammy felt a tremendous inner conflict. She respected and wanted to obey her parents; at the same time, she wanted the freedom enjoyed by most American college students.

She felt further trapped by her inability to discuss her feelings with anyone. It had been deeply ingrained in her that you should never talk to outsiders about your problems; you discuss them only with your family. But her family *was* her problem. How could she talk to them? It would be completely disrespectful.

I know of Tammy's situation because she was a student in one of my classes. As part of a class requirement, she had to keep a journal. There were several entries in which she discussed her dilemma and the fact that she had often considered suicide as a solution. When I read these entries, I immediately asked Tammy to come see me. I told her that I understood her situation, and strongly advised her to seek help at the student counseling center. Therapists who have worked with clients caught between cultures say that the most effective approach in dealing with such problems is a direct one: discuss the conflicts as resulting from cultural differences. It is not about being a "good" or "bad" person, but what is valued in different cultures.

The wise clinician will recognize the potential for such problems with their adolescent patients. The stress created by intergenerational, intercultural conflicts may be a complicating factor in presenting health problems. Social workers who are trained in cultural diversity may be needed. However, because people from many immigrant cultures have strong feelings against any kind of psychotherapy, either because "mental illness" is highly stigmatized or because personal problems should not be discussed with outsiders, any counseling sessions will have to be scheduled when other family members are not around. Because of the tendency to somaticize, physicians can play an important role in providing counseling, as does the Korean physician described above.

Key Points

- Because each culture values different behavior in its members, what is considered normal in one culture may be perceived as deviant in another.
- In many cultures, emotional stresses are converted to physical symptoms.
- Mental illness is highly stigmatized in Asian cultures.
- Remember to get the patient's point of view on his or her condition.
- In many cultures, people turn to family members or church for emotional support, rather than professionals, and may resist talking to health care providers about their personal problems.
- Acculturation can be a source of stress, as can intergenerational conflict.

Chapter 12

Traditional Medicine: Practices and Perspectives

People have been healing the sick long before the advent of biomedicine. Neanderthal burials from 65,000 years ago show evidence of healed wounds and the presence of plant pollen from species known to have healing properties. Even chimpanzees—our closest living relatives—have been observed chewing a particular species of leaf that appears to expel some sort of tapeworm.

Many people grow medicinal plants in their own gardens or obtain them from a neighborhood or professional healer. These plants may be used as first aid, to treat wounds and burns, aches and pains, upper respiratory infections, earaches, and chronic conditions. Most people will try home remedies, passed on from grandparents and parents, before coming in to the doctor. In many cases, home remedies are effective and save a trip to the physician. However, in other cases, they don't do the job, and the patient shows up in the emergency department or the physician's office. Because these remedies sometimes leave unfamiliar markings on the body, they can lead the clinician to a misdiagnosis. In other cases, they can have negative interactions with biomedicine. In rare cases, they may actually harm the patient.

It is the intent of this chapter to familiarize clinicians with some of the more common traditional remedies, along with a brief look at several traditional health care systems, including Ayurvedic medicine, Chinese medicine, Mexican folk medicine, and African American folk medicine. Also examined will be the kinds of errors that result from the fact that traditional remedies are often used differently from biomedical remedies. The examples of cultural competence in this chapter lie largely in the integration of traditional and biomedical approaches to healing.

Traditional or "Folk" Remedies

Coining

256

A Vietnamese girl named Kathy Dinh was in her first year at an American elementary school. She was not feeling very well one morning, so her mother rubbed the back of her neck with a coin. She then felt well enough to attend school. Later in the day, however, she began to feel worse and went to see the school nurse. When the nurse discovered the welts on Kathy's neck, she immediately assumed she was seeing a case of child abuse and conscientiously reported the Dinhs to the authorities. The situation was finally straightened out, but it created a great deal of needless embarrassment for Kathy's family.

Kathy had experienced a traditional Asian form of healing known as coin rubbing. There are several variations, including heating or oiling the coin or other metal object, such as a spoon, but they all involve vigorously rubbing the body with the metal object. This produces red welts on the affected area, which can distract health professionals from the real problem or be mistaken for abuse.

It is not that Asians never abuse their children, but rubbing them with coins is not the way they do it, any more than Americans abuse their children by having thin pieces of metal wrapped around their teeth and tightened until their teeth move out of place. Braces are often applied for primarily aesthetic reasons. Coin rubbing, at least, is an attempt to heal. Apparently, it often works; only the failures show up in the medical system.

Underlying this practice is the belief that the illness in the body needs to be drawn out. Rubbing the body with a coin produces a raised red area, giving the appearance that the illness has been brought to the surface of the skin. It is believed that red marks will appear only on people who are ill, which is seen as further support for the effectiveness of the technique. Many Asian Americans claim that they still practice coin rubbing because it brings relief from colds and other ailments.

257

While conducting a continuing medical education (CME) class for physicians, I showed a film on patient diversity that had a segment involving coining. A Vietnamese physician in the audience later shared with me that he had experienced coining the week before. The physician was born in Vietnam but came to America at a young age; he had no accent. He looked to be in his late twenties or early thirties. His medical training was in the United States. After my lecture, I asked him more about it. He said he had been experiencing migraine headaches, body aches, and general flu symptoms. First, he tried aspirin, but that didn't help. Next, he tried Naprosin. When that didn't work, he went to the strongest pain reliever he knew, Fiorinal. When that didn't help, he had his mother use coining on his chest. The coin was dipped in euca-lyptus oil and then rubbed until welts formed. He explained that if he weren't sick, no redness would appear. He claimed that the coining was effective whereas the other remedies were not; his symptoms were gone by the next day. He said that when he is ill, he tries Western medicine first. If that doesn't work, he turns to traditional medicine.

It is important that clinicians become familiar with the practice, lest they become distracted from the real problem or mistakenly make accu-sations of child abuse. When such welts are observed on an Asian patient, if the patient and family do not speak English, it would be a good idea to pull out a coin and mime rubbing the body with it. That, along with a questioning look, would probably convey the message. If the patient or family nods in agreement, the marks should be ignored. If it is necessary to write a report on the marks, a note should be made indicating that they may be the result of a traditional healing practice.

258   Claire, a nurse in one of my cultural diversity classes, helped avoid a potential problem in this way. Peter, one of the other nurses on the floor, asked her to take a look at one of his patients, an elderly Asian woman who presented with shortness of breath. Peter was concerned that his patient was being abused due to the marks all over her back. When Claire saw the marks, she suspected they were due to coining, which she then confirmed with the patient. She was able to identify coin-ing and taught Peter about this traditional Asian remedy for ridding the body of toxins. She felt quite pleased that she was able to use her knowl-edge to both identify the practice and teach a colleague about it.

Cupping

259   Another healing method that produces similarly misleading marks is cupping. John Bagdasarian, a forty-six-year-old Armenian man, was brought into the critical care unit with a diagnosis of acute myocardial infarction (heart attack). While doing a physical assessment, the nurse found round red marks all over his upper back that looked like burns. The staff speculated about the source of the marks. Theories ranged from birthmarks to some form of torture or sadism. An Armenian physi-cian finally cleared up the mystery. The marks were a result of cupping.

The patient's family had tried to cure him of his chest pains by heat-ing a glass and placing it on his body. The vacuum created under the glass caused the skin to rise and left the red marks. When cupping did not stop the chest pains, his family brought him to the hospital.

260   Amelia, one of my nursing students, reported that she had avoided a potential child abuse report with a Cambodian family, the Chhets. The child had suspicious burn marks on her body. Instead of assuming child abuse, she first interviewed both parents separately. Both explained that they had treated their child using cupping and coining to make her feel better and help her recover more quickly. Amelia then explained to her supervisor what she had learned from the parents, and they decided it was not a child abuse situation. The Bagdasarians and Chhets practiced the traditional form of cupping. A more modern version uses a suction pump to create a vacuum under the cups, and avoids the potential danger of burning the skin. In both cases, the skin is drawn up into the cup, increasing circulation and leaving a large, circular bruise. It is commonly used to treat sore muscles and respiratory problems.

Marianne Bernstein, a middle-aged Anglo American woman, was sick   261 with flu, bronchitis, and pneumonia. She could not stop coughing. She went to her physician for treatment, and took three rounds of antibiotics. Despite that, she continued to cough. She finally went to an acupuncturist who performed cupping on her. Her coughing relented that day and continued to improve. Although it may have been due to the antibiotics finally kicking in, or to the disease finally running its course, or perhaps to the Chinese herbs she took for the next week, Marianne was convinced that the cupping was primarily responsible.

I include this example for two reasons. One is to point out that traditional remedies may be used by patients from other than the "traditional" culture. Traditional Chinese medicine, for example, has experienced great popularity among upper-middle-class Anglo Americans. The second is to point out the possible efficacy of traditional "folk" remedies.

While discussing cupping in one of my medical anthropology classes, I shared with the class my only experience of cupping at that time, and commented on how painful it was. One of my Asian students raised her hand and said that it only hurt because I had a problem in the area where the cups were placed, and that the pain was a sign that it was working. She offered to bring in her set of cups to demonstrate. I accepted. The next class she brought in a set of the suction pump cups. She placed some near my neck, where I was experiencing chronic tightness, and some on my hip, which felt fine. As she predicted, cupping was painful only near my neck, not at my hip.

Cupping is said to be particularly successful for treating sore muscles and is frequently practiced for that purpose in many parts of the world, including Asia, Latin America, Russia, and parts of Europe, and it is taught in acupuncture colleges in the United States. As with coining, however, health care professionals who are not aware of the practice can easily misinterpret the marks it leaves.

Fevers

Current medical wisdom has it that the most effective way to reduce fever is to cool the body. This is done by removing regular blankets and placing an "ice blanket" under the patient. In contrast, many cultures believe that the best way to treat a high temperature is to sweat it out. These conflicting theories are the source of another common cultural conflict in the hospital.

262   Hiroshi Tomita, a Japanese business executive on a trip to the United States, was admitted to the hospital with a 102-degree fever of unknown origin. According to standard procedure, his nurse, Jean, removed the blankets from the bed, leaving only a sheet to cover him. She explained that it was to keep his temperature from going up. She gave him a glass of cold apple juice, but he only took two sips. At 9 P.M., the doctor examined Mr. Tomita and prescribed a mild analgesic every four hours for temperatures greater than 101 degrees and a cooling blanket for temperatures greater than 102 degrees. When his temperature rose to 103 degrees at 10 P.M., Jean ordered a cooling blanket, per the doctor's instructions. At this point, Mr. Tomita asked for his blankets, but Jean refused, once more explaining why. She put the ice blanket under him and left the room. In a few minutes, Mr. Tomita complained that the ice blanket was too cold and asked for his regular blankets. For the third time, Jean patiently explained the treatment. He did not say anything; he simply curled up under his sheet. When Jean returned a half hour later to check on him, he was sitting up in the chair with all the blankets wrapped around him, covered with goose bumps and shivering. By midnight, his temperature was up to 105 degrees. Jean gave him his second dosage of acetaminophen. Mr. Tomita continued to ask for his blankets and to get out of bed. Jean was at the point of putting restraints on him to keep him in bed.

She finally asked him why he did not want to stay in bed. He explained that in Japan, people with fevers were covered with warm blankets and given plenty of hot drinks. Cold juice was particularly inappropriate. This approach, found throughout Asia, is probably based on the Chinese notion of hot and cold balance, or yin and yang. Mr. Tomita was experiencing chills, which logically should be treated with heat, not cold. Furthermore, it is believed that fevers must be sweated out, again necessitating measures that produce greater warmth.

Reflecting on his comment, Jean asked herself what she did when suffering from a temperature and chills. She realized that she did exactly what her patient wanted—she piled lots of blankets on herself, turned the electric blanket to the maximum temperature, and drank hot liquids!

She then called a team conference. Most of her colleagues admitted to similar behavior, but no one wanted to take responsibility for going against medical orders. Realizing that she could no longer treat Mr. Tomita against his beliefs and wishes, Jean decided to call the admitting doctor. It was now 1 A.M. The physician was angry at being awakened. He impatiently listened to her story, was silent for a moment, and then agreed to a change in orders: discontinue the cooling blanket, adminis-ter analgesic tablets every three hours if the patient's temperature rose above 101 degrees, and keep the patient as comfortable as possible.

Mr. Tomita was extremely happy and grateful for the change in orders. His temperature came down after about three hours and he eventually removed the blankets on his own.

Interestingly, the field of Darwinian medicine, which looks at disease from an evolutionary perspective, sees fever as an adaptation to fight infection. Nesse and Williams (1994) don't advocate never trying to bring down fevers, but call for research to help physicians decide when treatment is useful and when it's not.

A similar case involved Rosa Torres, a twenty-nine-year-old Hispanic woman with a surgical infection. Her temperature was 104 degrees. She had piled six blankets on top of herself, curled up into a ball, and lay there moaning loudly. When Rebecca, her nurse, discovered the mound of blankets, she attempted to remove them. Ms. Torres vehemently refused. "No, I will get cold." Rebecca explained that the blankets were keeping her body temperature too high; she needed to remove them to reduce the fever. The explanation did nothing to change her mind, but Rebecca was determined and gently pulled off all but one blanket.

Shortly thereafter, Rebecca tried to take Ms. Torres's temperature rec-tally, per the doctor's orders. Again, she refused. She did not want her underwear removed and certainly did not want anyone to insert a rectal thermometer. Each of Rebecca's attempts to do so was met with screams. Rebecca tried to explain the importance of the greater accuracy of the rectal temperature, but Rosa did not care. Rebecca finally gave up, respecting Rosa's right to refuse. Another nurse on the unit, however, was not about to give in to the patient's desires and insisted that she remove her underwear. She managed to insert the thermometer despite Rosa Torres's cries and tears.

Although Rebecca did not understand the reason for Rosa's behavior at the time, she later learned from several Hispanic friends that it is believed that one of the greatest dangers during a fever is letting in cold air. Removing all the covers thus put the patient at risk. Second, the illness is seen as a kind of poison. Keeping the blankets on causes the body to sweat out the poison; thus, the fever goes down and the illness disappears. Ms. Torres's refusal to remove her underwear and have her

263

temperature taken rectally was probably due to the modesty typically found among Hispanic women, along with the discomfort and sense of indignity involved. Not to mention the cold that could enter!

Unlike the previous example, in which the nurse finally did respect the patient's wishes, in this case Western medicine won out. Rosa Torres was labeled a difficult patient because of her desire to adhere to her traditional beliefs regarding treatment of disease. Rebecca later suggested that the doctor could have been called to change the order from a rectal to an oral temperature. She still felt it was necessary to remove the blankets but thought that if she had understood Ms. Torres's reasons, she might have been more empathetic.

264   In another case, a Mexican American mother refused to use cooling measures in caring for her febrile infant, despite medical instructions to do so. Mrs. Lopez had called the hospital because her infant's temperature was very high. She was told to give the baby a mild analgesic and a cool bath and then to bring her in. Mrs. Lopez ignored both cooling instructions and, to the consternation of the medical staff, brought the child wrapped in several layers of blankets, outer garments, undershirt, and several pairs of socks. When asked why she did not follow the instructions given her, she replied, "He must sweat the fever out. Besides, he could get pneumonia from the night air and die."

Nurses who work in hospitals serving a large Hispanic population say that they see this behavior quite frequently. In fact, the sight of a family walking up to the registration window with a bundle of blankets in their arms usually prompts the nurses to prediagnose the child as having a fever and admit it right away. Immediate action is necessary to make sure the baby does not have a seizure while the family is registering.

Parents are generally willing to listen to the nurses' explanations on how to treat fevers in infants. The problem is often with their own parents. One young woman explained that she knew she should not wrap her baby so heavily, but her mother-in-law "made her do it." She had attended some parenting classes and knew the proper procedure, but felt it was too difficult to fight the whole family. Health education—with the key members of the family—is the only way to deal with such situations, but it will not be easy to overcome years of tradition.

265   Another example occurred with an African American woman and her tiny grandson. The child was brought into the hospital by his mother, Mary Wilson, and grandmother, Adele Wilson. The nurse explained that she would put the naked infant in a cool mist tent and bathe him in cold water to reduce his temperature. His mother was quiet, calm, and cooperative. She indicated her concern by asking several questions about her son's condition.

Adele Wilson, however, did not appear to be listening. She got up from her chair, looked into the tent, and said, "You forgot to give him a blanket. That thing is real cold inside." The nurse again explained that she was keeping him cool because of his high temperature. Mary Wilson tried to calm her mother-in-law, seeing that she was becoming hostile. "Mama, it's okay." Mrs. Wilson responded, "What you talkin' 'bout? They got you believing in this foolishness too. I'm gonna put his blanket on him 'cause he is cold. I raised all my nine children and I never put one in no icebox. You know you need to wrap him so he can sweat the fever out. Hot chamomile tea would bring that fever down."

Most of the nurses dealt with the grandmother by avoiding her. They could not talk to her without arguing. How might they have handled the situation? They might have begun by asking her how she would have treated the child. They could have acknowledged her approach, which comes from years of use of natural remedies within the African American culture. They might also have incorporated her recommendation of chamomile tea. Mrs. Wilson's hostility may have been a reaction to what she perceived as racism on the part of the white nurses. A bit more respect on the part of the nurses might have helped.

Medications

Applying the Medication Directly to the Site

A common source of cross-cultural misunderstandings involves the use of Western medications, which often differs from the application of traditional remedies. It is essential that complete explanations be given to patients regarding how to use medication. Florence, an African American nurse, was doing home care for a thirty-year-old Mexican woman named Lena Menendez, who had recently had a caesarean section. Mrs. Menendez spoke little English. Her mother, Gloria Flores, was staying with her to help with the baby. During her first visit, she wanted to make an assessment evaluation and change the dressing on the incision site.

When Mrs. Menendez removed her underpants, the first thing Florence noticed was the absence of a pad or gauze covering the gauze inside the wound. When she looked more closely, she discovered a bloody white cheesy substance on the gauze and in the corners and edges of the wound. Florence had no idea what it was. In her mind, she considered the possibilities: semen? intestines? When she removed the old dressing, she was relieved to find that it was not intestines. She could find no evidence of infection, and after cleaning the wound, decided it was just a dirty wound.

When Florence returned the next day, she noted more of the white, bloody, cheesy substance. This time, she asked Mrs. Menendez what it was. Her mother answered for her, replying, "Her medication—the one with the powder in it. The nurse said it was for infections." Florence was astounded. She explained that the medication was to be taken by mouth. Mrs. Flores said, "No, in my culture, we mix the powder and put it where the infection is. In order for the wound to heal, the powder goes in there." Florence then spent several minutes explaining to Mrs. Flores and her daughter the difference between American medicine and traditional Mexican medicine. It was unfortunate that the nurse who had originally given the medication to her had neglected to explain how it is used. Moreover, Florence should have asked about it on the first visit.

Do not assume that a patient will understand how to take the medication prescribed. Medicines are used in different ways in different countries, and confusion can result. Alternatively, people simply may be unfamiliar with the administration of medicinal products, as evidenced in the next two cases.

267   One nurse related the case of an angry Mexican woman who became pregnant even though she faithfully took her birth control pill every day. Questioning revealed that the woman had inserted the pills into her vagina. Her action may have seemed logical to her; unfortunately, it was not effective.

268   Another Mexican woman became pregnant while using contraceptive foam. Although the failure rate with foam is much higher than with birth control pills, that was not the cause of her pregnancy. No one had explained to her how to use the foam. Since the directions on the can were in English, which she did not understand, she and her husband did what made sense to them—they applied the foam to his penis before he inserted it into her vagina. Again, when giving information on the use of any kind of medication, it is extremely important to give clear and complete instructions on its use.

Filling a Prescription

269   Health care practitioners are often frustrated when patients do not follow through on their prescriptions. Sometimes this apparent lack of adherence can result from cultural factors. Serina, a home health nurse, was interviewing Huong Nguyen, a sixty-five-year-old Vietnamese refugee, regarding her condition and health care practices subsequent to her discharge for a gastrointestinal problem. Serina learned that Mrs. Nguyen was drinking rice water as a remedy for her gastrointestinal

tract. Although her physician had given her a prescription for medication, Mrs. Ngyuen was not familiar with the procedure of having a prescription filled, and had put the prescription with the rest of the indecipherable papers she had received at discharge.

There is an important lesson in this case. Realize that recent immigrants may not be familiar with the system of having prescriptions filled, since they may have always been given medications directly by the doctor. Be sure to explain the procedure.

Dangerous Substances

There is a long tradition of using folk medicine in many different cultures. Many current drugs, including digitalis, have been developed from native plants. Artemisinin, the main ingredient in several effective antimalarial drugs, was developed from a compound found in the wormwood plant and used to treat fever in China for 2,000 years. *Pasionara* (passion flower), a traditional Hispanic remedy for anxiety, is an effective sedative, and, if the right species is used, very safe. The same is true of *zábila* (aloe vera) when used externally to treat burns. The traditional Hispanic chili pepper is the source of the well-known pharmaceutical capsaicin, a topical cream used to treat arthritis pain, oral pain, and atypical facial pain. However, many traditional remedies can also cause problems, as the following case indicates.

Mrs. Jimenez brought her twenty-month-old infant to see the doctor because the baby was suffering from diarrhea. During the history, she mentioned that she had given her son a yellow powder that she got from a neighbor. She wasn't sure what it was, but said that it came from Guatemala and is used for stomach ailments. The powder was probably *azarcón* or *greta*, a compound that contains lead and can cause neurological disturbances including seizures, coma, and death.

While many traditional remedies are helpful, and many of those with no proven scientific benefit are at least not harmful, some can be considered dangerous. Sometimes this is due to inadvertent side effects caused by the potency of the main ingredient. For example, PC-SPES, a patent formula that contains eight different herbs and has been used to treat prostate cancer, has been shown to stimulate estrogenic activity, which has resulted in some patients having a pulmonary embolism. In other cases, the problem is that the medicine has become contaminated with heavy metals, pesticides, and pharmaceuticals, such as steroids and benzodiazepines. PC-SPES was taken off the market because some batches were found to contain unlisted prescription medicines, according to the National Cancer Institute.

270

In 1998, the California health department analyzed over 250 Chinese patent medicines containing premixed herbs compressed into pills or capsules (Chinese Herbs 2000). Nearly a third of the products were found to contain toxic ingredients, including high levels of lead, mercury, and arsenic. A little over 6 percent were spiked with pharmaceutical drugs. One of the problems is that some of the herbs grown in China become contaminated during the farming process, particularly when the herb fields are located next to factories and absorb the pollution. Some of the specific medications found to have problems are Ansenpunaw tablets, which are advertised as "a brain tonic and sedative medicine," and "Double Dragon Pills." The Chinese *ma huang* herb, which contains ephedrine and helps breathing problems, caused heart attacks and strokes among some Americans using it as a diet aid. *Kava kava*, a Pacific Island anxiety-relieving tea, has poisoned the livers of those drinking a concentrated form.

The use of herbal remedies has gained much popularity in recent years among several populations in the United States, including middle-class Anglo Americans. Unfortunately, many can interact with prescription drugs, by causing a synergistic effect, an antagonistic effect, or decreased bioavailability. *Danshen*, an herbal tea, can adversely affect heart rate, and if taken with digoxin, may cause heart failure. Seemingly innocuous herbs such as garlic, ginger, and licorice root can interfere with Coumadin, a prescription blood thinner. Ginkgo can increase bleeding and bruising when used with blood thinners, decrease the effectiveness of seizure medications, and increase the risk of side effects when used with monoamine oxidase inhibitor (MAOI) antidepressants.

271   Mrs. Raffetto, a sixty-year-old Italian women, was going in for colon cancer surgery. Her daughter-in-law Amanda was a nurse. Amanda was going through Mrs. Raffetto's medications to inform the doctor what she was taking. She was horrified to learn that her mother-in-law was taking 18 different herbal supplements, many of them combination pills that had the same ingredients. Some of these ingredients could cause bleeding, so Mrs. Raffetto needed to stop taking them several days before the surgery.

All this should serve to underscore the importance of discussing with *all* your patients the drugs, herbs, and other remedies they may be taking. It is incumbent on health care practitioners to ask their patients about this. It is also important to ask the right questions. Medical students are trained to ask patients what medications they're taking. But the word may mean different things to different people, as in the next case.

272   Fariba was asked to interpret for Fereydoon Jalili, an Iranian man who had come to the hospital with gastrointestinal bleeding. Mr. Jalili spoke

some English, and when the physician had asked him what medications he was taking, he told him he didn't take any. When Fariba was brought in to interpret, she began talking to him about his health. During their conversation, he admitted that he took vitamins to stay healthy and he was very proud of the fact that he had never been sick. He also mentioned that he took two aspirins a day for his heart after seeing a commercial on television which said it prevented heart attacks. When Fariba asked him why he didn't tell the doctor about the vitamins and aspirin, he said that he didn't consider anything he bought over-the-counter to be a "real" medication. Once the physician learned what he had been taking, he educated Mr. Jalili on appropriate aspirin consumption, since that was the likely cause of his GI bleed.

When asking patients about medications, it's best to be specific and mention herbs, vitamins, teas, and over-the-counter remedies. The challenge in asking about alternative treatments, particularly traditional remedies that may come from a neighbor or a *botánica* (a shop that sells folk medicine, religious candles, amulets, etc.), comes in keeping any criticism out of your voice. Many non-Anglo American patients have admitted to nurses that they don't usually tell the physician about traditional remedies because they don't want to be criticized. I once had a physician say to me, "You don't take any of that weird Chinese medicine, do you?" I do on occasion, but I found it exceedingly difficult to admit to it in the face of such obvious scorn. Keep in mind that if you convey any negativity, all you will probably do is alienate your patient. What you want to do instead is make sure they don't do anything harmful, and allow them to continue anything that may be helpful or at least neutral. Many treatments, even if they have no proven pharmacological value, may have psychological value, and allowing your patients to continue to use them will help you gain their trust. Let them know that your primary concern is their health and well-being, and that you will not look down on them or criticize them for anything else they do, as long as they tell you about it.

You might try saying something along the lines of, "Many of my patients also see traditional healers who prescribe herbal remedies, or use home remedies that have been passed down for generations. Often they can be effective, but sometimes they can cause problems, especially when mixed with other treatments. That's why it's important that I know everything that you are taking to treat this or any other problem." An attitude of respect, rather than derision, is crucial. As an added bonus, clinicians who ask such questions find they establish greater trust and rapport with their patients.

"Folk" Diseases

Folk diseases are those diseases that are specific to a culture. A number of common Hispanic folk diseases will be discussed later in the chapter. However, at this point, I want to discuss one that is found in numerous parts of the world: evil eye.

Evil Eye

Belief in the evil eye is widespread throughout Central America, the Mediterranean, the Middle East, much of Africa, and parts of Asia. Although the beliefs and associated practices vary, the concept generally includes an "evil" that one person puts on another that causes the victim to fall ill. The motive is usually envy.

273   Jen, a second-year medical student, was on a pediatrics visit learning how to perform a newborn exam. As she followed the attending into the patient's room, she noticed that the baby's mother was sitting on the side of the crib talking in Spanish to her husband. The attending started to explain to Jen what is important to notice about a baby and what to look for on the physical exam, and proceeded to ask her questions about the causes of pneumonia and meningitis in the newborn period. As they were talking, the infant's mother came over to the crib. In an attempt to welcome her into their conversation, Jen said "hello," and proceeded to compliment her on her beautiful child. As soon as she finished the sentence, the mother said "thank you," but frowned, and her demeanor changed slightly—she stopped smiling, and looked nervous.

Jen wondered what she had done wrong, and suddenly realized that the family was Mexican, and her complimentary words, intended as a tool to gain the mother's trust, resulted in causing her distress. Remembering what she had learned about Mexican culture and *mal de ojo* (evil eye), she touched the baby's hand, and looked back at the mother. The change was remarkable—the mother smiled back at her, and nodded her head. She did not say anything, but her smile and nod tacitly communicated her gratitude for preventing *mal de ojo.* Jen later commented to me that during the challenging period in medical school, while the medical student is learning to become a doctor, it is often easy to focus on studying diseases, and to approach a patient with the perspective of having to figure out what is wrong and how to fix it. What medical students and doctors often forget is that patients' belief system may be a very important part of their lives, and unless this aspect is respected, they will not form a coalition with the doctor to help solve the mystery of their own sickness. She emphasized that knowledge of culture is an essential tool that should be understood and remembered alongside anatomy, pathology, and other important traditional medical school subjects. I agree.

Anthropologists have explained the evil eye curse in terms of the "theory of limited good," which is based on the idea that there is a limited amount of good things in the world, whether beauty, intelligence, wealth, luck, or health. If one person gets more, there is less of it in the world for others. Envy may dictate giving someone the evil eye. The victim's ensuing illness somehow helps even things out.

Belief in the evil eye can create distress and confusion between Mexican and American mothers. In traditional Mexican culture, babies are considered weak and extremely susceptible to the power of an envious glance. It is not even necessary to wish a child harm; a simple compliment, unaccompanied by a touch, can bring on the evil eye. Touching the person while complimenting him or her, however, neutralizes the power of the evil eye.

Americans are raised to believe that germs cause disease. Mothers are uncomfortable when people get too close to their infants, especially when ill. Traditional Mexican mothers, in contrast, may worry when strangers admire their babies without touching them. The very act that is believed to *protect* a child from illness in one culture is thought to *cause* illness in another.

Each culture that believes compliments can cause the evil eye also has ways to neutralize it or protect against it. Putting a bit of saliva on one's finger and making the sign of the cross on a child's forehead when giving a compliment can prevent the evil eye in some (but not all) parts of the Philippines. In parts of Ethiopia, spitting on a child while remarking on its good looks will prevent an inadvertent casting of the evil eye. Babies may wear special amulets to protect them against the evil eye. In Mexico, a "deer's eye"—a large seed pod with a bit of red yarn—may be used; in Greece and Turkey, a blue glass "eye" charm; in Italy, an animal's horn; and in the Middle East, a hand. Not all members of these cultures adhere to the belief, however, so it is important to pay close attention to nonverbal cues from the mother. Does she appear uncomfortable when you compliment her child? If so, she may believe in the evil eye, as in the case described above.

Ronnie first learned about the evil eye when her attention was drawn to a baby brought to the clinic where she worked. The infant had a blue "eye" amulet with small blue beads attached to his clothing with a diaper pin. When she asked the mother about it, she was told that it was to protect her baby from the evil eye. Ronnie told me that in the past she would have been reluctant to ask about the amulets for fear of offending. She now realized that she was less likely to offend if she simply asked. This is an important lesson for those who are learning to be more culturally competent. Most people are proud to share information about their culture with those who are truly interested. The trick is in how you ask.

Traditional Healers

Most cultures have traditional healers. Although their actions are based on a model of health and illness different from biomedicine, they can often be effective. The question many health care practitioners may have is, *why* are they effective? They operate outside the realm of Western biomedicine. Can it be that there is some validity to other healing models? For those who have difficulty accepting this possibility, consider the fact that the mind has a powerful influence over the body. The placebo effect has long illustrated that belief in the power of a "sugar" pill to heal, or faith in the abilities of a physician, can result in actual healing. Such power may be at work in the case of traditional healers. Culturally competent practitioners realize that collaboration between traditional healers and biomedical doctors can often result in better care for their patients, as the next three cases illustrate.

275   Daniel, an eighteen-year-old Igbo (his tribe) Nigerian boy who had been living in the United States since he was nine, was admitted to the ICU due to an acute sickle cell crisis. He had suffered from sickle cell disease since childhood, but had not had a major crisis since he had moved to the United States, and only one minor crisis. His mother was frantically crying, and kept repeating that the curse of Daniel's Ogbanje had finally caught up with him. According to Igbo belief, the spirit of a dead child may reenter the mother's womb to be reborn in the next child. Daniel's mother had had a miscarriage before becoming pregnant with Daniel, and that child's spirit was thought to be possessing Daniel. Ogbanje children generally don't live very long. From a medical perspective, many of these children are thought to be suffering from sickle cell disease. Traditional treatment involves taking the child to a medicine man, who attempts to cajole the Ogbanje spirit into leading him to his spiritual paraphernalia. The medicine man then creates a charm out of the paraphernalia to give to the parents, or the objects are ritually destroyed. In Daniel's case, each time he had had a sickle cell crisis, or, in their view, each time the Ogbanje appeared, the spirit refused to show the medicine man where his paraphernalia were buried. It wasn't until Daniel was nine years old that the medicine man was able to locate the snail shells that had been buried in a corner of Daniel's house. Once they were destroyed, Daniel's parents took the additional step of moving to the United States, where the medicine man promised

the curse would not follow. It seemed to work . . . until the night his parents had to bring him to the emergency department.

While the medical team worked on Daniel, his father consulted with an Igbo medicine man over the telephone. Daniel's eldest uncle asked the nurse if he could bring in a special lotion of olive oil and tea tree oil to rub on his body and keep evil spirits from entering. Daniel's nurse, Keisha, who happened to be from Cameroon and thus more familiar with traditional African beliefs than most nurses, consulted with the doctor and got permission for him to do so. The entire family surrounded Daniel in his bed and prayed for him. Despite the fact that they held traditional beliefs, they were also Christian. And although she understood the disease process of their son's illness—it had been diagnosed during a minor crisis shortly after they arrived in the United States—his mother believed that the Ogbanje curse had returned to haunt them. She appreciated how much biomedicine could help her son's condition, but in the case of evil spirits, she also wanted the help of an Igbo medicine man and Jesus.

When Daniel's father finally reached the medicine man in Nigeria, he advised them to put salt paste on the soles of Daniel's feet to help drain out any remnants of the Ogbanje curse. Back in Nigeria, the medicine man performed the necessary rituals.

The combination of the medical treatment, traditional rituals, and Christian prayers worked; by the end of the week, Daniel was extubated, breathing normally, completely off sedation, and eating food his mother had brought in for him. His family was grateful to the medical staff for allowing them to incorporate some of their traditional healing practices.

An eighty-three-year-old Cherokee woman named Mary Cloud was brought into the hospital emergency room by her grandson, Joe, after she had passed out at home. Lab tests and x-rays indicated that she had a bowel obstruction. After consulting with Joe, the attending physician called in a surgeon to remove it. Joe was willing to sign consent for the surgery, but it would not be legal; the patient had to sign for herself. Mrs. Cloud, however, refused; she wanted to see the medicine man on the reservation. Unfortunately, the drive took an hour and a half each way, and she was too ill to be moved. Finally, the social worker suggested that the medicine man be brought to the hospital.

Joe left and drove to the reservation. He returned three hours later, accompanied by a man in full traditional dress complete with feather headdress, rattles, and bells. The medicine man entered Mrs. Cloud's room and for forty-five minutes conducted a healing ceremony. Outside the closed door, the stunned and amused staff could hear bells, rattles, chanting, and singing. At the conclusion of the ceremony, the medicine man informed the doctor that Mrs. Cloud would now sign the consent

276

form. She did so and was immediately taken to surgery. Her recovery
was uneventful and without complications.

What was responsible for her recovery? The hospital staff were sure it
was the skill of the surgeon; Mrs. Cloud was convinced it was due to the
power of the medicine man. In any case, without the medicine man, she
would not have agreed to the surgery or, if she had, her attitude might
have been so poor as to interfere with recovery. This is a perfect example
of how traditional healers and physicians can successfully work together
in the care of patients.

277   Another case involving a successful collaboration between traditional
and Western medicine occurred in a prison health facility, thanks to the
cultural competence of the prison nurse. Amy was assigned to care for
Edgar Manuelito, a thirty-eight-year-old Native American. Although very
ill, he was refusing food and medication, and did not allow the nurses
to bathe him. His physician and most of the nursing staff expected him
to die shortly. When Amy learned that he was Native American, she
asked him if he would like a medicine man to come pray for him. His
face lit up at her question. He asked if it would be possible for her to
arrange it. It took Amy ten phone calls, but she finally located a medicine man who was associated with the prison. She contacted him, and
he said he would be happy to pray for Mr. Manuelito. The medicine
man also told her about the seldom-used sweat lodge the prison had for
its Native American inmates. A sweat lodge is used in a traditional Native
American ritual. It is like an outdoor sauna, often made with tree
branches. Stones are heated and water poured on them. There are usually several rounds of prayers in this purification ritual. With some difficulty, Amy and the medicine man were able to convince the prison
guards that it was important for Mr. Manuelito to visit the sweat lodge.
The medicine man performed a traditional ritual involving burning
incense and chanting. Mr. Manuelito then spent half a day in the sweat
lodge. Although the other nurses thought Amy was "crazy" for arrang-
ing all this, Mr. Manuelito suddenly began to eat and take his medication. His health started to improve and he eventually recovered. Amy's
culturally competent approach to his care probably saved his life.

One nurse, Leila, after taking a course in cultural competence, said
that when she has a Mexican patient, she always asks whether the patient
is following the advice of a *curandero* or *yerbera* (herbalist). If the patient
replies affirmatively, she'll ask if she or he is following any special recommendations or taking any herbal remedies. Most of the Mexican patients
she has treated thus far have been fairly acculturated, and none have
replied "yes" to her questions. It is likely, however, that one day someone will. Such questions should be a standard part of the intake interview. The fact that none have said "yes" should also be a reminder not

to stereotype individuals. Leila begins with the generalization that Mexicans may consult a traditional healer before seeing a physician, and then asks the individual to verify if the generalization can be appropriately applied in each specific instance.

Traditional Medical Systems

It is not uncommon for individuals to seek out multiple health care practitioners for the same problem without sharing this information with their medical practitioners, because they fear offending them or being ridiculed by them, or because they don't think the information is important. This can lead to problems, especially if they are taking herbs or treatments that interact with medical treatment. An East Indian patient may be receiving treatment from an Ayurvedic practitioner while being treated by a medical doctor. A Chinese patient may be taking herbs prescribed by a traditional Chinese physician and medication prescribed by a family practice physician. A Mexican patient may be visiting a *curandera* or taking traditional home remedies for a problem also being treated by her doctor. It is important that health care providers have some knowledge of traditional medical systems and inquire about them. Again, however, it is imperative that such queries be made nonjudgmentally. If patients feel that they will be ridiculed, they will simply withhold information, information that may be crucial for the physician to know. It is important, also, to have a basic understanding of some of these systems.

Ayurvedic Medicine

Ayurvedic medicine is a traditional Hindu system. *Ayurveda* (a Sanskrit word meaning "Laws of Health") is the title of one of the four sacred Hindu texts known as the Vedas. The notion of the whole person is emphasized, including the physical, psychological, and spiritual aspects—in other words, body, mind, and spirit.

To summarize and simplify an incredibly complex system, according to Ayurvedic theory the universe is composed of five elements—earth, water, fire, air, and ether. The human body also has three humors, or *dosha*, which relate to different aspects of bodily function: (1) respiratory system—air; (2) digestive system (which produces heat)—fire; and (3) moisture in the body—water. These must be maintained in a state of balance. If this balance is lost, then treatment might include foods, minerals, and herbs of the proper forces to restore balance.

For example, if someone had a condition in which the element of "air" was excessively dominant, the Ayurvedic physician would prescribe a diet that excludes "air" foods such as rice and spices, and would use a remedy that stimulated the other two forces, fire and water. When diagnosing and prescribing, the physician also takes into account the patient's character, age, nationality, and life and family circumstances.

Good health is maintained by paying attention to the five natural elements, and the life force, known as *prana*, which can be channeled to help or heal. *Prana* can be thought of as "energy." It is similar to the Chinese notion of *chi*. The Ayurvedic worldview can be best understood through yoga, through which *prana* is received, transmuted, and transmitted to various parts of the body via the seven chakras, or "wheels of energy." They can be opened through yoga, meditation, and chanting or rhythmic breathing.

A student from India shared that medical treatment for children is largely based on Ayurvedic home remedies, passed on by family elders. Such traditional remedies are often given precedence over Western biomedicine. However, when traditional remedies do not work, they will turn to biomedicine.

Traditional Chinese Medicine (TCM)

Chinese medicine has received a great deal of attention and interest in the United States over the past several decades. It has had a major influence on nearly all medical systems throughout Asia. The worldview that humans are a part of nature is reflected in the Chinese health care paradigm. Rather than try to control nature by destroying germs as the Western health care system does, it seeks to restore a person's natural place in the natural system. It is based on the principle of harmony and balance.

According to TCM, the two opposing principles in the universe are *yin* and *yang.* Yin is the female principle; it represents cold, darkness, and other qualities. Yang is the male principle; it represents heat, light, and so forth. When yin and yang (or cold and hot) are in balance, the individual is healthy. When they become out of balance, illness results. The goal of treatment is to restore balance, which can be achieved through acupuncture (a cold, or yin treatment, used for yang ailments) or moxibustion (a hot or yang treatment, used for yin ailments), and/or herbs.

278   Dak-Ho Yi, an elderly Korean man, was admitted for depression. The staff became concerned because he refused to take any of his medications. His family finally explained the problem. The nurses had been giving him juice or water to take his pills. That violated the hot/cold

balance. Once they gave him hot tea instead, he took his medication without incident. It was a simple adjustment for the staff to make, once they understood the problem.

A diagnosis is made through an examination of the tongue and the pulses. Chinese medicine recognizes twelve pulses (readings are taken at three depths on each of the two pulses in each wrist), each associated with a different organ or system. Ted Kaptchuk's book, *The Web That Has No Weaver* (1983), is one of the better texts explaining Chinese medicine for the layperson. The title comes from the fact that Chinese medicine is less concerned with the *cause* of disease than with the pattern of disharmony. Kaptchuk describes how the Chinese, if they were to see a web, would ask different questions from those an American would ask. Westerners are concerned with origins and issues of control. The Judeo-Christian Bible, for example, begins by answering the question "who created the universe?" Science addresses the same question, albeit with a different answer. Traditional Chinese religions do not have a god in the sense of a creator of the universe. In their view, it doesn't matter who created the universe; what is important to understand is the patterns that exist and constantly repeat themselves. If they saw a web, they would be more interested in the pattern of the web; most Americans who would want to know who created the web. For the Chinese, the universe is a web that has no weaver.

Kaptchuk gives the example of six patients with stomach pain. The Western physician would order upper-GI x-rays or endoscopy using a fiber-optic scope, and might diagnose all six patients as having peptic ulcers. Because they all have the same disease, they would all be given the same treatment.

The traditional Chinese physician might examine the first patient and find that pain increases at touch (by palpations) but diminishes with the application of cold compresses. He has a robust constitution, reddish complexion, and a full, deep voice. He seems assertive and aggressive. He is constipated and has dark yellow urine. His tongue has a greasy yellow coating. His pulse is "full" and "wiry." The diagnosis: Damp Heat affecting the Spleen. He might observe the second patient to be thin, with an ashen complexion and ruddy cheeks. She reports that she is constantly thirsty, and has sweaty palms. She has a tendency toward constipation, insomnia, and night sweats. She appears to be nervous and fidgety. Her tongue is dry and slightly red. This patient may be diagnosed with Deficient Yin affecting the Stomach. The third patient, with different signs and symptoms, might be diagnosed with Exhausted Fire of the Middle Burner, sometimes called Deficient Cold affecting the Spleen. All six patients would be given different treatments, according to their pattern of disharmony.

The bottom line is that Western medicine is concerned with the dis-ease agents, which it tries to change, control, or destroy. Traditional Chinese medicine looks for patterns of disharmony that it tries to return to a state of balance. It's as though the Chinese are looking at the entire tree, while Western medicine is focusing on an insect on one of the leaves of the tree. Both approaches have value; they are different and reflect alternate worldviews. Some say that biomedicine excels with more acute problems, TCM with chronic problems. They can often be used as adjuncts, for example, using Chinese medicine to treat the side effects of chemotherapy—as long as both practitioners are aware of what the other is doing.

Hispanic Folk Medicine

One important aspect of Hispanic folk medicine is based on the theory of hot/cold body balance, as discussed in earlier chapters. Food, ill-nesses, and emotions are all thought to have the quality of being hot, cold, or neutral. What is considered hot and what is cold can vary from culture to culture, however. Often, diseases associated with vasoconstric-tion and low metabolic rates are considered "cold," while those associ-ated with vasodilation and a high metabolic rate are considered "hot." Hot conditions include pregnancy, hypertension, diabetes, and acid indigestion. Cold conditions include menstrual cramps, pneumonia, and colic. To prevent illness, one should avoid extremes in diet and emotion. To treat illness, food or medicines with opposite qualities are used. It should be noted that this system is thought to derive from the Chinese system of body balance.

Traditional Remedies

279

Although it's not clear whether the following example is based on hot and cold theory, it reflects the importance of food in the treatment process. It also serves as a good example of cultural competence. Andrew, an RN, said that the majority of his Hispanic patients use herbal treatments. The one he hears about most frequently is *nopales* (cactus). He shared the example of Mrs. Gutierrez, a diabetic patient. She told Andrew that eating *nopales* would lower her blood sugar, and pointed to the evidence in her lowered blood sugar measurements. Andrew, curi-ous to learn more, interviewed Mrs. Gutierrez. He learned that when she eats *nopales* with eggs at breakfast, she eats fewer tortillas. *Nopales* is a non-starchy vegetable that is also high in fiber. This causes her to get full more quickly, and thus eat fewer tortillas. Substituting fiber for starch is good for her diabetic condition, so Andrew congratulated her on increasing the fiber in her diet and for eating more vegetables.

Rather than challenge her interpretation, he encouraged her to eat *nopales* and other non-starchy vegetables. In this way, he was able to incorporate traditional diet into a culturally appropriate dietary plan for diabetes. Interestingly, a scientific study (Bacard-Gascon 2007) found that adding *nopales* to the traditional Mexican breakfast results in a reduction of glucose concentration in diabetics.

Luz Castillo, a thirty-five-year-old recent immigrant from Mexico, was in the hospital recovering from a repeat caesarean section. She was upset because the staff would not allow her to give her newborn *manzanilla* (chamomile tea) to treat his colic. She was afraid that without it, her infant would suffer. According to a pediatrician I consulted, the only danger would be if parents used too much in place of higher-calorie breast milk or formula so that the baby didn't get enough calories. Allowing Mrs. Castillo to give the baby the tea, while cautioning her not to give too much, would have been a much more culturally competent approach.

Manzanilla tea is commonly used to treat other ailments, including indigestion, cramps, and stomach problems. Arturo Romero, a Mexican patient in his fifties, was hospitalized with a stomach problem. He wanted to take *manzanilla* tea to help treat it. When his nurse saw what he was drinking, however, she immediately took it away from him and told him not to take *anything* the doctor had not ordered. Although I'm sure the nurse was trying to protect Mr. Romero's health, given the large number of Mexicans in the United States and the prevalence of the use of herbal teas, it would be helpful for health care providers to learn something about the more commonly used herbs.

Folk Diseases

A number of folk diseases are recognized in the Hispanic culture. Folk diseases, also known as culture-bound syndromes, are a constellation of symptoms recognized as a disease in one culture but not in others. Some Hispanic folk diseases are of natural origin, others are of supernatural origin. Some of the more common "natural" folk diseases include *caída de mollera* (fallen fontanelle) and *empacho* (blocked intestine). *Caída de mollera* would generally be diagnosed as dehydration. It is commonly thought to be caused by the child falling or being dropped or bounced, or by pulling the nipple out of the child's mouth too vigorously. Symptoms include colic, listlessness, inability to suck, loss of appetite, vomiting, diarrhea, and fever. Traditional treatments include pushing the palate back in place by pushing on the upper palate; holding the child upside down over a pan of water; and applying a poultice, usually of fresh soap shavings, to the depression.

282   Alicia, a Mexican American student, shared that when she was a sixteen-year-old mother, her infant would not stop crying one night. His soft spot was sunken, and he would not eat. She went to see her sister Graciela, who was ten years older, had three children, and had grown up in Mexico. Graciela took Alicia's baby and massaged his upper palate, abdomen, and back. Alicia was a bit disconcerted to see Graciela then swing her baby upside down. She wanted to tell her to stop, but she didn't want to hurt Graciela's feelings. She was surprised to see that her infant soon began to nurse and then fall asleep for the entire night.

Symptoms of *empacho* include indigestion/upset stomach, constipation, diarrhea, dizziness, nightmares, and migraine headaches. The treatment involves rubbing the stomach or pinching the back to dislodge the bolus of food. A purgative or tea may also be given. Physicians should note that *azarcón* or *greta* might be given to children suffering from *empacho*. These can be dangerous, because they contain lead and mercury oxides. Physicians should be sure to ask about them in a nonjudgmental manner, and calmly explain the dangers if being taken.

Common "supernatural illnesses" include *mal de ojo* (evil eye) and *susto* (fright/shock). *Mal de ojo*, as discussed earlier in this chapter, is caused by admiration or jealousy of a person with "strong eyes." It most commonly affects infants. Touching a child while complimenting him prevents giving the evil eye. Symptoms include a sudden reversal in the physical or emotional well-being of an infant, vomiting, fever, crying, restlessness, or nervousness. Treatment consists of a *limpia*, or cleansing, by sweeping the body with a raw egg to extract the "heat."

283   Sue Ramis, a home health nurse, received an angry call from Juanita Garcia, a Mexican American woman whose house she had visited the day before. As Sue was leaving, she innocently remarked that Mrs. Garcia's child was adorable. The next morning, the infant was crying and feverish. When Mrs. Garcia recalled Sue's compliment and the fact that she had not touched the child, she concluded that Sue had given him the evil eye. Being Anglo, Sue had no knowledge of the evil eye. She was innocent, except in the mind of Mrs. Garcia.

Susto is also known as "soul loss." It is caused by a traumatic experience, which can be major (e.g., witnessing a death) or minor (e.g., being startled). Symptoms include malaise, fever, insomnia, irritability, nightmares, depression, and anxiety, and can occur anytime from immediately after the fright or up to months later. The treatment, done by a *curandero*, involves a *limpia*, or "cleansing," and prayers.

284   Rowena first encountered *susto* several years earlier. She was treating Concepcíon Montes, a Hispanic patient who had been diagnosed with Bell's palsy. A few days before the paralysis occurred, Mrs. Montes had suffered a great emotional shock and she was convinced that the shock

had brought on her symptoms. Rowena spent a great deal of time trying to convince Mrs. Montes that the symptoms were *not* caused by *susto*, but were more likely a viral infection or immune disorder. Now, after taking a course in cultural diversity, Rowena realized that her approach might not have been the best one. She said that if this were to happen now, she would probably concede that the shock the patient had suffered (the *susto*) had weakened her immunity and made her more susceptible to the illness. This is a much more culturally sensitive solution, and is likely to increase the patient's faith in the caregiver.

Trust is a key factor in health care, because a lack of trust can lead to lack of adherence and poorer outcomes. Cultural sensitivity generally results in greater trust, which is why I've emphasized the importance of respecting the patients' beliefs, even if they conflict with your own and that of biomedicine. For an example of why this is so important, see the next case study.

Silvia Evangelista came to the United States from Mexico when she was twelve years old. Now in her fifties, she was going over her past medical history with her new physician, Dr. Miles. She mentioned that she had had an emergency caesarean section years earlier. When Dr. Miles asked why she needed it, she explained that she had experienced *susto*, and her family had rushed her to the hospital. When she arrived there, she was so sick from the *susto* that she was immediately taken into surgery. Dr. Miles told Mrs. Evangelista that the scenario she had just described did not make any sense, and that it was medically impossible to believe her. Furthermore, he said, there was no such thing as *susto*. Mrs. Evangelista said she felt "dumb and belittled" by him, and refused to answer any more questions. It was the last time she saw Dr. Miles. It might have been the last time she saw *any* physician.

285

Traditional Healers

There are a number of traditional Hispanic healers. They include *curandero/as*, *parteras*, *sobadoro/as*, and *yerbero/as*. A *curandero/a* uses diet, herbs, massage, and rituals to treat illnesses. A *partera* is a midwife. A *sobador/a* is a folk "chiropractor" who treats the patient by manipulating bones and muscles. A *yerbero/a* is an herbalist who treats both natural and supernatural ailments.

Taryn was working in the emergency department when Mr. and Mrs. De Canul, a young couple recently emigrated from Mexico, brought in their one-year-old son. Mrs. De Canul had accidentally slammed the door on the baby's right index finger. The father was concerned over whether Antonio would suffer from *susto*. Fortunately, Taryn was taking a class on cultural diversity and knew that *susto* was commonly treated by a *curandero*. She told the parents that they should not worry about it,

286

but if it would make them feel better, they could take Antonio to see a *curandero*. They thanked Taryn profusely and told her that in the past, other nurses had told them they were crazy for taking their children to a *curandero*. By acting in a culturally competent manner, Taryn was able to build rapport with this family. If they had been in a more long-term setting, such trust would likely have led to increased adherence and better patient outcomes.

It is important, however, to remember not to stereotype patients. Just because someone is Hispanic does not mean they will utilize traditional healers. As one nurse shared, she often asks the family if they would like to have a *curandero* visit the patient. Often they tell her, "That was only in the old country." Others inform her that they already consulted one before coming to the hospital. Use such information to generalize, not to stereotype. Keep in mind the possibilities for any particular ethnic group, and then see whether they apply to the individual in question. In the above case, the fact that the family were concerned about *susto* and had recently immigrated from Mexico made it more likely that they used traditional healers, but should never be assumed to be the case.

A word of warning. Health care providers should be aware that in Mexico it is common for pharmacists to prescribe drugs, and thus many patients are used to buying drugs from storefront *botánicas*. Unfortunately, there are a lot of unscrupulous fraudulent doctors and pharmacists selling drugs that may not be up to Federal Drug Administration (FDA) standards. Dosages may vary considerably, and there may be a problem with counterfeit drugs. However, these drugs are often cheaper than reputable pharmaceuticals, which contributes to their appeal. It's therefore extremely important that you make your patients feel comfortable enough to share information about all the medications they are taking.

Traditional African American Health Beliefs and Practices

Loudell Snow (1983) writes about traditional health beliefs and practices among lower socioeconomic class African Americans in the South. She found that illnesses were classified as either "natural" (based on how God intends the world to be) or "unnatural" (the work of the Devil). Physicians can cure only natural illnesses. Illness is generally seen as an attack by outside forces, which can be cured by the proper remedy, right physician, or more powerful healers. God can cure anything, if the patient's faith is strong enough.

287   As you may recall from case study #5, Emma Chapman was a sixty-two-year-old African American woman admitted to the coronary care unit because she had continued episodes of acute chest pain after two

heart attacks. Her physician recommended an angiogram with a possible cardiac bypass or angioplasty to follow. Mrs. Chapman refused, saying, "If my faith is strong enough and if it is meant to be, God will cure me."

When Judy, her nurse, asked her what she thought had caused the problem, she said she had sinned and her illness was a punishment. According to her beliefs, illnesses from "natural causes" can be treated through nature (e.g., herbal remedies), but diseases caused by "sin" can be cured only through God's intervention. Remember, treatment must be appropriate to the cause. In addition, Mrs. Chapman may have felt that to accept medical treatment would be perceived by God as a lack of faith.

Mrs. Chapman finally agreed to the surgery after speaking with her minister, whom Judy called to the hospital. Another approach would have been to talk with Mrs. Chapman about her faith, emphasizing that God works through doctors and nurses as well as the patient directly. Utilizing the patient's belief system generally leads to better communication. In this case, medicine could not offer Mrs. Chapman a certain cure; it offered only the possibility of symptom relief and life extension. Someone could have suggested that if she prayed and had enough faith, God would see to it that the operations were successful. She might also have been told the following story:

A huge flood came and destroyed a tiny village. Almost everyone managed to escape in time except for one very religious man who believed that God would save him. He climbed onto his roof to wait. Soon a rescue boat came to help him, but he turned it away, saying, "God will save me." The next day, a second boat came, but again he refused to leave. He said, "My faith in God is strong; He will save me." On the third day, a helicopter flew by to rescue him, and again he turned it away. "God will save me." On the fourth day, the waters rose above his roof and he drowned. When he reached heaven, he demanded to see God. "Why didn't you save me?" he asked. "You've never had a more faithful or loyal servant than I." God responded, "What do you mean? I did try to save you. I sent two boats and a helicopter."

In her research, Snow found that diet and emotional shock were believed to cause two conditions in the blood: high blood and low blood. High blood would indicate too much blood, low blood not enough. Eating too many rich foods was associated with high blood, and not enough red meat with low blood. Treatment generally involved diet and home remedies. Clear and white foods, such as lemon juice, pickle juice, and garlic, were thought to lower high blood, while red and rich foods were thought to raise low blood.

Ryan shared the case of Mrs. Washington, an older African American patient who had presented with two to three days of nausea and vomiting. She had been diagnosed six years earlier with high blood pressure, 288 but had not been taking any medication to treat it. When Ryan explained why it was important to both keep her blood pressure in the normal range and to see her physician periodically to help monitor her blood pressure, she revealed that she had been drinking vinegar to lower her blood pressure (in her mind, she had high blood). It turned out that the vinegar consumption has caused the gastrointestinal symptoms.

Summary

Most medical personnel believe that Western scientific medicine is superior to all other medical systems. In many cases, this may be true. It is important to remember, however, that medical practitioners in other cultures have been treating patients with some success for centuries. Several modern drugs, including quinine, were discovered in native "medicine kits." Furthermore, scientific medicine has been notably unsuccessful in curing many ailments, including the common cold.

Even in cases where Western scientific medicine is superior, if the patient believes it is insufficient for treating the problem, it probably will be. The mind has a powerful effect on the body and can influence both illness and health. To treat patients successfully, it is extremely important to consider their beliefs regarding the cause of the disease, how the disease should be treated, what behavior is appropriate when ill, and how the body is to be viewed.

Ideally, medical professionals everywhere will recognize the value of what other systems have to offer. They can then take the best of each and reach the ultimate goal of providing effective health care for all.

Key Points

- If you see unfamiliar markings on a patient's body, ask about them rather than assuming they are a sign of abuse or a medical symptom.
- Be sure to give clear instructions on the use of medications; nonadherence may simply reflect a lack of understanding.
- Many traditional remedies are helpful, and many with no proven scientific benefit are at least not harmful. Allowing your patient to continue to use them will help you gain their trust and increase the chances they will listen to you when you tell them something *is* harmful.

- It is common for individuals to seek out multiple health care practitioners for the same problem without sharing this information with their medical practitioners because they fear offending them, or being ridiculed by them, or because they don't think the information is relevant. It is important to ask respectfully.
- You can say something along the lines of: *Many of my patients also see traditional healers who prescribe herbal remedies, or use home remedies that have been passed down for generations. Often they can be effective, but sometimes they can cause problems, especially when mixed with other treatments. That's why it's important that I know everything that you're taking to treat this or any other problem.* An attitude of respect, rather than derision, is crucial.
- Collaboration between physicians and traditional healers is often in the best interests of the patient.
- Not everyone will adhere to traditional health care practices.
- Respect your patients' beliefs, even if they conflict with your own and that of biomedicine.

For more on pain medications, see Chapter 3.

Chapter 13

Improving Adherence

A common problem referred to throughout this book is lack of adherence. According to the World Health Organization, 50 percent of patients in developed countries with chronic diseases do not adhere to treatment recommendations (WHO 2003). And as Surgeon General C. Everett Koop famously put it, "Drugs don't work in patients who don't take them." As a side note, the WHO prefers the term "adherence" to the more commonly used "compliance." Adherence assumes patient-centered care—that the patient is "sticking to" the treatment plan created with the clinician. Compliance assumes more paternalistic care—that the patient is following the orders of the physician.

Poor adherence leads to both poor health outcomes and higher medical costs. By improving adherence, providers can make a difference both in their patients' health and in their own level of professional satisfaction. This chapter will examine some of the causes of lack of adherence, and suggest solutions. Sometimes the causes are related to cultural issues; sometimes they focus on basic communication and teaching skills.

Lack of Understanding

Sometimes, the patient doesn't understand the instructions. The first step to ensuring understanding is to make sure that the patient has a good command of English; otherwise, a professional interpreter—not a family member—should be used. If the patient is fluent in English, lack of adherence can be due to poor teaching skills on the part of the health care provider or hesitancy on the part of the patients to admit they don't understand. This hesitancy may be due to embarrassment—fear that they will appear "stupid." This is especially common in Asian cultures where self-esteem is a major value, but can—and does—appear in any culture. Or it may be due to respect; the patient may not want to even *imply* that the provider did a poor job of explaining something. A nurse shared that one of her Latina patients confessed that she says *yes* to everything a medical professional tells her because to say *no* would be disrespectful. To deal with that possibility, the provider can normalize *not* understanding by saying something along the lines of, "I know this can be confusing; most of my patients have trouble understanding at first. It will help me enormously if you can tell me what you find most confusing, so I can try to explain it another way."

Insufficient Instruction or Explanation

In many cases, lack of adherence stems from insufficient instruction or explanation.

My mother, an eighty-eight-year-old native born English speaker, had a leg infection that required frequent dressing changes. I was with her when the nurse showed her how to do it. The "teaching" consisted of the nurse changing the dressing on her leg and saying, "This is how you do it." What the nurse *should* have done is demonstrated it once, and then had my mother do it while she watched. She could have then observed any confusion or misunderstandings she had, and corrected them. She might have also asked me to demonstrate it as well, so that I could help my mother if she forgot. At the end, rather than asking, "Do you have any questions?" she might have asked, "What questions do you have?" This implies the assumption that *of course you will have questions*, and this may make people feel more comfortable in asking. Although it may take more time, in the long run, it will save time since it reduces the chances that patients will have to return to the office for more instruction or suffer the consequences of not properly adhering to instructions. After we left, my mother had no clue as to how to change her own dressing.

Bodenheimer, MacGregor, and Sharifi (2005) outlined what I believe is an excellent approach to providing information to patients called "Closing the Loop." Specifically, the provider asks the patient to repeat back the information so that s/he knows that it's clear. Tone of voice is important; you don't want to make the patient feel like a child. But making sure the patient understands is a crucial step in patient adherence. Jesus Garcia, the patient in case study #76, would not have taken an overdose of pain medication had someone gone over the instructions with him.

Spending a little time up front can also save the clinician a lot more time in the end, as was evident in case study #33, where the physician had to deal with calls from confused family members and needed to

289

schedule a family conference in order to explain the patient's condition. Had he made sure the patient understood the situation when he originally spoke with her, he could have avoided the phone calls and conference.

Unclear Rationale

Sometimes patients fail to adhere because the reason for the instructions is unclear.

290   Angie Morrison, a highly educated, Anglo American woman in her thirties, made an appointment for an ultrasound to look for uterine fibroids. At the time she called the clinic to make the appointment, the receptionist told her to drink four to five glasses of water right before coming in. What she neglected to tell Angie was that the reason for drinking the water was to expand her bladder and thus move it out of the way so that the technician could see her uterus. Angie's appointment was in the late morning. Before her appointment, she followed her usual routine of going to the gym and working out. She then drank the water as instructed, and went to the imaging center. When the technician tried to do the ultrasound, he couldn't see her uterus; her bladder was in the way. The water she had drunk merely replaced the fluids lost during her workout. Angie ended up having to drink several more glasses of water, causing her to have to urinate every few minutes. In the end, the technician had to use an internal probe, making the procedure more uncomfortable and something he had hoped to avoid. All this could have been avoided if the receptionist had added a one sentence explanation of *why* she was to drink several glasses of water before coming in. Angie would have gone to the gym *after* her ultrasound, rather than before. The problem was created not by a language problem or an unwillingness to follow instructions, but simply by a lack of explanation. There will be times when a health care provider may instruct a patient to do something unpleasant or that conflicts with the way s/he normally does things. Explaining the reason for the instructions will go a long way toward insuring adherence.

Recall case study #74 of the woman from India who stopped taking her pain medication as prescribed following knee replacement surgery. This resulted in increased pain which kept her from doing the rehabilitation exercises necessary for recovery. Had the physician explained *why* it was necessary to take pain medication—and addressed her and her son's concerns about addiction—she would have been more adherent.

Similarly, one of the most common cases of "noncompliance" involves taking medications only when symptoms are present.

An Anglo American nurse named John was caring for an older African   291
American patient named Robert Williams. Mr. Williams had been admitted for congestive heart failure. Apparently, he had not been taking
several of the medications his doctor had prescribed. When John asked
why, he explained that he only took his "breathing pill" (digoxin) when
he became short of breath. He did not see why he had to take it every
day, even when he had no symptoms. It is important that health care
providers explain the reason for taking each medication, particularly
those that have a preventive function. Specifically addressing the reason
why the medication should be taken even in the *absence* of symptoms is
crucial, particularly when the patient has a present time orientation.

Conflict with Cultural or Religious Beliefs or Practices

Sometimes patients do not comply because the recommendation conflicts with cultural or religious beliefs or practices, or is impractical given
the patient's life circumstances. Recall case study #124, in which the
Arab student refused to change his colostomy bag. His "noncompliance" was not due to an unwillingness to change the bag, but the fact
that it required him to use *both* hands, and he was forbidden by his
culture to "dirty" his right hand (the one meant to be used for eating)
in that way. Also remember case study #111, in which a Filipina patient
refused to eat during the day and would not take her medications at the
assigned time. It turned out her "noncompliance" was adherence to
the rules of her Muslim faith during Ramadan. Adherence to religious
dictates can sometimes have major consequences, as in the case below.

Aarash Sahar, the sixty-year-old Muslim man from Afghanistan pro-   292
filed in the documentary film *Worlds Apart: Mohammad Kochi's Story*
(2005), had stomach cancer. Following surgery, his oncologist, Dr. Jeffries, recommended chemotherapy. The oncologist assured him that
treatment would be simple; they would insert a catheter into his arm
and then a small pump would drip the chemotherapy into his body 24
hours a day. Mr. Sahar told Dr. Jeffries that he didn't want chemotherapy; pills or shots would be fine, but no pump. Furthermore, he said he
believed the day of his death had already been chosen and could not be
changed. At each visit, his physician recommended chemotherapy, and
each time he refused, saying, "No pump." Several months later, he was
losing weight and experiencing discomfort. Scans showed that the cancer had spread. Mr. Sahar's adult daughter came to see Dr. Jeffries. She
was angry and upset that her father hadn't received chemotherapy. The
oncologist shared the conversation he had had with her father. The
daughter suddenly understood what had happened. Her father had *of*

course refused chemotherapy because it had been offered as a continuous infusion. Muslims must be clean in order to pray. If something is being continuously injected into his body, he is considered unclean and thus unable to pray. If Dr. Jeffries had used the 4 C's and asked what *concerned* Mr. Sahar about "the pump," he would probably have offered other alternatives. But he didn't, nor did Mr. Sahar offer an explanation, and thus the recommendation of chemotherapy went unheeded. Had Mr. Sahar begun chemotherapy after his partial gastrectomy, he might have lived longer. It's unclear how his fatalistic attitude toward the day of his death might have figured in.

293   Carmen was instructing Raul Gallegos, a Latino man in his fifties, how to perform intermittent catheterization—inserting a catheter to empty the bladder, and then removing it. After he demonstrated his ability to do so in the clinic, she felt confident he would be able to do it at home so she discharged him. Two days later, Mr. Gallegos returned to the clinic confused and upset. "Esta cosa no sirve!" (This thing doesn't work!) Carmen took him into an exam room and asked him to show her what wasn't working. As he undressed, she noticed the catheter coming from his perineal area and taped to his leg. This was *not* how it was intended to be used. He responded that since he had to work, he thought it would be easier to leave it in. As a result, he had been urinating all over his pant leg. Under the circumstances, Mr. Gallegos might have been better off with a leg bag. The nurse should have discussed all the alternatives with him to figure out which would be most appropriate given his lifestyle.

Regarding the point about making sure the instructions are practical given the patient's life circumstances, I'll never forget an article I read while preparing for my doctoral exams. Unfortunately, I no longer remember the author or any of the details, but I do remember the lesson. Some public health workers were in a small village somewhere in a mountainous region of Latin America. They concluded that many of the villagers' health problems could be avoided if they simply boiled their water. A simple solution, right? Wrong. It turns out that in order to obtain the wood to make the fire, they would have to walk several miles, and carry it back the same distance. This would consume many hours of their day, and they were already spending several hours collecting wood for cooking. Their "stoves" had room for only one pot; therefore, they would have to choose between boiling water and cooking food. A health recommendation that seemed so simple—boil your water—was actually incredibly impractical given their life circumstances.

An obvious aspect of life circumstances is financial. Sometimes patients don't take their medication because they simply can't afford it, but are embarrassed to say so. My grandfather used to take his blood pressure medication every *other* day to save money. Ideally, physicians will acquaint themselves with the cost of the drugs they recommend, and come up with alternatives if they are expensive. At the same time, they need to explain *why* the medications need to be taken on the schedule in which they are prescribed.

Belief in a Different Disease Paradigm

As discussed in Chapter 1, there are a number of different disease paradigms. Medical recommendations assume a belief in the biomedical model of disease, something all patients may not share. Recall case study #278 about the Korean man admitted for depression who refused to take his medications. The problem was he had been given water or juice to take his pills, and this violated hot/cold principles. When they gave him hot tea, he took his medication. He believed in the holistic model of disease, and wouldn't adhere to recommendations that violated the paradigm of body balance. Adjusting the treatment so it fit the model made all the difference.

Another good example of this explanation for lack of adherence is case study #287 in which an African American woman believed her chest pains were due to punishment by God for sins she had committed in the past. The culturally competent approach taken by her nurse used her belief in the magico-religious model of disease and brought in a member of the clergy to talk with her.

Mrs. Minh Tran, a fifty-six-year-old Vietnamese woman, wasn't taking her diabetes medication because she believed that, like all Western medicine, it was "too hot" (yang). She clearly believed in the holistic model of disease. When the doctor asked her if there was anything she could take it with to cool it down, Mrs. Tran thought a minute, and said she had a tea that was yin (cold). The doctor then suggested she take her medication with the yin tea and she agreed. It was a simple compromise by a physician who was willing to work within the patient's disease paradigm while still following the biomedical model.

294

Knowledge of Someone Who Had a Bad Outcome

Sometimes patients are nonadherent because a friend or relative who did what the provider is recommending had a bad outcome. Recall the case of Mr. Valdez (case study #9). He refused to take insulin because both his mother and uncle went blind after taking the drug. He assumed that the insulin caused the blindness, a not illogical assumption. It is always a good idea to ask your patient whether they know anyone else who has taken this medication or had the procedure and what was their experience with it.

Lack of Trust

Sometimes the patient doesn't trust the health care provider. This can be due to many factors. Older African Americans, for example, may carry the knowledge of the Tuskegee experiment (see Chapter 1), or having experienced prejudice and discrimination, not trust a white physician or "white" institution.

295   Mr. Harris, a sixty-eight-year-old African American man, was scheduled to have his cancerous prostate removed at a government hospital. Two days after scheduling the procedure, he called Karen, his nurse, in a panic. He had spoken to several friends about his upcoming surgery and now wanted to know about various forms of alternative treatments. Karen spent about an hour on the phone with him and gave him a great deal of information as well as phone numbers he could call to learn about other options. She realized that he was probably overwhelmed and frightened about his diagnosis.

Right before hanging up, Mr. Harris said, "You know I trust *you*, Karen; I just don't know if I trust the hospital to take care of me. I have older friends who were subjected to government studies without knowing it back in the '40s and '50s." Karen suddenly realized it wasn't just the cancer he feared, but what a white institution might do to him, an African American man. The Tuskegee experiments done with syphilitic black men who were left untreated in order to study the course of the disease are infamous.

Sometimes it's not that patients specifically distrust the physician, but that they place greater trust in people they know—or feel they know—personally. In the past several years, there has been much concern about a connection between childhood vaccines and autism. Although numerous scientific studies have proved that there is *no* relationship between the two, many parents still refuse to vaccinate their children. Their refusal generally stems from the trust they place in their friends and some celebrities who say that vaccines cause autism, over the word of their physician.

Lack of trust can also derive from the clinician having a different personal style than what is expected. If they expect a physician who is warm and friendly and cares about the patient's personal life—someone with *personalismo*—and instead they are they are treated by one who is impersonal and "professional," they may not have as much trust in that provider as they would otherwise. Recall case study #30, of the middle-aged

Hispanic woman who left her physician for a *curandero* because the physician didn't greet her or seem to care about her as an individual. Contrast this with case study #31, where a different middle-aged Mexican woman with diabetes and renal failure became much more adherent to diet and fluid restrictions when her nurse demonstrated a personal interest in her.

Dealing with trust issues can be difficult. There are many ways to gain a patient's trust. Show that you care about the individual. It can often be helpful to show some interest in a patient's culture. There are numerous books, websites, and courses on culture that can provide you with a starting point. Sometimes just listening to a patient can improve trust. Be open to your patient's beliefs and practices. Be willing to compromise, as did the physician in case study #294.

Present Time Orientation

As discussed in Chapter 2, another cause of lack of adherence, particularly with preventive medicine, can be a present time orientation. Extra time spent on patient teaching and tying adherence to something they value, such as holding a grandchild, can often help improve adherence.

Summary

Lack of adherence, a common cause of poor health outcomes and higher health costs, can result from a number of factors. Sometimes the patient doesn't understand the instructions, but is too embarrassed or respectful of the health care provider to say so. Other times the provider has given insufficient instruction or explanation to ensure understanding; asking if patients "have any questions" isn't enough. Or the underlying reason for the recommendation may be unclear. The recommendation may conflict with cultural or religious beliefs or is impractical given the patient's life circumstances. Sometimes the patient has a friend or relative who did what the provider is recommending and had a bad outcome. Commonly the patient doesn't have enough trust in the health care provider to follow his or her recommendations. Many of these barriers to adherence can be overcome by following the key points listed below.

Key Points

- Make sure your patients understand your instructions by having them demonstrate and explain them to you.

Chapter 14

Making a Difference

In addition to looking at the ways in which cultural differences can lead to conflict and misunderstanding, this book has emphasized the things clinicians can do to provide more culturally sensitive care for their patients. Individual doctors and nurses can make a big difference, as will be demonstrated, but for cultural competence to become an integral part of health care, hospitals and clinics must make changes as well. I'm delighted to report that many already are. In this chapter, I want to focus on some of the things various hospitals and clinics are doing to provide more culturally sensitive care, as well as things they *could* be doing. It is my hope that health care facilities around the country will be inspired to adopt some of these changes and come up with more of their own. Making such changes may cost money in the short term, but in the long run, it should save money by reducing errors, increasing adherence, improving patient health, and building good will (which, incidentally, can result in fewer lawsuits). Hospitals that earn a reputation for providing more culturally appropriate care will also attract a larger client base. Hospitals have the opportunity to do well by doing good.

In my nursing class on cultural diversity, I assigned the students to interview at least three patients and/or family members of a single ethnic group and to find out what the hospital could do to provide more culturally appropriate care. I also challenged them to make those changes by involving the appropriate departments or administrators. I'm pleased to say that many of them did. You will read about some of the success stories here. The assignment also had an unexpected benefit. Hearing something from a patient/family member made a much stronger impact on the nurses than did hearing it from me. I recall one class in particular in which we had had a long discussion about being more flexible in allowing visitors. The majority of the class were opposed to the idea, citing how much more difficult it would make their job to have family members underfoot. Several weeks later, after the students completed their assignment, the topic arose again. This time, they were overwhelmingly in favor of expanding visiting hours and allowing more visitors, since this was the one point that came up over and over again in their interviews. Hearing their patients and family members talk about the importance of family made a much greater impression on them than hearing me talk about it. The broader lesson to be taken from this is the importance of patient-centered care. Talk (listen) to your patients. Get *their* perspective. Use the 4 C's . . . and any other questions that will help you better understand them. Satisfied patients are easier patients, which will make *your* job a whole lot easier. One nurse shared that she received a letter of appreciation from the daughter of a patient she interviewed. The daughter thanked her for taking the time to get to know her mother. The nurse added, "That not only made me feel good, but it was a big plus on my employee profile." Win-win.

Of course, not every nurse is going to feel that way. Rebecca observed that her new attention to cultural care has brought comments from other staff members on her unit. They've told her she's spending too much time concerning herself with cultural needs, and it's a luxury to offer "special" care to these patients. Rebecca points out to them that they would benefit from and expect the same care if they were hospitalized in another country. Yes, *all* patients should be treated this way.

Language

As discussed in Chapter 2, CLAS standards instituted in 2001 require language access services in all federally funded health care facilities. Thus, patients are to be provided access to live or remote interpreter services 24 hours a day, seven days a week. One hospital in the Midwest has a Refugee Health and Interpreter Services department and its own on-site full-time interpreters. This is the ideal situation, but, unfortunately, it is not always feasible. Having bilingual staff can help as well, although it is important that such staff receive training to be competent interpreters. They should also be remunerated for doing double duty because it can stress a work load that is already often filled to capacity. A list of staff who can provide interpretation services when professional interpreters are unavailable should be posted on every unit.

All hospitals should have signs and forms in multiple languages reflecting the populations served. Facilities that want to show they truly value the populations they serve can also provide television channels in multiple languages. For example, one hospital in a predominantly Chinese neighborhood has a 24-hour Chinese language news channel in patient rooms. Another hospital, which serves a Russian community, provides magazines and literature in Russian. Most of the Russian-language magazines are donated. Even if they are slightly out of date, patients and family members appreciate them. Hospitals can post signs in family waiting rooms, requesting donations of magazines in various languages.

Diet

Hospital food is infamous for being bad, but it doesn't have to be that way. Some hospitals have begun buying food from local farmers, which means fresher, healthier food, often at lower cost. Others shop at Asian and Hispanic markets to get food for their Asian and Hispanic patients. Many hospitals have added ethnic foods to their menu. For example, a hospital in an area with a large Chinese population now serves *jook*, an easily digested rice porridge. Another hospital, also in a Chinese neighborhood, serves Asian-style porridges and stews, buying ingredients from a nearby Hong Kong market. Chopsticks are included with meals. A hospital with a predominantly Mexican immigrant population has menus printed in Spanish and English and offers pork chile verde, enchiladas, and burritos. Another hospital has menu selections for Russian, Jewish, Italian, and Hispanic foods, since they serve those populations. Dietitians download culturally specific recipes and incorporate them into the menu.

A hospital in Brooklyn, New York, has done much to incorporate cultural competence into its meal service. They include food items that their Hispanic, Chinese, Russian, and Arabic patients prefer when they are ill, such as rice porridge for Chinese patients. The menus, translated into different languages and accompanied by pictures, are available on each patient's television. For religious Jews and Muslims, kosher and halal meals are available.

As discussed in Chapter 9 on Birth, many cultures have dietary prescriptions and prohibitions following delivery. Dietitians at some hospitals are making sure warm teas are available for new mothers as an alternative to ice water. Other hospitals offer traditional foods such as *miyeok-guk*, a Korean seaweed soup rich in iron and protein and traditionally served to women after giving birth. Many hospitals are being more flexible about allowing family members to bring in food for their patients. Ideally, patient rooms would have a small refrigerator and microwave to accommodate that, along with culturally appropriate utensils, such as chopsticks.

Tamara worked as a nurse at a very small hospital serving, among others, an Afghani population. While interviewing several Afghani

296

patients and family members for a class project, she learned that due to the restrictions of their Muslim religion, they do not eat pork. She also discovered that their concern for getting a possibly "contaminated" item is so strong that they will usually request a vegetarian meal. Family members expressed concern that patients might not be getting enough nutrients. So Tamara arranged a meeting with the director of food services to discuss their concerns. The director had no idea it was an issue. When they examined the menu items for the vegetarian tray, they discovered that only ten food items were used, so often the same items would be served for both lunch and dinner, day after day. This led to another meeting with a nutritionist, and a committee was formed to see how they could better serve both their Afghani patients and any vegetarian patients. These meetings have had several positive outcomes. They have enlarged their menu, and have looked into allowing family prepared meals, since nutritional status can be better maintained when the patient eats meals he or she prefers. A nutritionist is now on call to meet with the family and help them provide a balanced menu should they want to bring in meals from home, taking into account the patient's illness, baseline nutritional status, and ability to eat. A physician's order is required, but most, if not all the physicians have been quite positive about this change.

Respecting Cultural and Religious Beliefs and Practices

An excellent way to demonstrate a commitment to serving culturally diverse populations in a sensitive manner is to provide amenities that respect cultural and religious beliefs and practices. However, before a facility can attend to a patient's spiritual, religious, and cultural needs, it has to learn what they are.

Intake Questionnaire

297   Pedro was a member of the Policy and Procedure Committee at the hospital where he worked as a nurse. Part of his job was to research and review policies and update protocols on nursing procedures. Based on what he learned in his cultural diversity class, he proposed additional questions to be added to the hospital's medical history questionnaire. At the time, the only questions relevant to the patient's spiritual, religious, or cultural needs were whether they wanted a pastoral or social worker consult. He added the question, "Are there any religious, spiritual or cultural practices you would like to observe while in the hospital?" Pedro was also working on developing questions to address the needs of the gay, lesbian, bisexual, and transgender communities that would help patients feel open enough to honestly share pertinent information. A hospital in Portland, Oregon, has made significant strides in that area, as will be discussed later.

Modesty

As discussed in earlier chapters, modesty—especially for women—is very important in many cultures. The typical hospital gown, which is quite revealing with the open ties in the back, can create a great deal of discomfort for modest patients. One hospital found that many of their female Muslim patients were either canceling or not showing up for their appointments as a result. In response, they designed a new two-piece gown that covers the legs, back, and arms. It buttons up the side, rather than tie in the back, for greater modesty. The gowns are available to patients on request; it's important, however, to let patients know this. Signs placed in every patient room announcing the availability of "modest gowns" would be helpful. At least one hospital has instituted a policy that also helps respect patient modesty: "knock, wait, and enter" rather than the usual "just enter" policy.

Numbers

One hospital took an unusual step to demonstrate sensitivity to the beliefs of its Chinese population: changing the main telephone number. The old number, which the hospital had had for several decades, contained the number 4 several times. As discussed in Chapter 10, the character for the number 4 is pronounced the same as the character for "death," and thus has the same negative connotation. The new telephone number has the number 8 three times; 8 represents good luck and wealth.

Keeping Warm

While doing interviews for a class assignment, Roberto discovered that many of his Filipino patients believed that heat loss can lead to illness and that by covering their head they can prevent illnesses caused by cold temperatures and exposure to outside air. He then took the initiative to contact the volunteer services manager. The solution they came up with was to offer knit stocking caps to the patients. Because the hospital was unwilling to take on the expense, the manager contacted several hospital volunteers who knit as a hobby. They were delighted to help out, and volunteered to keep the hospital supplied in brightly colored knit

298

stocking caps at all times. Roberto then printed up a flyer to inform the staff of their availability. The caps are now offered to patients when they are admitted. Not only has they brightened up the unit, but patient and family satisfaction has improved. This excellent example of how one person can make a significant difference in a hospital also serves as a reminder that money needn't necessarily be a deterrent to offering culturally sensitive care. Volunteers can be used to creatively help cut expenses.

Games

In a clever nod to traditional games, a hospital serving a large Chinese population has mah-jongg, a Chinese game using small tiles, in the exercise room. Doctors use the game to work on patients' motor skills.

Postpartum: The Placenta

As discussed in the chapter on birth, women from a number of cultures may want to take home the placenta after they give birth; unfortunately, this conflicts with most hospitals' infection control policies. A hospital serving a large African population worked with the health department and hospital infection control to find a way to make this possible. They are now able to store the placenta in the hospital for the mother until she goes home and can take it with her.

Cultural Bridges

Some hospitals have hired "cultural concierges" or "advocates" or "patient navigators" to provide a bridge between the hospital and the communities it serves. They help educate staff about cultural beliefs and practices, while at the same time helping the communities be less wary of American hospitals. Sometimes they give tours of the hospital to members of the ethnic community to help educate the community. One "cultural ambassador" program for nurses has a representative from each ward of the hospital volunteer for a program that provides quarterly trainings on cultural issues. They then serve as mentors and resources on cultural issues.

In doing research for this chapter, I learned that the notion of concierge services is very popular in medical tourism. However, they often do not serve the needs of the patients in the way I would advocate. The "concierge" is generally an expatriate from the same country who also speaks the language of the country. His or her job is to pick patients up at the airport, get them settled in the hotel, transport them to medical appointments, and interpret. Most are not trained in either cultural competency or medical interpreting. It's a start, but it doesn't go far enough.

Policy for Traditional Healers

A hospital in an area serving a large Hmong population has developed a "shaman policy" that recognizes the important cultural role traditional healers play. The policy includes a list of nine approved ceremonies they can perform, including "soul calling" and chanting in a soft voice. Many of the ceremonies have been modified to avoid disturbing other patients. In order to become part of the hospital program, the shamans go through a seven-week training program to learn about Western medicine. Traditional healers who have been thus certified are given official jackets and badges and have the same unrestricted access to patients as more traditional clergy. It's hoped that the program will help increase the trust between physicians and the Hmong community, and alleviate some of the fears they have about medical treatments.

Prayer and Religious Icons

There is probably no time that prayer is more important than when one is ill. Therefore, providing what is needed to assist in a patient's or family's ability to pray can be essential. A hospital serving a large Muslim population provides prayer rugs in the chapel/meditation room. However, again, it is important that hospital personnel make such amenities known to patients; otherwise, they will go unused. Signs on the walls of patient rooms informing them of the amenities available would be helpful. It is important, however, not to mention specific ethnic or religious groups on the signs, lest other groups feel slighted.

As discussed in the chapter on religion, any religious icons (such as crosses) that are hung on patients' room walls should be able to be easily removed. Space should be made for patients' own religious symbols.

Ideally, each hospital will have a chapel where patients or family members can go for contemplation and prayer, but when that isn't possible, there are inventive solutions, such as Brittany came up with for the Gomez family.

Juan Gomez faced imminent death. The family was Catholic, and Mr. *299* Gomez's granddaughter asked for a place the family could pray. Brittany's first step was to move him to a single room large enough to accommodate his large family. One of the other nurses on the floor went to the hospital gift shop and purchased a small crucifix and picture of Our Lady of Guadalupe. Another bought religious candle holders and battery-operated tea lights from a local market. The family were then able to gather round their beloved father/grandfather and pray for him. Mr. Gomez died peacefully, surrounded by his loved ones. The family were very grateful for what the staff had done, and thanked them profusely for their efforts and compassion. Afterward, the crucifix, picture, and candles were stored in the nurses' lounge for future use.

Brittany then spoke to the house supervisor about turning the small quiet room near the emergency department into a makeshift chapel for families who request a place to pray. The house supervisor agreed, saying she thought it was one of the staff's better ideas.

Visitors

One of the simplest and most effective things hospitals can do to accommodate patients from diverse cultures is to extend visiting hours. They can also provide reclining chairs for visitors to spend the night. Although many nurses may resist having family members underfoot, as described in Chapter 6, there are effective ways to involve family members that will help lighten their load. Of course, without private rooms, this will be problematic, but most newer hospitals are building private rooms, and enterprising nurses can create private rooms when space is available.

300   Elizabeth spoke with several families of patients from Afghanistan as part of a school assignment to find out how to provide more culturally appropriate care. One of the points that came up repeatedly was the desire to have more family members involved in the patient's care. The rules in place at the time in her critical care unit (CCU) allowed only two visitors at a time, no one under age fourteen, and no overnight visitors. Furthermore, those interviewed were concerned that when the nurses were going to provide care to their loved one, family members were asked to leave the room. They didn't understand why they couldn't stay. What was happening that the nurses didn't want them to see? They wanted at least one family member to stay and help with the care. In most cases, the care being provided was not technical care requiring an RN, but nontechnical care such as bathing, oral care, and changing bedsheets. Although sometimes nursing assessments were conducted during these procedures, there was no real reason family members couldn't help out.

Elizabeth decided to look up hospital policy regarding visitation and learned that one reason to limit visitors was to protect the privacy of other patients' information, which could be an issue in an open unit. However, she could find no hospital policy with regard to the family caring for patients. She went to the manager and the director of the unit to ask what problems could arise from allowing family members to stay with patients at night and to help administer care. After some discussion, it was brought to the staff. Most of the nurses hadn't realized that their restrictions were creating a problem for some of their patients and acknowledged that they could involve families more in patient care. They were, however, concerned about having eight critically ill patients plus possibly eight family members at night, since they had a much smaller staff on night shift. Some research was done in the facility to compare outcomes of patients who had family members involved in their care and those who did not. The results showed unequivocally that patients responded better when a trusted family member stayed with them overnight and helped administer care. Family members were able to explain procedures to the patients and the patients could thus rest easier. They generally responded to treatment faster, and hospital stays were reduced by 2.8 days. The hospital administration became involved and a certified nurse assistant (CNA) was hired for the night shift in the CCU to help with family members. This freed up the RNs, because the family and CNA were able to provide much of the nontechnical care. In the end, the hospital was able to reduce costs while increasing patient satisfaction. Win-win.

Flexible Scheduling

As discussed in Chapter 2, many people from developing countries have a present time orientation. That, along with other socioeconomic factors, often results in patients who are late for appointments. The consequence is generally anger and frustration on everyone's part. Practitioners often feel insulted and taken advantage of when patients arrive late for their appointment and yet still expect to be seen. Patients resent being scolded for tardiness and often don't understand the source of the practitioner's hostility. When one of the nurses in my class learned about time orientation, she had an epiphany . . . and suggested and implemented a successful plan at the clinic where she worked.

Rather than have a specific appointment time, patients are given an appointment for either the morning or afternoon of a specific day. Within that time frame, they are to be seen in the order in which they sign in. The morning session is from 8 to 11 A.M. Patients arriving by 11:00 are seen by 12:30. Those arriving after 11:00 are seen in the afternoon session, from 2 to 4 P.M. Since this new policy was instituted, clinic patient satisfaction has increased and practitioner frustration has decreased.

LGBT

A hospital in Portland, Oregon has made a giant commitment to be LGBT affirming, in terms of both patients and staff. Their visitation policy grants same-sex couples the same access as different-sex couples and next-of-kin, as well as giving same-sex parents the same access as different-sex parents for visitation of their minor children. They offer comprehensive reconstructive and cosmetic procedures for transgender patients, and comprehensive fertility services to same-sex couples. In addition, they offer LGBT-specific and sensitive mental health and addiction counseling. All these policies and services are spelled out clearly in waiting room brochures.

The commitment to be LGBT affirming extends to the staff as well. Employees receive transgender inclusive health care benefits; all transgender surgeries, hormone therapies, and sex-reassignment are covered. Guidelines have been developed around employees transitioning at work, and help them navigate the transition, including bathroom access and paperwork for changing identification and gender.

Showing Commitment to Cultural Competence

It is one thing to espouse an interest in cultural competence. It is another to truly support it, as described for the Portland hospital above. Facilities that are serious about providing culturally competent health care to their patients can demonstrate their commitment in several ways.

Educate Staff

The first is to provide education and training in language and culture for the staff. Continuing education courses can be offered on-site. Grand rounds can include topics on cultural issues. Monthly lunchtime discussion of culturally relevant topics can be organized. A bulletin board in the break room can include information about different cultures and health beliefs. If clinical staff members get involved in posting the information, it will increase the learning potential.

Motivate Staff

Clinical staff may need to be motivated to provide culturally competent care. One way to do this is to require that culture-specific nursing interventions be part of nursing care plans. Physician bonus pay can be made contingent on participating in cultural competence training. Clinicians who provide culturally competent care and are specifically mentioned in the cultural competence category of patient satisfaction surveys should be publicly recognized and perhaps given a small award, such as movie tickets. Cultural assessments should be part of the patient intake form. This information should be included on the charge sheet to ensure that it gets passed on from one shift to the next. (Remember that sensitivity in asking such questions is essential, lest people fear you are going to stereotype them.) If cultural competence is made part of the job description and thus part of the yearly evaluation, staff will be much more likely to pay attention to such issues.

At the same time, it's best to motivate clinicians by helping them see the importance of culturally sensitive care. They should be encouraged to share cultural aspects of their cases with their colleagues during rounds or shift report. A "Cultural Questions Box" at the nursing station can be a place to post questions to discuss at staff meetings. Because many of the staff at most hospitals are ethnically diverse, they should be encouraged to share information about their own cultures. A monthly potluck lunch in which staff members bring ethnic foods (remember, Anglo American counts as an ethnicity) and talk about and answer questions about their own cultures can be a fun and tasty way to learn. It might also help ease culturally based tensions among staff.

Make Information Available to Staff

It is important that clinical staff have easy access to resources with cultural information. There are some excellent books and resources available. A copy of *Culture and Clinical Care*, edited by Lipson and Dibble (2005), belongs at every nursing station. Computers can be bookmarked with links to sites that provide information on cultural issues (see my website www.ggalanti.org/resources for a list of recommended websites). Inexpensive pocket guides (such as my *Cultural Sensitivity: A Pocket Guide for Health Care Professionals*) can be provided for staff members. Information on how to contact an interpreter or cultural resource person should be in clear view at every nursing station.

Show Patients Your Commitment to Cultural Competence

Signs and forms should be printed in the languages of the ethnic groups served, as well as in English. Patients should be surveyed and interviewed regarding how well their cultural and religious needs were met. A category regarding culturally competent care could be added to patient satisfaction surveys. And, most important, hospital policies can be modified to accommodate different ethnic and religious groups—for example, regarding visiting hours, dietary practices, and so on.

Summary

There is much that can be done to make hospitals more welcoming to patients from a multiplicity of cultures. It is basically a matter of taking individuals and their families into account. *All* patients, not just those of color. Some of the recommended changes cost money, but most expenses can be recovered in the savings from reduced errors and lawsuits, as well as from increased business once the facility gains a reputation for culturally competent care. Other changes cost little, or can use the skills and resources of volunteers. Providing culturally competent care doesn't have to be difficult. And there is much satisfaction to be gained, on everyone's part.

Key Points and Suggestions for Hospitals

- Train bilingual staff to serve as interpreters; post a list on every unit of staff who can provide interpretation services.
- When using telephonic interpreters, use dual receivers/handsets, or, if unavailable, speaker phones.
- Have signs and forms in multiple languages reflecting the populations served.
- Offer television channels in multiple languages.
- Ask families to donate books and magazines in their language.
- Serve ethnically appropriate foods and utensils.
- When medically appropriate, allow family members to bring food from home and provide facilities for storage and reheating.
- Offer more modest patient gowns to women.
- Make sure any religious icons on the wall can be removed.
- Allow a place for patients to place religious symbols.
- Extend visiting hours and add visitor chairs.
- Survey and interview patients regarding how well their cultural needs were met. Add a category regarding culturally competent care to patient satisfaction surveys.
- Allow for flexible scheduling in clinics.
- Educate staff on cultural competence.
- Provide on-site continuing education on cultural diversity issues.
- Create a bulletin board in the break room with information about different cultures and health beliefs.

- Motivate staff to become culturally competent.
- Make cultural assessments part of the intake form. This information could be included on the charge sheet to help ensure that the information gets passed on from one shift to the next.
- Require culture-specific nursing interventions be part of nursing care plans.
- Make cultural issues a regular topic for discussion at staff meetings.
- Create a "Cultural Questions Box" for nurses to post questions that could be discussed at staff meetings.
- Make cultural competence part of the job description, and thus part of the yearly evaluation.
- Organize potlucks in which each person brings something from his or her own culture, and describes any associated traditions or significance.
- Publicly recognize clinicians who provide culturally competent care. If a nurse's name is specifically mentioned by a patient in the cultural competence category of patient satisfaction surveys, he or she could receive a small reward.
- Have resources easily available for staff to access cultural information.
- Post information at nursing stations on how to contact an interpreter or cultural resource person.

Appendix 1

Cultural Profiles

It is with some trepidation that I have included cultural profiles for a variety of broad culture areas. It is obvious to all that there are tremendous differences within a single family; it would be ludicrous to assume that every member of a culture would think or act identically. Factors such as religion, class, socioeconomic status, age, gender, education, and time in the United States will often affect their beliefs and behaviors as much as their culture. However, some cultural patterns are common enough to warrant mention. They might serve as useful guideposts for health care providers. It is important to remember, however, that they are merely *generalizations*, meant to be used as starting points, not as something to *stereotype* individuals. They might help health care providers understand behavior in those instances when it deviates from the expected in a culturally consistent direction.

The material contained in these profiles is taken from Galanti (2012), *Cultural Sensitivity: A Pocket Guide for Health Care Professionals.*

Cultural Profile: African Americans

Caution: These are broad generalizations and should not be used to stereotype any individuals.

VALUES, WORLD VIEW, AND COMMUNICATION
- African American patients, especially older ones, may not trust hospitals. This is due to a long history of racism and discrimination. Another reason lies with current studies showing racial disparities in health care, as well as the notorious Tuskegee experiment initiated by the U.S. Public Health Service in 1932. In this case, African American males with syphilis were left untreated to observe the course of the disease. Results were observed on autopsy. The hundreds of men who "participated" in the experiment were never informed, but merely told they had "bad blood."

- African Americans may be very sensitive to discrimination, even when it is not intended. For example, do not use the term "gal" to refer to a woman. It has the same connotations as "boy" for an African American male. Address the patient as Mr., Mrs., or Ms., or by professional title and last name. As with all patients, be sure to apologize and explain if a patient is kept waiting. It may be interpreted as a sign of disrespect or discrimination.
- Religion is important to many African Americans. Clergy should be allowed to participate when appropriate. Privacy for prayer is important and quiet time should be allowed for it. Health care practitioners may offer to pray with a patient if all parties are comfortable. It is customary for clergy and acquaintances from the patient's place of worship to visit the sick on Sundays, often directly from church.

TIME ORIENTATION
- Those of lower socioeconomic status may be present-time oriented, which may impede preventive medicine and follow-up care. Explain the need for preventive medication (such as for hypertension) or to finish antibiotics even when symptoms disappear. Explanations may be important. Due to time orientation and/or economic factors, some may delay seeing a physician until symptoms are severe.

PAIN
- Expression of pain varies widely. It is equally acceptable to be expressive or stoic.

FAMILY/GENDER ISSUES
- Family structure may be nuclear, extended, or matriarchal. Close friends or church members may be part of a kin support system and even referred to by terms like "sister" or "brother." Households headed by women are common. In such cases a grandmother or aunt may be the patient's spokesperson. Often, the father or eldest male may take this role.
- Generally, women are considered equal to men. Many women achieve higher socioeconomic status and educational levels than men.

PREGNANCY AND BIRTH
- Prenatal care is common.
- Traditionally, only females attended birth, but this now varies. Today, a male partner often assists the delivery.

END OF LIFE

- The incidence and death rates of some forms of cancer, including prostate and cervical, are particularly high among African Americans. This may in part be due to the fact that lack of trust for the health care system leads to delays in screening.
- May be reluctant to sign DNR for fear that physicians will withhold beneficial treatment. This can be addressed directly by asking, *"Some patients don't like to talk about these issues because they're afraid their doctors may withhold treatment that might be beneficial to them. Is this something that you're concerned about?"*
- Reluctance to remove life support may be due to belief that miracles are always possible. The thought may be that only God knows for sure if a situation is hopeless. Additionally, patients and caregivers may not trust the medical community, again due to historical experiences with racism.
- Some consider it taboo to donate organs or blood except to a family member, for fear it will hasten one's own death.

HEALTH BELIEFS AND PRACTICES

- Beliefs about the cause of disease include biomedical beliefs and divine punishment. If lack of adherence stems from a belief that disease is due to punishment for sin, it may be helpful to involve clergy or to have the patient pray for God to guide the physicians.
- In rural areas of the South, rich foods (red) may be thought to cause "high" blood, which may be confused with high blood pressure among older African Americans. Attempts may be made to treat "high" blood with clear, white foods to "lower" the blood. Since white foods can include things high in sodium, this should be discussed with the patient. "Low" blood is thought to result from too much vinegar, lemon juice, and garlic, and not enough red meat. Be sure to clarify the difference among "low" blood, low blood count, and low blood pressure.
- The African American culture has a rich tradition of herbal remedies. Be sure to discuss the use of home or herbal remedies to prevent potential drug interactions.

Note: Material is drawn from the work of Snow (1973, 1983, 1993) on lower SES African Americans in the rural South, as well as Waters and Locks (2005) and National Cancer Institute Fact Sheet on Cancer Disparities.

Cultural Profile: Anglo Americans

Refers broadly to those of Northern European descent.

Caution: These are broad generalizations and should not be used to stereotype any individuals.

VALUES, WORLD VIEW, AND COMMUNICATION
- Independence is valued, so patients are likely to be receptive to self-care.
- Both direct eye contact and emotional control are expected. However, try to avoid excessive direct eye contact with members of the opposite sex to avoid any hint of sexual impropriety.
- Privacy is important, yet the patient may want/expect nurses to provide psychosocial care.

TIME ORIENTATION
- Lower-income people tend to be present-oriented; middle-and upper-class individuals tend to be future-oriented.

PAIN
- Patients will tend to be stoic although most will want pain medication.

FAMILY/GENDER ISSUES
- Generally, family size is small and "immediate family" generally refers to spouse, siblings, parents, and children. Families are often spread out and patients may have fewer visitors than those of other ethnic groups.
- Among gay and lesbian patients, friends may take on the role of family.
- Husbands and wives usually have equal authority, with either parent making decisions for the child.

PREGNANCY AND BIRTH
- Prenatal care is generally sought.
- The husband or domestic partner, regardless of gender, is usually the preferred labor partner.
- Hospital births are generally preferred, even if an alternative birthing center is used. This may be related to a cultural desire to control events.
- There are no postpartum rituals other than those associated with specific religions.
- Breastfeeding may be practiced for 3 to 6 months or more.

PEDIATRIC
- Some upper-middle-class parents believe there is a link between childhood vaccinations and autism and refuse to get their children vaccinated.

END OF LIFE
- Patients will generally want to know their diagnosis and prognosis.
- Many want "everything done," but hospice is an acceptable alternative, although often hospice is not seriously pursued until the last few days before death.
- Stoicism is valued when someone dies.
- Organ donations and autopsies are usually acceptable, as are cremation or burial unless forbidden by the patient's religion.

HEALTH BELIEFS AND PRACTICES
- A patient may prefer to be left alone when ill.
- Patients generally prefer an aggressive approach to treating illness.
- Biomedicine is preferred, although many may also use complementary and alternative medicine. Be sure to inquire about the use of herbal medications.
- Germs are thought to cause disease and patients expect treatment to destroy germs. Antibiotics are often requested, even for treating viral illnesses. Be sure to explain the difference between treating viral and bacterial conditions. Explain why antibiotics must be finished, even once symptoms subside.
- Middle-class patients commonly use the Internet to obtain information and may want to dictate specific treatment based on what they learn there.

Cultural Profile: Asians

Caution: These are broad generalizations and should not be used to stereotype any individuals. Statements are most applicable to the least acculturated individuals.

VALUES, WORLD VIEW, AND COMMUNICATION
- Harmony and avoidance of conflict are highly valued. For this reason, patients may agree to things on which they have no intention of following through. Similarly, agreement may be offered out of respect. Make sure the reasons for adherence to any directives or recommendations are explained and stressed. Avoid asking questions requiring a "yes" or "no" response. Find a way to have the patient demonstrate an understanding of what you expect.

- Filial piety (respect for and duty to one's parents) is an important value.
- As a sign of respect, patients may avoid direct eye contact. Do not immediately assign other meanings to this.
- Avoid hand gestures in case they are offensive. For example, beckoning with the index finger is insulting to Filipinos and Koreans.
- Giggling at "inappropriate" times usually indicates nervousness or discomfort.
- Make offers several times as patients may refuse at first to be polite.
- Pronouns do not exist in most Asian languages so patients may confuse "he" and "she."

Time Orientation
- Traditional Chinese patients may be past-oriented, placing a heavy value on tradition. Filipinos may be both past- and present-oriented, and may not always adhere to "clock" time. Japanese may be both past- and future-oriented, and generally adhere to clock time. Many Koreans are future-oriented and adhere to clock time for appointments, but not social events.

Pain
- Stoicism is highly valued. Pain may be expressed only by a clenched jaw. Offer pain medication when the condition warrants it, even if the patient does not request it. When it is medically necessary, explain why and insist on giving it.
- Filipinos may be particularly concerned about addiction to pain medication.

Family/Gender Issues
- Most Asian cultures tend to be hierarchical, with the elderly afforded more respect than younger people, and males more than females. Accept that wives may defer to husbands in decision-making and that sons may be valued more than daughters.
- Allow family members to spend as much time as possible with the patient, as many consider it their familial duty. Involve the family in decision-making when it comes to the patient's care.

Pregnancy and Birth
- Traditionally, the birth partner is the mother-in-law or another female relative.
- Because pregnancy is thought to be a *yang* or "hot" condition in traditional Chinese medicine, birth is believed to deplete the body of heat. Restoration of warmth is important. With this in mind, offer

new mothers liquids other than ice water, which may be deemed too *yin* or "cold." There may be traditional soups or foods the new mother may desire. Offer them, if possible, or allow family members to bring them in. Also respect postpartum prescriptions for rest.
* Traditionally, bathing is avoided for a month after giving birth. If patient is reluctant to shower, offer a sponge bath.
* Parents may avoid naming the baby for up to 30 days. Traditionally, a child is given an unattractive nickname before then so as to avoid attracting the attention of spirits who might want to steal the child.

PEDIATRIC
* A great deal of pressure is often put on children to succeed in school.
* "Mongolian spots" are common and should not be misinterpreted as a bruise. This congenital birthmark, not uncommon in Asian births, usually fades as the infant grows into childhood.

END OF LIFE
* When a patient is diagnosed as terminal, family members may wish to shield him or her from that fact. On admission (or before the need arises, if possible) ask patients to identify how much information they want to be given regarding their condition, or to whom the information should be provided. If the patient requests that all information be given to a family member, be sure to investigate the legal implications of doing so.
* Patients and their families may not want to discuss end-of-life issues in advance. One approach is to ask, *Some (Chinese) families do not like to discuss these issues in advance. Is this something that you feel comfortable discussing with me?*
* Cancer is both highly feared and stigmatized. If it has been agreed that the patient *not* be informed of a cancer diagnosis, subsequent discussions should involve terms such as "growth" or "lesion" rather than "cancer," and "medication" rather than "chemotherapy."
* Due to the high level of respect for parents and the elderly, some adult children may be reluctant to withdraw life support for fear of giving the appearance of not honoring their parents.

HEALTH BELIEFS AND PRACTICES
* In China and Korea, coining and cupping therapies are traditional medical practices and not forms of abuse, despite the marks they may leave on a patient's body.
* Fevers are often treated by covering the patient in warm blankets and offering warm liquids.

- Avoid giving ice water without asking whether the patient prefers it to water at room temperature. Patient may prefer hot liquids, such as tea.
- The use of herbs is common. Be aware that if patients have only used traditional Chinese herbs, they may not know how to take Western medications, since the herbs are usually boiled in water and then drunk.
- Avoid the number 4. Because the character for the number 4 is pronounced the same as the character for the word "death" in several Asian languages, avoid putting these patients in rooms or operating rooms identified with that number if possible.
- Mental illness can be highly stigmatizing in Asian countries. Patients with emotional problems are likely to present with physical complaints. They may be reluctant to discuss emotional problems with anyone outside the family, including health care professionals.

Cultural Profile: Hispanics/Latinos (Primarily Mexicans)

Caution: These are broad generalizations and should not be used to stereotype any individuals. Statements are most applicable to the least acculturated individuals.

VALUES, WORLD VIEW, AND COMMUNICATION
- Personal relationships are valued. Asking about the patient's family and interests before focusing on health issues will generally increase rapport and trust.
- May have a fatalistic view of the world, which can interfere with preventive behavior.

TIME ORIENTATION
- Many have a present time orientation, which may impede preventive medicine and follow-up care. Explain the need for preventive medication (such as for hypertension) and to finish antibiotics even after symptoms have disappeared. Tie adherence to something they care about (e.g., dancing at a daughter's wedding or holding a grandchild).

PAIN
- While patients may tend to be expressive (loud) when in pain, males may be more expressive around family members than around health care professionals. Remember, however, that just because it is acceptable to be loud, it does not mean there is not a real medical problem.

Family/Gender Issues

- Large numbers of family may visit the patient. It is a cultural way to express love and concern. Allow family members to spend as much time as possible with the patient. Allow them to assist the patient with the activities of daily living if the patient is reluctant to do self-care.
- Realize that patients may not want to discuss emotional problems outside the family.
- Modesty is important, especially among older women; try to keep them covered whenever possible.
- Accept that older, more traditional wives may defer to husbands in decision-making, both for their own health and for that of their children. When patients come in, find out with whom they may want to consult before making decisions.

Pregnancy and Birth

- Pregnancy is seen as a normal condition so prenatal care may not be sought.
- The woman's mother may be the preferred birthing partner.
- Laboring women may yell out "aye yie yie!"—a loud form of controlled breathing. Others may be stoic.
- Traditionally, new mothers avoid cold, bathing, and exercise for six weeks postpartum. Respect postpartum prescriptions for rest. Sponge baths may be preferred.
- Pregnancy is considered a "hot" condition; birth is thought to deplete the body of heat.
- Restoration of warmth is important. Offer liquids other than ice water, which may be deemed too "cold."

Pediatric

- There are a number of folk diseases that affect children, including *mal de ojo* (evil eye), *caída de la mollera* (fallen fontanelle, often caused by dehydration), and *empacho* (stomach pain).
- "Evil eye" is generally believed to be caused by envy when someone compliments a child. Be sure to touch the child when complimenting him or her to prevent this. The child may be wearing a red string or "deer's eye" (a large brown seed with red string) to prevent it.
- Herbal remedies are often used. Be sure to ask about them. Chamomile tea (*manzanilla*), used to treat colic, is generally safe and sometimes helpful. However, *greta*, a yellow to grayish-yellow powder, and *azarcón*, a bright reddish-orange powder, both used to treat *empacho* (stomach pain), contain lead and can be dangerous.

- A chubby baby is seen as a healthy baby, so additional teaching regarding diet and diabetes may be warranted.
- A baby who has a fever will often be bundled up, which may run counter to the use of cooling measures that may have been instructed. It is important to include the grandmother in patient teaching since she may have the most say in terms of day-to-day health care issues, especially if she lives with the family.
- Belly button binders may be used to prevent an "outie." Your concerns should be with the cleanliness of the coin and the tightness of the binder. Instead of advising caregivers not to use a binder, teach them to make sure the coin is clean and that the binder is not too tight.

END OF LIFE
- When a patient is diagnosed as terminal, family members may wish to shield him or her from that fact. On admission (or before the need arises, if possible) ask the patient to identify how much information they want to be given regarding their condition, or to whom the information should be provided. Family members may resist hospice for fear it will emphasize the fact that their loved one is dying and thus encourage the individual to give up hope and the will to live.
- The family of a terminal patient may be reluctant to remove life support lest it be seen as encouraging death. If the illness is determined to be "punishment by God," life support may be considered interfering with the opportunity for the patient to redeem his or her sins through suffering. At the same time, however, traditional respect and courtesy toward physicians may lead the patient or the patient's family to agree with a doctor who suggests removing life support, even when they are opposed to it.

HEALTH BELIEFS AND PRACTICES
- A predominant theory of illness is that it results from an upset in body balance. Patients may refuse certain foods or medications that upset the hot/cold body balance, even if they do not verbalize it as such. With this in mind, offer alternative foods and liquids. Ask if they prefer water with ice or at room temperature.
- Among those following traditional cultural practices, fat is seen as healthy. Many Mexican foods are high in fat and salt. Because of this, nutritional counseling may be necessary for diabetics and individuals with high blood pressure.
- Ask what remedies the patient tried before coming in. Ask in a way that implies that *all* of your patients attempt self-treatment before

coming in, and that you need to know what those attempts were to avoid prescribing something that could result in a bad interaction. Do not let patients believe you are criticizing them for trying home remedies or seeing other healers. Doing so might lessen their trust in you.

Cultural Profile: Middle Easterners

The following includes Arabs and Iranians (Persians). Although most Middle Easterners are Muslim, there is a large population of Jewish Iranians who fled Iran after the Islamic revolution in 1979. Most live in greater Los Angeles, California, and in Great Neck, New York.

Caution: These are broad generalizations and should not be used to stereotype any individuals. Statements are most applicable to the least acculturated individuals.

VALUES, WORLD VIEW, AND COMMUNICATION
- Effective communication is often assumed to be two-way. You may need to share information about yourself before these patients will share information about themselves. Health care providers may be expected to take a personal interest in their patients.
- Female patients may avoid direct eye contact with health care providers of the opposite gender to avoid any hint of sexual impropriety.
- Islam is a dominant force in the lives of many Middle Easterners. Give patients the opportunity to pray privately several times a day, facing east toward Mecca. Many have a fatalistic attitude regarding health (it is all in Allah's hands), so they may see their health-related behavior as being of little consequence. *Inshallah* means "God willing."
- Repetition of demands is often made to show emphasis, as is a loud tone of voice.
- For many Iranians, "thumbs up" is a rude gesture and should be avoided.

TIME ORIENTATION
- Arabs tend to have a past and present time orientation. Human interaction is usually given higher priority than "clock" time; so if being on time is important, be sure to emphasize it.
- Iranians tend to be more future-oriented, although a fatalistic attitude can interfere with adherence to preventive medicine. Social time can be flexible.

Pain

- Patients tend to be very expressive about pain, especially in front of family members. Pain is greatly feared and should be minimized as much as possible. Explaining the source of pain and prognosis may improve these patients' ability to cope with it.

Family/Gender Issues

- Middle Easterners are very family-oriented. The family is seen as more important than the individual. Expect large numbers of familial visitors to see the patient.
- Be patient with "demanding" family members. They may see it as their job to make sure that the patient gets the best care possible. It is usually appropriate to speak first to the family spokesman.
- Personal problems are usually taken care of within the family. They may not be receptive to counseling.
- Traditionally, the eldest male is the decision-maker. Even among the more acculturated, the entire family (including extended family) may participate in decision- making.
- Sexual segregation can be extremely important, especially for Muslim women. Assign same-sex caregivers whenever possible, and respect a woman's modesty at all times.
- Accept the fact that women may defer to husbands for decision-making about their own and their children's health. In fact, the husband may answer questions addressed to his wife. This, in itself, should not be taken as a sign of abuse, but try to talk to the wife alone when possible.
- Middle Eastern cultures are patriarchal and men receive more respect and status than women. Thus, male physicians may be accorded more respect.

Pregnancy and Birth

- Arab women may delay prenatal care since pregnancy is seen as a normal condition.
- There may not be any plan for birth since planning can be seen as challenging the will of Allah.
- Women in labor tend to be vocally expressive of pain. Iranian women often receive a gift of expensive jewelry to compensate for their "suffering."
- A female relative may be the birth attendant; Arab men are not expected to participate. However, acculturated Persian men are more likely to participate.
- Colostrum is believed to be harmful to the baby, so breastfeeding is often delayed for the first few days. Education regarding the benefits of early breastfeeding is important.

END OF LIFE

- When offering chemotherapy, be sure to offer all options for administration. While an implantable pump may seem the most convenient, it may be determined that it has rendered a Muslim "unclean," thus preventing him or her from praying.
- When a patient is diagnosed as terminal, family members may wish to shield him or her from that fact. On admission (or before the need arises, if possible) ask patients to identify how much information they want to be given regarding their condition, or to whom the information should be provided.
- They may not want to plan for death, since doing so can be seen as challenging the will of Allah. You might approach them by saying, *Some [Muslim] families feel that making such decisions is interfering with the will of Allah. Is this a belief you share, or do you want to begin discussing the decisions that need to be made?*
- Avoidance of planning for death may also interfere with acceptance of hospice care. Another factor contributing to lower use of hospice is the belief that the family should be the one to care for the patient. When discussing hospice, be sure to explain that it can be done at home.
- Muslims may not allow organ donation, as tradition dictates that the body should be returned to Allah as it was given: whole. Those who are in favor of it say that because it can save a life, it falls under the Islamic doctrine that "necessity allows the prohibited." For the same reason, they may be reluctant to allow an autopsy, but will if required by law.

HEALTH BELIEFS AND PRACTICES

- Muslims may not take medications, eat, or drink from sunrise to sunset during the month of Ramadan. This period of fasting, self-sacrifice, and introspection is based on the Islamic calendar and thus occurs at a different time each year. Although they may be exempt during illness or pregnancy, Muslims may have to make up for it later on, which is much more difficult since no one else will be doing so at that time.
- They may see the expectation of self-care as a lack of caring. Family members and caregivers are often expected to take care of them. Because of this, include family members in any patient education.
- Injections may be preferable to pills based on the belief that injections are more effective. Offer options when available.
- Damp, cold, and drafts may be thought to lead to illness. Strong emotions are also suspect. For example, the "evil eye" (envy) may be thought to cause illness or misfortune. Amulets to prevent this

may be worn and should not be removed. Amulets include the *hamsa*, which looks like a hand with a blue stone in the palm, and a round blue stone with a blue and white "eye" in the center.
- The patient may feel slighted if not given a prescription.
- When providing meals, be aware that observant Muslims and Jews do not eat pork. Muslims are also expected to abstain from alcohol, which may be found in cough medicine. Medications that contain gelatin may also be a problem.
- If a patient offers you food, it may be perceived as rude to refuse it. The second time it is offered, it is best to accept it.

Note: Some of this information is based on material from Meleis (2005) and Hafizi (2005).

Cultural Profile: Native Americans

Caution: These are broad generalizations and should not be used to stereotype any individuals. There are over 500 different tribes, each with its own culture and variations within each.

VALUES, WORLD VIEW, AND COMMUNICATION
- Anecdotes or metaphors may be used by the patient to describe his or her own health status. For example, a story about an ill neighbor may be the patient's way of saying he or she is experiencing the same symptoms.
- Long pauses often indicate that careful consideration is being given to a question. Do not rush the patient.
- Both loudness and a firm handshake are often associated with aggressiveness and should be avoided.
- Lack of direct eye contact may be a sign of respect, or possibly a desire to avoid loss or theft of one's soul. Do not misinterpret it as lack of interest or evasiveness.
- Due to a history of misuse of signed documents, some Native American patients or their caregivers may be unwilling to sign informed consent or advanced directives. In fact, some may display hostility toward health care providers due to the history of poor treatment of Native Americans.
- The names of deceased relatives may be avoided, though a relationship term (e.g., brother, father, sister) may be used.

TIME ORIENTATION
- A present time orientation is common. Patients are generally oriented to activities rather than to the clock.

PAIN

- These patients generally tend to be stoic, not expressing pain other than by mentioning, "I don't feel so good" or "Something doesn't feel right." Offer pain medication when the condition warrants it, even if the patient does not appear to be in pain.

FAMILY/GENDER ISSUES

- Extended family is important, and any illness concerns the entire family.
- Decision-making varies with kinship structure. Patients will generally make their own decisions.

PREGNANCY AND BIRTH

- Prenatal care is uncommon.
- A female relative may be the birth attendant. Stoicism is encouraged during labor and delivery.
- Postpartum, the mother and infant may stay inside and rest for 20 days or until the umbilical cord falls off, depending on custom. Some may want to save the umbilical cord because it may be seen as having spiritual value.

PEDIATRIC

- In some tribes, long thick hair is the sign of a healthy child; cutting it is taboo and believed to lead to illness or even death.
- Teen pregnancy rates are high, and may be more culturally acceptable than in other populations.

END OF LIFE

- Some tribes may prefer to avoid discussion of terminal prognosis or DNR orders because they believe negative thoughts hasten death. Others will use the information to make appropriate preparations.
- Some tribes may avoid contact with the dying, while others will want to be at the bedside 24 hours a day. Visitors may display a jovial attitude so as not to demoralize the patient. Mourning is often done in private, away from the patient.
- After death, wailing and shrieking may occur.
- Some may want to leave a window open for the soul to leave at death; others may orient the patient's body to a cardinal direction before death.

HEALTH BELIEFS AND PRACTICES

- Before cutting or shaving hair, check to see if the patient or family want to keep it. Realize that in some tribes, cutting hair is associated with mourning.

- A medicine bag may be worn by the patient. Do not treat it casually or remove it without discussing it with the patient. If it is absolutely necessary to remove it, allow a family member to do so, keep it as close to the patient as possible, and return it as soon as possible.
- Food that is blessed (in a traditional religion or Christianity) may be thought to be harmless. Nutritional guidance should take this into account. Many traditional foods are high in fat.
- Similarly, tobacco is seen as sacred and has important ceremonial use in some tribes. This may provide a challenge when counseling against smoking.
- A traditional ritual that may be used for healing is the sweat lodge. It is akin to an outdoor sauna, and involves long rounds of prayer while sweating.
- Traditional healers may be combined with the use of Western medicine. Allow traditional healers to perform rituals whenever possible.

Note: Much of the material contained in this profile is adapted from Kramer (1996) and Palacios, Butterfly, and Strickland (2005).

Cultural Profile: Russians

Caution: These are broad generalizations and should not be used to stereotype any individuals. Statements are most applicable to the least acculturated individuals.

VALUES, WORLD VIEW, AND COMMUNICATION
- To help allay the anxiety of family members, provide frequent updates on patient treatments and progress. These patients may expect nurses to be friendly, warm, and caring—that is, to "feel" for them.
- Family members and friends are expected to visit patients in the hospital; they may participate in providing care. Family may want to stay overnight.
- They may speak loudly and seem abrasive; this was likely necessary in Russia to get attention in the health care system.
- Make direct eye contact, be firm, and be respectful. Use hand gestures and facial expressions when English proficiency is minimal. Address patients using their last names preceded by Mr., Mrs., or Ms.
- They tend to be very direct and straightforward, and do not spend time on small talk.

RESPONSE TO PAIN
- Patients generally tend to be very stoic. Coupled with fear of drug addiction, it may be necessary to discuss with them the importance of pain medication. Pre-medicate for dressing changes or daily care that causes discomfort.

TIME ORIENTATION
- Patients are mostly future-oriented and punctuality is valued. They may arrive early to appointments in an effort to be seen first or late so as not to waste time waiting.

FAMILY/GENDER ISSUES
- Patients often have a strong extended family, with mothers and the elderly often well-regarded.
- The gender of the provider is usually not an issue, but a patient may prefer to have a family member of the same gender present when receiving personal care.

PREGNANCY AND BIRTH
- Exercise and lifting heavy objects are often avoided during pregnancy for fear of harming the unborn baby.
- A female relative is often the preferred labor and delivery partner.

END OF LIFE
- Autopsies and organ donations may be refused due to what may be considered the sacredness of the body.
- When a patient is diagnosed as terminal, family members may wish to shield him or her from that fact. On admission (or before the need arises, if possible) ask patients to identify how much information they want to be given regarding their condition, or to whom the information should be provided.
- These patients generally accept hospice care.

HEALTH RELATED BELIEFS AND PRACTICES
- Choosing among various treatment options may be challenging since some patients may be used to a system that offered no choices.
- Generic drugs may be refused due to the low quality of Soviet-made substitutes provided by Soviet pharmacists.
- Many, especially the elderly, believe illness results from cold. Therefore, keep a patient covered, close windows, keep the room warm, and avoid iced drinks, especially if the patient has a fever. These patients may also prefer sponge baths to showers.

- They may not like taking a large number of pills. Space out medication administration so that as few pills as possible are given at one time.
- They may prefer nonpharmacologic interventions for nausea, including lemon slices, ginger ale, mineral water, or weak tea with lemon.
- They may practice cupping therapy, so any resulting marks should not be misinterpreted as abuse or a symptom.

Note: Information for this profile is based on the work of Peter Anderson, RN, and from Evanikoff del Puerto and Sigal (2005).

Cultural Profile: South Asians

Includes Hindus, Sikhs, and Muslims from India, Pakistan, Bangladesh, Sri Lanka, and Nepal. Some may still use the term East Indian interchangeably for South Asian, but the latter is currently the preferred term.

Caution: These are broad generalizations and should not be used to stereotype any individuals. Statements are most applicable to the least acculturated individuals.

VALUES, WORLD VIEW, AND COMMUNICATION
- Hindus and Sikhs may believe illness is the result of karma, due to actions in a past life. Those who follow Ayurvedic medicine may see it as resulting from an imbalance in bodily humors.
- Patients may not express feelings openly, so observe facial expressions closely.
- Direct eye contact may be considered rude or disrespectful, especially among the elderly.
- Silence often indicates acceptance or approval. With some South Asians, a side-to-side head bob may indicate agreement or uncertainty. An up-and-down nod may indicate disagreement, while acknowledging what the speaker is saying.
- Some patients may not want to sign consents, as they may consider health care professionals to be the authorities and thus may prefer to have them make the decisions.

PAIN
- These patients generally tend to be stoic, except during childbirth.

- There is a great concern regarding drug addiction and thus there may be a reluctance to take pain medication. When pain medication is necessary, explain why. Muslims may not want narcotics for anything other than severe pain.
- Some Pakistani Muslims may prefer injections to pills.

TIME ORIENTATION
- This group is generally future-oriented. Some, including some Pakistanis, may not be oriented to "clock time."

FAMILY/GENDER ISSUES
- Women are often modest and may prefer a gown that provides better coverage. Many may prefer female caregivers as well.
- Male health care providers should not shake hands with a female unless she offers her hand first.
- Close female family members may insist on remaining with the patient. Family members may take over the activities of daily living for the patient, such as feeding, grooming, etc. Because of this, do not insist the patient practice self-care unless medically necessary.
- The father or eldest son usually has decision-making power, but generally family members are consulted before decisions are made. Husbands may answer questions addressed to the wife.

PREGNANCY AND BIRTH
- Pregnant Hindu women are often encouraged to eat nuts, raisins, coconuts, and fruits in the belief that doing so will lead to a healthy, beautiful baby. Dried ginger powder, celery seeds, nuts, and puffed lotus seeds may be given to a new Hindu mother in an effort to cleanse her system and restore her strength.
- Moaning and screaming are acceptable during childbirth.
- Traditionally, female relatives served as labor partners, though it is becoming more common for the husband to assist.
- South Asian women may practice a postpartum lying-in period. While they are expected to feed the baby, everything else is done for them. Traditionally, female relatives take over. If none are around, the patient may expect nurses to do this.
- Baby naming may be delayed for a week among Hindu Indians. It should not be misinterpreted as a lack of bonding.

END OF LIFE
- When a patient is diagnosed as terminal, family members may wish to shield him or her from that fact. On admission (or before the need arises, if possible) ask patients to identify how much information

they want to be given regarding their condition, or to whom the information should be provided.
- Most family members will not allow autopsy unless absolutely necessary.

HEALTH RELATED BELIEFS AND PRACTICES
- Use of home and folk remedies is common, but may not be disclosed to physicians. Explain in a nonjudgmental way that most patients try home remedies first and why it is important you know what self-treatment regimens they have tried.
- Sikhs are required not to cut their hair or shave their beards. Their hair will usually be worn in a turban. Consider this before cutting or shaving any hair in preparation for surgery.
- Observant Hindus will generally not eat meat or fish; some may not eat eggs. Observant Muslims will not eat pork.
- Muslims may not take medications, eat, or drink from sunrise to sunset during the month of Ramadan. This period of fasting, self-sacrifice, and introspection is based on the Islamic calendar, and thus occurs at a different time each year.
- Those who practice Ayurvedic medicine (Hindus, Sikhs, and some Muslims) classify food in terms of hot or cold, based on qualities inherent in the food rather than on its temperature. "Hot" foods, including meat, fish, eggs, yogurt, honey, and nuts, are encouraged for "cold" conditions, such as fever or in anticipation of surgery, especially in winter. "Cold" foods like milk, butter, cheese, fruits, and vegetables are encouraged during the summer and for "hot" conditions, including pregnancy.

Note: Some material adapted from Zachariah (2005), Hashwani (2005), and Rajwani (1996).

Cultural Profile: Southeast Asians

Caution: These are broad generalizations and should not be used to stereotype any individuals. Statements are most applicable to the least acculturated individuals.

VALUES, WORLD VIEW, AND COMMUNICATION
- Keep in mind that many Southeast Asians are refugees who fled to the United States to save their lives rather than simply to improve them.

- Many Southeast Asians are Buddhist and believe in reincarnation. Many traditionalists are animists, believing that spirits inhabit objects and places, and that ancestors must be worshipped so their spirits do not harm their descendants. It is not unusual for members of this cultural group to practice Christianity, however.
- Modesty is highly valued, and this value may interfere with some screening procedures, such as pap smears and colonoscopies. Clinicians may need to take extra time to explain procedures and to accommodate modesty concerns as well as possible.
- Giggling at "inappropriate" times usually indicates nervousness or discomfort.
- Realize that it may be difficult to obtain an accurate health history as patients have rarely been told the name of illnesses, medicines given, or procedures performed.

Time Orientation
- Present time orientation is common, though emphasis on remembering ancestors reflects a past time orientation as well.
- Older, less acculturated members may not be oriented to "clock" time and may thus arrive early or late for appointments.

Pain
- This group is generally stoic. Pay attention to nonverbal indications, such as a clenched jaw. Anticipate the need for pain medication, even if a patient does not ask for it, and explain that the doctor ordered it.

Family/Gender Issues
- Great respect for elders is common. Adult children are expected to care for their parents.
- Among older generations, men are the decision-makers and either the husband or eldest son (if his father is deceased) may take on the role. Note that the family spokesperson may not be the decision-maker, but merely the one who speaks English.
- When a patient is accompanied by relatives, address the eldest person present—especially if male.

Pregnancy and Birth
- Either the mother or the husband may be the preferred labor partner. When asked, they may not give an accurate count of pregnancies because many count only live births.
- Some Hmong new mothers may want to take home the placenta for burial.

PEDIATRIC
- A baby may not be seen as "human" until several days old—a tradition that probably developed to discourage mothers from bonding too closely in an environment with high infant mortality rates.
- The head is the seat of life and is thus considered very personal, vulnerable, honorable, and untouchable (except by close intimates), so avoid putting intravenous lines in an infant's scalp unless necessary, and then only with explanation.
- Some Vietnamese mothers may appear to have difficulty bonding; this is an illusion. If they pay little attention to their newborns, it is probably out of fear that if they call attention to how attractive their infants are, spirits may want to steal the child, which could result in the child's death.
- Children may wear "spirit-strings" around their wrists or "neck rings." Neither should be cut or removed as some consider these to carry the children's life-souls.

END OF LIFE
- When a patient is diagnosed as terminal, family members may wish to shield him or her from that fact. On admission (or before the need arises, if possible) ask patients to identify how much information they want to be given regarding their condition, or to whom the information should be provided. Be aware that in most parts of Southeast Asia, diagnoses are usually given to the family, who decide whether or not to tell the patient.
- Some may believe that at death parents and grandparents become ancestors who should be worshipped and obeyed. Since these ancestors shape the well-being of living descendants, a child (regardless of age) may have trouble agreeing to terminate the care of a parent.
- Family may want to wash body at death and some may want to place a coin in the deceased's mouth, according to custom.
- Hmong may refuse autopsies and organ donations because they believe that whatever is removed from the body will be missing when they are reincarnated.

HEALTH BELIEFS AND PRACTICES
- Patients (especially rural non-Christians) may fear surgery because many believe that souls are attached to different parts of the body. They feel a surgical procedure might sever this connection, thus causing illness or death. Some may believe that if the body is cut or disfigured or parts are amputated, the patient will remain in a state

of imbalance for life. It is felt that this will trigger frequent illnesses and render the person physically incomplete in his or her next incarnation.

- Some Hmong believe that when people are unconscious their souls can wander, so anesthesia is dangerous.
- Some believe that verbal statements in and of themselves can cause illness or death, and for this reason may not want to discuss potential risks and dangers. Less acculturated patients may want to consult a shaman.
- Therapies like cupping and coining (or coin rubbing) are traditional remedies, not forms of abuse. So ascertain how and why any observed markings on a patient's body were made before reporting them.
- Some patients may have concerns about blood being drawn. They may fear it will sap their strength, cause illness, force their souls to leave their bodies, or that it will not be replenished. If a patient is anxious, ask about his or her concerns so they can be addressed.

Note: Information for this profile was adapted from several sources, including Kulig and Prak (2005), Johnson and Hang (2005), and Muecke (1983). Additional information on Hmong beliefs was taken from Fadiman (1997).

Selected Religions

Just as culture can have an enormous influence on behavior, so can religion. Although there are differences within the various sects of each religion, and people vary significantly with regard to how closely they adhere to the tenets of their faith, knowledge of religious beliefs and practices may be useful to the clinician. It is important to remember, however, that the information presented in this appendix should be used as *generalizations*, not as something to *stereotype* individuals.

Rachel Spector (2000) and Lynn Stoller were important sources for the information presented in this appendix.

BAHA'I

Autopsy	Acceptable with medical or legal need
Diet	No alcohol or drugs
Disposal of the body	Burial preferred; cremation strongly discouraged
Healing beliefs	Harmony between religion and science
Healing practices	Prayer
Medications	Narcotics with prescriptions
Organ donation	Permitted
Right-to-die issues	Life is unique and precious, so do not destroy

BUDDHISM

Autopsy	Matter of individual practice; some Buddhists believe consciousness remains in the body for up to three days after the patient stops breathing so an autopsy would not be appropriate in that time frame
Diet	Many do not eat meat
Disposal of the body	Burial or cremation, depending on the wishes of the family; cremation common; belief in reincarnation

Healing beliefs	Illness sometimes seen as an imbalance of energy
Healing practices	No restrictions; may perform rituals to promote healing; some use of herbal remedies
Medications	Some abstain from "intoxicants" that could cloud the mind, including pain medication; some may object to medications with animal by-products
Organ donation	Considered act of mercy; if hope for recovery, all means taken
Right-to-die issues	Personal choice in time and manner of death is of extreme importance; death should be with a clear mind, even if it means experiencing pain
Sabbath	None
Spiritual practices	Daily chanting or meditation

CATHOLIC

Autopsy	Permissible
Disposal of the body	Usually burial, although cremation is now acceptable
Euthanasia	Direct life-ending procedures forbidden
Healing beliefs	Belief in the power of God to heal
Healing practices	Sacrament of sick (includes anointing, communion if possible, and blessing by a priest), candles, laying-on-of-hands
Health care issues	Birth control, abortion, in vitro fertilization and sterilization are forbidden; birth control pills may be allowed when they are necessary for medical reasons (most commonly for endometriosis)
Medications	May be taken if benefits outweigh risks
Organ donation	Justifiable
Right-to-die issues	Obligated to take ordinary, not extraordinary, means to prolong life
Sabbath	Sunday
Spiritual/religious items	Crucifix, rosary beads, scapular

CHRISTIAN SCIENCE

Autopsy	Not usual; individual or family decide
Diet	No alcohol or tobacco
Disposal of the body	Burial or cremation

Healing beliefs	Accept physical ("mechanical"—like a broken arm or intestinal blockage) and moral healing; they believe that humans are not matter but spirit, and therefore illness, injuries, and suffering are not "real" and can be overcome through faith and prayer.
Healing practices	Utilize full-time healing ministers known as Christian Science Practitioners who heal through "prayer"; may use physicians for childbirth and setting broken bones.
Medications	None
Organ donation	Individual decides
Right-to-die issues	Unlikely to seek medical help to prolong life

HINDUISM

Autopsy	Varies; for some it is acceptable; for others it could be problematic since opening the body is believed to be disrespectful to the dead
Diet	Many are vegetarian
Disposal of the body	Cremation
Healing beliefs	Some believe in faith healing
Healing practices	Traditional faith healing system; many practice Ayurvedic medicine
Medications	Acceptable, unless they contain animal products
Organ donation	Acceptable
Disposal of the body	Cremation common; believe in reincarnation
Other practices	Note that many follow the cultural practice of using the right hand for eating and the left hand for toileting and hygiene
Right-to-die issues	No restrictions
Sabbath	None
Spiritual/religious items	Some may wear a thread around wrist or body; do not remove

ISLAM/MUSLIMS

Autopsy	Permitted for medical and legal purposes; otherwise forbidden
Diet	No pork or alcohol; food should be *halal* (permissible according to Islamic law),

which also takes into account the method of slaughter; daylight fasting during the month of Ramadan

Disposal of the body	Cremation forbidden; body must be washed by same sex Muslim at death; burial usually within 24 hours
Healing beliefs	Faith healing generally not acceptable
Healing practices	Some use of herbal remedies
Holy Days	The month of Ramadan (which varies each year) is a time for reflection; during this time, Muslims are required to fast from sunrise to sunset
Medications	No restrictions, although there may be some concern around those made with animal products
Organ donation	Varies according to interpretation
Other practices	Note that many follow the cultural practice of using the right hand used for eating, left for toileting and hygiene
Right-to-die issues	Attempts to shorten life prohibited
Sabbath	Friday
Spiritual practices	Prayer five times daily, facing Mecca; boys usually circumcised

JEHOVAH'S WITNESSES

Autopsy	Acceptable if required by law
Diet	No tobacco; moderate alcohol allowed
Disposal of the body	Burial or cremation
Healing beliefs	Faith healing forbidden
Healing practices	Reading scriptures can comfort the individual and lead to mental and spiritual healing
Health care issues	No blood or blood products allowed; the use of derivatives of primary blood components is left up to individual choice
Medications	Accepted except if derived from blood products
Organ donation	Individual decision; all blood must be removed beforehand
Right-to-die issues	Use of extraordinary means an individual's choice
Sabbath	Sunday

JUDAISM/JEWISH (APPLIES LARGELY TO ORTHODOX JEWS)

Autopsy	Permitted if required by law
Diet	Kosher laws for orthodox and some conservative Jews forbid pork, shellfish, and mixing of meat and dairy products; separate (or disposable) dishes and utensils must be used for meat and dairy; fasting on Yom Kippur
Disposal of the body	Cremation inappropriate; someone should sit with body after death; burial within 24 hours; all body parts including bloody clothing and amputated limbs should be buried with body
Euthanasia	Prohibited
Healing beliefs	Under *Halacha* (religious law) it is the duty of followers to do what they can to preserve and protect their lives
Healing practices	Prayers for the sick
Holy Days	Yom Kippur (the date of which varies from year to year) is the Day of Atonement during which Jews are to fast and do no work from sunset the evening before, to the following sundown.
Medications	There may be concerns around medication being kosher (medications with porcine components); while insulin is no longer made with porcine products some patients may still have that concern; others might be concerned with use of gelatin tablets
Organ donation	Complex issue; some practiced
Right-to-die issues	There is an obligation to preserve and protect life; withdrawing a "cyclical" treatment such as chemotherapy may be permitted whereas withdrawing life support (a "continuous" treatment) is generally problematic
Religious practices	Boys circumcised on eighth day of life
Sabbath	Sundown Friday to one hour past sundown Saturday. Orthodox Jews will avoid all "work" (activities that are "creative" or that exercise control or dominion over one's environment) including ringing the call button, signing forms or exchanging money.

| Spiritual/religious items | Orthodox men may wear prayer shawl, *yarmulka* (skull cap), and *tfillin* (black strings) on arms and forehead while praying |

MORMONS (CHURCH OF JESUS CHRIST OF LATTER-DAY SAINTS)

Autopsy	Permitted with consent of next of kin
Diet	No alcohol, tobacco, coffee, or tea
Disposal of the body	Cremation discouraged; burial common
Euthanasia	Humans must not interfere in God's plan
Healing beliefs	Power of God can bring healing
Healing practices	Anointing with oil, sealing, prayer, laying on of hands
Health care issues	Birth control, abortion, in vitro fertilization and sterilization strongly discouraged
Medications	No restrictions; may use herbal remedies
Organ donation	Permitted
Religious practices	Baptism after age eight; not in infancy or at death
Right to-die issues	If death inevitable, promote a peaceful and dignified death
Sabbath	Sunday
Spiritual/religious items	"Garment"—a type of underwear that is considered sacred; individuals may not want to remove it

SEVENTH-DAY ADVENTIST

Autopsy	Acceptable
Diet	Vegetarian diet encouraged; alcohol, coffee, tea prohibited
Disposal of the body	Burial or cremation
Healing beliefs	Divine healing
Healing practices	Anointing with oil and prayer
Medications	No restrictions
Organ donation	Acceptable
Right-to-die issues	Follow the ethic of prolonging life
Sabbath	Sundown Friday to sundown Saturday

SIKHISM

Autopsy	Permitted
Diet	Intoxicants, including tobacco, forbidden; many do not eat beef due to a ban on eating meat that has been ritually slaughtered or prepared for another religion (e.g., kosher

	or *halal* meat); some Sikhs extend this rule to all meat and meat products, and even eggs, fish, and dairy products; when Sikhs are confused with Muslims they may be offered *halal* food by well-meaning staff; this can be problematic
Disposal of the body	Cremation generally preferred
Healing practices	Prayer; playing of sacred music
Health care issues	Their bodily hair is not to be cut or shaved; daily washing appreciated; culturally, same-sex providers often preferred
Medications	No restrictions
Organ donation	Acceptable
Right-to-die issues	Death is a natural process and God's will
Disposal of the body	Cremation preferred
Sabbath	None
Spiritual/religious items	The Sikh articles of faith include the *Kesh* (uncut hair), which is kept covered by a distinctive turban, the *Kirpan* (sword), *Kara* (metal bracelet), *Kanga* (comb), and *Kaccha* (undershorts)

Appendix 3

Dos and Don'ts of Providing Culturally Competent Care

Don'ts

- Don't stereotype people. Remember that the information given for each culture group is meant to be a broad general guideline, to serve as starting points. Find out whether or not the individual fits the generalization.
- Don't judge a patient's level of pain based on his or her expressiveness. Some cultures encourage expressiveness, others encourage stoicism.
- Don't wait to offer pain medication until a patient asks for it; many Asian and Native American patients will suffer in silence.
- Don't assume lack of eye contact indicates lack of interest, guilt, or some other negative point. For Asians, it may be a way of showing respect; for Middle Easterners, a way of maintaining propriety.
- Don't judge people as "pushy" or "cold" based on how close they stand to you.
- Don't expect that all patients will make their own decisions. In cultures where the family is the primary unit, important decisions may be made by the family. In cultures where males are dominant, the husband may make the final decisions regarding the health care of his wife and children.
- Don't offer ice water as the only liquid. Many will prefer room temperature or warm liquids.
- Don't confuse traditional health care practices such as coining and cupping with abuse.
- Don't assume that a patient's appetite is based solely on feelings of hunger; some foods prepared by the hospital may violate rules of body balance or religious prohibitions, or may simply be unfamiliar to the patient.
- Don't assume the patient wants to be informed of a terminal diagnosis. Ask the patient on admission (or before, if possible) to whom he or she would like information about his or her condition to be

given. Often family members will want to shield patients from a terminal diagnosis.

Dos

- Do remember to ask the right questions of all your patients: the 4 C's of Culture (What do you *call* your problem? [i.e., What do you think is wrong?] What do you think *caused* it? What have you done to *cope* with it? What *concerns* you about it? What *concerns* do you have about my recommended treatment?)
- Do ask your patients how much information they want about their condition, especially at the end-of-life.
- Do ask your patients if they want to make decisions about their treatment or prefer to consult with (or defer to) other family members, especially around end-of-life care.
- Do try to understand people's values, since they will influence their behavior.
- Do realize that not all patients believe germs caused their disease. Again, ask them what they think caused their illness.
- Do recognize that people with a present time orientation (most poor people, many people from agriculturally based countries) may have difficulty with preventive health care. Make an extra effort to explain the importance of preventive health care, and why it is necessary to continue medication even after the symptoms have disappeared.
- Do try to allow a patient as many visitors as she or he would like to have, as long as others are not disturbed.
- Do distinguish the degree of self-care necessary for recovery from that which is merely an imposition of the value of independence.
- Do include family members in the patient teaching, if a family member will be caring for a patient at home.
- Do respect a woman's concern for modesty; try to keep her covered.
- Do try to assign same-sex health care providers when possible, especially for Middle Eastern patients.
- Do be sensitive to the fact that most African Americans have been subjected to much racial prejudice and discrimination.
- Do respect patients' religious beliefs; involve clergy in their care when appropriate.
- Do learn about the beliefs and practices of the patient populations you serve.
- Do keep in mind that there is always individual variation within a group.
- Do develop a tolerant accepting attitude about views different from your own.

- Do make sure your patients understand your instructions by having them demonstrate and explain them to you.
- Do explain the rationale for your instructions.
- Do find out if your instructions/recommendation conflict with their religious or cultural beliefs or practices, or with their life circumstances.
- Do what you can to develop trust.
- Do be curious about other cultures. Ask questions of your patients and co-workers. People generally like to talk about their culture.

Appendix 4

Tips for Working with Interpreters

These guidelines were developed by medical anthropologist M. Jean Gilbert and are included with her gracious permission.

- Brief the interpreter before the encounter if possible; give him/her relevant information about the patient and/or purpose of the conversation.
- When possible, choose an interpreter whose age, gender, background, etc. make it easiest to work with the patient or family.
- Place the interpreter behind the patient or behind you. Never place the interpreter between you and the patient/family.
- When talking, look directly at the patient and speak in first person: "Mrs. Jimenez, I will need to have you go to the lab for a couple of tests." Don't tell the interpreter to "Tell Mrs. Jimenez she'll need to go to the lab . . ." Ask the interpreter to speak in the first person for you and for the patient instead of saying, "The doctor says . . ." or "Mrs. Jimenez says . . ."
- Don't talk for long without letting the interpreter interpret what you are saying.
- Let the interpreter know that s/he can request clarification from you whenever it's needed.
- Pursue seemingly unconnected issues that the patient raises. These issues may lead to crucial information or uncover difficulties with the interpretation.
- Come back to an issue if you suspect a problem and get a negative response. Use related questions, change the wording and come at it indirectly.
- Learn basic words and sentences in the target language. Asking interpreter about words that have not been translated prompts attention to detail.
- Make sure the interpreter conveys everything the patient says and doesn't abbreviate or paraphrase.

Following these tips keeps you in charge of the encounter and prevents the interpreter from inadvertently taking control. Using first person will seem more natural to the patient and will help you develop and maintain rapport.

In addition to Gilbert's guidelines, you might also want to discuss with the interpreter whether you expect his or her role to be that of a "conduit," merely interpreting the words from one language to the other, with no additions, omissions, or editing, or that of a "culture broker," who provides the cultural information necessary for understanding the message. According to the Cross Cultural Health Care Program, since the goal of interpretation is to facilitate understanding between two people who are speaking two different languages, the latter role might be particularly relevant when the clinician has little understanding of the patient's culture. However, the clinician's expectations for the interpreter should be discussed in advance.

Appendix 5

Summary of Case Studies

Note: Cases demonstrating cultural competence are in italics.

Chapter 1. Basic Concepts

(1) American female physician brought to an Islamic Arab nation to care for a member of the royal family tried to respect Arab dress for women but found that it was not wanted.

(2) American anthropologist (the author) forgot that people in the American South are more religious and neglected to wait for "grace" before eating.

(3) Young Mexican boy presents with symptoms consistent with *susto*, but physician is unaware of it, thus missing a possible opportunity to develop rapport.

(4) Mexican woman came to emergency department with epigastric pain. Nurse used the 4 C's to learn patient thought it was due to stress and had stopped her anti-anxiety medication the day before the pain started.

(5) African American woman refused an angiogram for acute chest pain because she believed it was punishment for her sins and that only God could cure her. (See also case #287)

(6) Nurse used 4 C's to learn postsurgical Hispanic male patient believed he developed pneumonia because he wasn't wearing socks during surgery. This knowledge leads her to discuss temperature management with all her patients prior to surgery.

(7) Hispanic woman refused pain medication but was in too much pain for physical therapy until culturally sensitive nurse asked her what she had used to cope with the pain before surgery. She had been using herbal teas from a curandero. *After discussing it with the pharmacist, the nurse told the patient's daughter to bring in the tea, after which the patient returned to physical therapy.*

(8) Nurse used 4 C's to learn that pediatric Hispanic patient suffering from Kawasaki Syndrome did not experience peeling skin due to use of snake oil cream.

Since peeling skin is an important symptom for the differential diagnosis, it was helpful that the nurse asked what the patient had been using to cope with his symptoms.

(9) Culturally competent physician asked her Latino patient the right question and learned he didn't want to take insulin because he feared it caused blindness; both his mother and uncle went blind after going on insulin.

(10) Physician used 4 C's with Vietnamese patient, which caused her to lose faith in the doctor. She saw it as the physician's job to know what is wrong and how to treat it, not to ask her opinion.

(11) African American patient deemed a "frequent flyer" by emergency department personnel and thought to be drug seeking, turned out to have a rare form of meningitis and died.

(12) Physician stereotyped mother of Hispanic infant as non-English speaking and called for an interpreter, thus offending the bilingual woman.

(13) Nurse stereotyped a Middle Eastern patient for being loud and later learned that the patient was riddled with cancer.

(14) Nigerian nurse refrained from stereotyping an African American male patient as drug seeking, due to cultural sensitivity training. It was fortunate he reassessed the patient, because he needed immediate medical intervention.

(15) African American woman assumed the physician was being racist when he asked if she wanted her tubes tied after her twelfth pregnancy.

(16) African American woman assumed racism when case manager told her that five-months post-op pain for carpal tunnel release was too long. The case manager's cultural competence skills restored the situation.

(17) Nurse used understanding of Hispanic patient's fatalistic worldview to adjust education regarding his uncontrolled diabetes. Rather than "lecture" him, she explained everything to him and his wife and discussed with them how to make gradual changes in his diet.

Chapter 2. Communication and Time Orientation

Language Issues

(18) Chinese doctor unfamiliar with the American idiom "cold feet" ordered vascular tests for his patient.

(19) Korean physician didn't understand the idiom "kick the bucket" and responded affirmatively when his patient asked if that would be the result of his surgery.

(20) English couple were amused when female patient was instructed to slide her fanny up to the middle of the bed. In England, "fanny" is a crude term for a woman's vagina.

(21) Mexican parents misunderstood the word "puto" when used by a Filipina pediatric nurse. They thought she was having sexual relations with a prostitute; she was referring to the rice cake she was having for lunch.

(22) A Cuban male ends up quadriplegic in part due to confusion over the word "intoicado."

(23) Hispanic male patient accidently took a drug overdose when he misinterpreted the written instructions to take the medication "once" a day. *Once* in Spanish means eleven.

(24) African American man threw a plate of food at a white Canadian nurse when she politely asked, "Do you boys mind if I sit down here?" The term "boy" doesn't have the same connotation in Canada as in the U.S., due to our history of slavery.

(25) Filipina patient and husband said they understood the nurse's discharge instructions when in fact, they didn't because they wanted to preserve self-esteem.

(26) Chinese women hospitalized with an acute evolving heart attack agreed to the physician's recommendation that she return in two weeks for a follow-up visit, even though she had no intention of doing so. She felt that to refuse would have been disrespectful.

(27) Hmong patient respectfully agreed with a physician's recommendation to have surgery, even though she had no intentions of undergoing the knife.

(28) Deaf gay male assumed the best when told that his HIV test had come back "positive." "Positive" and "negative" have different meanings outside of medicine.

Communication Style

(29) A linguist solved the problem of "rude" cafeteria workers in England by discovering that in their native language they asked questions, not by raising their voice at the end of the sentence, but by adding a word. When he trained them to change their tone at the end of the sentence, they were perceived as friendly.

(30) Hispanic woman was treated professionally, but without the personal warmth (*personalismo*) valued in Hispanic cultures, so she did not return.

(31) Diabetic Mexican clinic patient on dialysis became more compliant when treated with personalismo.

(32) Culturally competent nurse utilizing personalismo *was one of the few staff members not named in a lawsuit by a Latino patient's family after the woman died with end-stage renal disease.*

(33) Hispanic family didn't want to "bother" the physician with their questions, and told him they had none. Instead, they questioned the nurse.

(34) African American woman came to the emergency department with chest pain. Physician was led to wrong diagnosis by asking leading questions. Nurse corrected the situation by asking more open-ended questions.

(35) Anglo American woman was misdiagnosed by ophthalmologist as possibly having diabetes due to marked change in her vision a few weeks after her eye exam. The problem was not diabetes, but that rather than allowing her time to respond during the original vision test, he fed her the answers.

(36) New nurse working in a psychiatric hospital was so intent on getting through the patient intake questionnaire that she neglected to follow up when the patient answered "yes" to the question, "Do you still think about killing yourself?"

Names

(37) African American patient didn't respond when nurse called her by her first name, but did when the nurse showed her respect by calling her by her last name.

Interpreters

(38) Vietnamese patient who hadn't been eating any of her meals avoided a nasogastric tube when an interpreter discovered that the patient's daughter had been bringing her food.

(39) Spanish-speaking woman kept returning to the clinic to treat her abdominal pain. When the staff finally used a professional interpreter rather than the woman's young daughter, it came out that she needed treatment for a sexually transmitted disease, something she couldn't say in front of her child.

(40) Gay patient was abandoned when a family member was used to interpret the patient's HIV diagnosis and prognosis.

(41) Deaf teenage girl refused to respond to the psychiatrist's questions when she was brought her into the emergency department after threatening suicide. The reason she wouldn't respond is that her parents were used as interpreters and they were the source of the girl's problem.

(42) Mexican home hospice patient didn't want her family to know she was having a difficult time, so she withheld this important information when the hospice nurse used family members to interpret for her. It was much better when a professional interpreter was brought in.

(43) Arab mother-in-law refused to translate contraception information for her daughter-in-law, who had just given birth; she wanted more grandchildren.

(44) Korean daughter did not pass on information to her father about his stroke or instructions given by the nurse because she didn't want to reveal a negative diagnosis and did not feel comfortable telling her father what to do.

(45) Hispanic parents declined the physician's offer of an interpreter to sign consent for their son who needed surgery. However, the father then misinterpreted what the physician said and became outraged, thinking the surgeon was going to kill his son.

(46) A bilingual Mexican medical technician was unable to pass the test to become a Certified Healthcare Interpreter. Special training is needed to be a professional interpreter.

(47) Adult daughter of a Latino patient was offended when the hospital wanted to use a professional interpreter rather than let her interpret for her mother.

Dealing with Silence

(48) Navajo woman left long silences when nurse asked her questions while taking a medical history, not because she didn't hear or understand the nurse, but because, in the Navajo style, she was giving thoughtful consideration to her answers.

Informed Consent

(49) Middle Eastern man was reluctant to sign informed consent for heart catheterization, believing that since the physician was the one with the expert knowledge, he should take responsibility for making the decision.

(50) Cambodian woman delayed signing consent for a skin graft, probably due to fear stemming from the time of the Khmer Rouge war, when signed life histories were required from those who were later executed.

(51) Chinese man signed consent for an angiogram out of respect for the physician, who mistook smiling and nodding for understanding, when in fact the patient spoke no English.

(52) Right before Hispanic patient was to have back surgery, nurse discovered he didn't understand what was to be done in the surgery. A family member rather than a professional interpreter had been used to get informed consent. Once the patient understood, he canceled the surgery.

Nonverbal Communication

(53) Navajo patient avoided making eye contact with nurse while she was giving diabetic health teaching; he wanted to show respect and perhaps to avoid soul loss or theft.

(54) Hmong girl avoided making eye contact with nurse case manager while she was doing health teaching following the birth of the girl's child; she was doing so to show respect.

(55) Rabbi ignored the proffered hand of a family member (the author) when he was making a hospital visit to a Jewish patient because among ultra-Orthodox Jews it is forbidden to touch the opposite sex unless you are married to the person.

(56) Filipina nurse became angry when a patient beckoned her by motioning with his right index finger because in the Philippines that gesture is used to call dogs and is thus insulting when used with a person.

(57) Filipina nurse was hurt when she motioned in the Filipino manner for an Anglo aide to come assist her, and the aide simply smiled and waved at her because she had no idea what the gesture meant.

Time Orientation

(58) Filipino patient was upset when clinic refused to see him after he arrived 30 minutes late. Filipina nurse provided a culturally competent resolution—she spoke to him respectfully, explained the reason for the clinic policy, and made an appointment for him the next day.

(59) Mexican woman with kidney failure and diabetes was often late to clinic appointments. Nurse provided a culturally competent resolution—she took the needs of the family into account when scheduling appointments and stressed the importance of clock time when specific timing was required.

(60) Latino patient failed to adhere to his physician's instructions to take medication for congestive heart failure and hyperkalemia because he stopped experiencing symptoms, and thus had an early, unscheduled return to the hospital.

Chapter 3. Pain

Expression of Pain

(61) Nicaraguan patient recovering from coronary bypass surgery was very expressive of his pain.

(62) Chinese patient recovering from coronary bypass surgery was very stoic.

(63) Mexican woman recovering from femoral bypass surgery complained loudly about pain. Nurse stereotyped her as a loud Mexican patient, but it turned out that she was bleeding internally and in a great deal of pain.

(64) Indian doctor didn't understand the significance of a normally stoic Irish woman's complaints about pain prior to surgery, assuming that because most women from India were loud and expressive, *all* women were. He thus did not see the need to operate sooner than planned, and the patient died on the operating table.

(65) A culturally competent nurse calmed a dramatic Italian woman by speaking calmly, explaining to the patient and her family what to expect, and giving her non-narcotic pain medication.

(66) A Jewish woman feared that a minor pain in her finger signaled the advent of crippling arthritis, thus illustrating greater concern for the meaning and significance of pain than for the pain sensation.

(67) A young Anglo American girl sat stoically through a painful examination, waiting to cry until the physician left the room.

(68) Culturally competent triage nurse no longer focuses on appearance to determine who needs to be seen most urgently, recognizing that people express pain differently.

(69) Hmong teenage girl, suffering from painful bone cancer, was very stoic and did not ask for pain medication until the pain was excruciating.

(70) Young Jewish girl was culturally atypical in being very stoic during her first urinary catheter insertion.

Pain Medication

(71) Stoic Muslim Nigerian farmer never asked for pain medication following knee surgery, instead offering his pain to Allah.

(72) Filipino patient didn't want to bother the nurse by asking for pain mediation after a shoulder repair.

(73) An Asian patient didn't request pain medication postoperatively, but his culturally competent nurse noted nonverbal signs of pain and educated him on the importance of pain medication.

(74) East Indian woman, on the advice of her physician son, stopped taking her pain medication following a total knee replacement, despite levels of pain that kept her from doing rehab exercises. He didn't want his mother to become addicted, but was in fact, impeding her recovery.

(75) Egyptian patient receiving home hospice care for advanced lung cancer preferred injections or IV infusion to oral medication, even though the pills were working. He believed that the more intrusive the procedure, the more effective it was.

(76) Hispanic man nearly died of an overdose of pain medication because no one took the time to explain how to take it; since he was told he could take up to six tablets a day, he assumed it would be more effective if he took them all at once.

(77) Anglo American woman did not comply with referral to the pain team, despite severe leg pain, because she misunderstood the meaning of "pain team"; she felt she had enough pain and did not need more.

(78) Filipina nurse halved the doctor's prescribed dosage of medication for her dying mother because she feared her mother would become addicted to the medication.

Chapter 4, Religion and Spirituality

Religious Practices

(79) Buddhist monk from Cambodia became greatly distressed when a female nurse touched his shoulder because it violated the rules of his religion, which required sexual segregation.

(80) Culturally sensitive nurse followed through on a Catholic patient's request for a priest.

(81) Christian Scientist with colon cancer allowed doctors to perform a colonoscopy and colostomy, but refused the surgery that would have saved her life because it violated her religious beliefs. Physicians accepted her decision and did what they could to help her while staying within the bounds of her beliefs.

(82) Spiritual leader of an Indian Orthodox Christian church had to delay open-heart surgery while he underwent a purification ceremony after non-Orthodox Christians performed some medical procedures and a female operated the x-ray machine in the catheterization lab.

(83) Patient called nurse when he saw his roommate on the floor, thinking he had had a seizure. He hadn't; he was Muslim and was on the floor to pray.

(84) Jehovah's Witness patient's doctor decided to transfuse her and was later sued for assault and battery because he violated her express wish to adhere to her religion's rule against receiving blood.

(85) Jehovah's Witness who began bleeding heavily after giving birth eventually changed her mind at the last minute and agreed to a blood transfusion.

(86) Culturally competent nurse spoke with wife of a Jehovah's Witness who had refused even albumin for her critically ill husband. By telling her he respected and understood her beliefs and explaining why her husband needed albumin, she agreed to allow it.

(87) Jewish father requested the bloody scrubs of the nurse who tried to save his daughter after she was hit by a car. According to Jewish tradition, the individual must be buried whole and the blood was considered part of her body.

(88) Culturally sensitive nurse allowed adult son of Orthodox Jewish man to stay with his father's body until it was picked up by the mortuary because according to Jewish custom the body of the deceased must not be left unattended.

(89) Orthodox Jewish man brought his wife to the hospital in labor during the Sabbath, and then could not leave or buy food due to Sabbath laws.

(90) Sikh from India refused to have any of his hair shaved prior to heart catheterization because the Sikh religion forbids cutting or shaving any body hair.

(91) Culturally competent nurse took the time to explain to Sikh mother and child why she wanted to shave the child to prep him for an appendectomy and allowed the family to make the decision.

Sacred Symbols

(92) Culturally competent nurse arranged for Latina patient to wear rosary beads into surgery.

(93) Italian Catholic woman became upset when her soiled gown was thrown into the laundry without removing her scapular, an important spiritual symbol.

(94) Culturally competent nurse convinced other nurses to allow patients to keep religious statues in the room when Mexican patient explained how important they were to him.

(95) Buddhist Cambodian woman was disturbed by the crucifix on the wall of her hospital bed.

(96) Mormon woman refused to remove her long underwear because "the garment" signifies adult religious status in the church and is considered sacred; the surgeon refused to operate unless she did. Eventually, he relented.

(97) Culturally competent ICU nurse hung a "soul catcher" over the bed of a Native American from the Hoopa Valley Reservation when the patient's granddaughter brought it in. It provided psychological comfort to the patient and his family.

(98) Cambodian mother became very upset when the nurse first tried to remove the strands of dark brown strings on her infant's wrists, and then inserted an IV line in the infant's scalp. The head is thought to be the seat of life, and holes could allow the child's soul to escape. The strings are thought to "tie in the soul."

(99) Chinese Buddhist wanted to cancel major surgery because the hospital insisted she remove her "protection" bracelet. A compromise was

reached by putting it in a sterile specimen bag and placing it in the pocket of her gown.

(100) Culturally competent nurse prevented nursing assistant from removing a sacred string from Hindu patient's wrist.

Spiritual Beliefs and Practices

(101) Filipina woman was upset when the nurse did not respond for several days to her request for a chaplain to bless her daughter who was ill with sepsis and possibly dying.

(102) African American woman complied only with procedures and medications she believed were ordered by God.

(103) Hispanic woman stopped taking her diabetes medication because a curandera *told her that God had cured her; however, her symptoms had returned. Culturally competent physician suggested that God might have taken away her diabetes for a while, but had now brought her to the doctor to treat it with medication. He encouraged her to pray and she agreed to take her medication.*

(104) Culturally competent nurse allowed Mexican family to pray together in private before patient had a colonoscopy.

(105) Culturally competent nurse, observing that a fearful Hispanic patient was wearing a cross, calmed her down by encouraging her family to pray with her.

(106) Family of Hmong teenage girl with appendicitis refused to allow her to have surgery for fear that cutting her open would risk having an evil spirit enter her body. Her appendix burst and she became septic and died.

(107) Navajo boy was upset when nurse took his photograph because he believed it would steal his soul.

(108) Mien man refused to have his blood drawn for diabetes test for fear that it would sap his strength and could result in soul loss.

(109) Culturally sensitive nurse took the time to explain to a Cambodian patient the need to draw blood, in case she held traditional beliefs regarding blood loss.

Chapter 5. Activities of Daily Living and the Body

Eating

(110) Culturally sensitive nurse realized it was Ramadan, and apologized to Egyptian Muslim patient with diabetes for eating in front of her. This opened up communication and led to improved health for patient.

(111) Nurses were annoyed at Filipina patient's apparent noncompliance regarding eating and taking medications. Culturally competent nurse learned that the patient was Muslim and following the customs of Ramadan.

(112) A variety of Orthodox Jewish patients refused foods that violated kosher dietary laws.

(113) Hindu man in the emergency waiting room angrily refused the hamburger a nurse had gotten for him because cows are considered sacred and not eaten.

(114) Pakistani woman hospitalized with tuberculosis refused many of the foods served to her because they violated rules of "hot" and "cold."

(115) Chinese patient with lung cancer ate only the foods his family brought because, unlike hospital meals, they were consistent with yin/yang *(cold/hot) principles. Staff accommodated him.*

(116) Mexican woman with diabetes and kidney failure ate only the foods that fit her notion of hot/cold body balance, many of which were bad for her. Nurses handled the situation with cultural competence by emphasizing that she eat large amounts of the "cold" foods lower in dangerous minerals and smaller amounts of those high in them. They also adjusted her dialysis.

(117) Staff was concerned about a Korean woman with congestive heart failure who had not been eating. When the nurse interviewed her, she learned it was because the food was bland and unappealing and she did not like to eat in bed, preferring to eat with her family. Culturally competent nurse made accommodations so she would eat.

(118) Vietnamese refugee receiving palliative care for cancer would not use dietician's recommended liquid dietary supplement because it was in a taste pleasing to the American palate but not hers. Home health nurse found a substitute more suitable to the Asian palate. (See also case #269 involving the same patient.)

(119) Saudi Arabian patients on dialysis refused to stop eating potassium-rich dates. They believed that Allah determined whether or not they lived or died, that what they ate was irrelevant.

(120) While discharging a Filipino patient on Coumadin, a blood thinner, a culturally competent nurse realized that she needed to consider their typical ethnic diet when educating patients about what foods to avoid with certain medications.

Bathing and Toileting

(121) Homeless patient would not bathe because he believed dirt would protect him from illness.

(122) Filipino patient refused to use a bedpan because he did not want to "dirty" his bed and made a mess of the bathroom because he was used to backyard pit toilets, which are rinsed with a bucket of water.

(123) Anglo American woman teaching kindergarten in a Mexican neighborhood didn't realize that students were likely throwing toilet paper on the floor instead of the toilet because they assumed the plumbing couldn't handle it.

(124) Arab man would not change colostomy bag, probably because it required two hands and many Arabs follow the culture practice of using the left hand to clean oneself after defecating; the right hand is used for eating out of communal bowls.

Hair and Body

(125) Native American woman took her grandchild out of hospital against medical advice after a nurse cut the child's hair to attach IV lines, believing cutting the child's hair would cause her to become sick or die. After the child was readmitted, she brought in a medicine bundle to protect her; the nurses didn't want to allow it, but finally relented.

(126) Nigerian patient was upset because his knee surgery left scars that were too small. How would others know how much he had suffered and thus offered to Allah?

(127) Overweight Anglo nurse was humiliated when her Panamanian boyfriend's family kept telling her how fat she was. They were delighted; it meant she could have lots of babies.

Chapter 6. Family

Decision-Making

(128) Latina woman with diabetes would not agree to take insulin without first consulting with her family.

(129) Twenty-two-year-old Mexican patient refused to sign consent for a kidney biopsy, saying his older brother must make that decision in the absence of his father, who was in Mexico.

Role of the Family

(130) Although the eldest male is often the family spokesperson in Hispanic families, in this case, the youngest daughter was responsible for making medical decisions for her mother. Once the staff realized this, things went much more smoothly.

(131) Young African American boy with uncontrolled asthma kept returning to the clinic until the physician involved the boy's grandmother in his care.

(132) Staff members were confused when two women both claimed to be the mother of a little girl who had almost drowned. They were lesbians.

(133) Nurse handled the 20–30 emotional family members of Hispanic patient with cultural competence by involving them in the patient's care and bending the visiting rules.

(134) Culturally competent labor and delivery nurse found that having family members assist with patient care is often successful when dealing with large numbers of visitors.

(135) Culturally competent nurse handled the problem of large numbers of Mexican family members by asking the patient's eldest son to be in charge of the room and to decide which two family members could be in the room at which time.

(136) Anglo American student, injured while in Spain, was attended constantly by friends, who couldn't believe she would want to be left alone.

(137) Sephardic woman (the author) was hurt that only seven relatives accompanied her to the hospital to have a 12-minute outpatient breast biopsy.

(138) Nurse discovered that the Hispanic patient who came to express her complaints was much less angry and more relaxed when treated with cultural competence.

(139) Japanese stroke patient in rehab refused to perform self-care when his family was present because it was their duty to obey and care for him.

(140) Mexican burn patient's wife continued to feed him, even after being told not to, because that is how love and concern are demonstrated.

(141) "Tough" Sephardic man with leg amputation subsequent to diabetes insisted his daughter (the author) feed him the watermelon she brought for him. She realized this was a more passive way for him to remain in charge.

(142) Culturally competent nurse recognized that a Muslim family were being so demanding because this was their way of showing they loved and cared for their family member. Once she arranged for them to have a private room so they could pray together and for the patient to have food that was halal *under Muslim law, they were very grateful and much easier to deal with.*

(143) An Iranian man explained why Iranians can be so demanding of staff by telling the story of when his grandmother was in the hospital in Iran. His mother kept watch over her. One night she noticed that her mother wasn't getting oxygen; the man in charge of changing the oxygen tanks had fallen asleep. If she hadn't woken him up, her mother could have died.

(144) Large Sephardic family (the author's) were "easy" with the ICU nurses who took the time to show they cared about their ill family member as an individual, and "difficult" with those who did not.

(145) Culturally competent nurse spoke to Korean patient's adult son to find out if patient knew of his cancer diagnosis, rather than assume that he did.

(146) Pakistani family withheld news of their brother's death from their mother for fear that the news would kill her.

(147) Japanese patient with uncontrolled diabetes gave her nurse a beautiful beaded necklace she had made to thank her for taking the time to show her how to check her glucose level. When the nurse refused due to hospital policy, the patient was clearly hurt. The nurse then remembered the importance of reciprocity in Japanese culture and suggested that she fill out a "gratitude card" instead. Both were pleased with the cultural compromise.

Chapter 7. Men and Women

Sex Roles

(148) Pediatric nurse tried to get Middle Eastern father involved in the care of his young daughter, newly diagnosed with type 1 diabetes, but he would not consider it; it was a job for a woman. When the nurse involved the girl's grandmother, all went well.

(149) Mexican mother would not sign consent for her ill infant to have a spinal tap in the emergency department, preferring to wait for her husband to make the decision.

(150) Female resident who couldn't get Hispanic mother to sign consent for child's procedure called on older male physician to speak to child's mother. He got her to agree.

(151) Indian woman would not agree to an epidural, even though she wanted one, because her husband would not allow it. Culturally competent nurse respected the authority structure in the family and spoke with husband; he soon decided she should have the epidural.

(152) Husband of an Indian patient refused to accept discharge instructions from any of the female nurses, only from the male physician.

(153) Iranian couple whose child had Wilms's tumor (a childhood cancer) became very uncooperative when assigned a female oncologist because they couldn't accept a woman making life-and-death decisions for their son.

(154) Father of a twenty-seven-year-old Saudi Arabian woman refused to allow her to sign consent for a possible hysterectomy prior to surgery because if she couldn't have children she wouldn't marry and would thus be a burden to her family.

(155) The husband of an Iranian woman who had just given birth would allow no one in the room, answered questions put to her, and told her when to eat and bathe.

(156) Physician was frustrated by a middle-aged Armenian woman who always deferred to her husband or son when asked a question. She eventually reached a compromise by first addressing questions to the husband and son and then asking the patient if there was anything she wanted to add.

Female Purity

(157) Husband of Iranian woman with serious heart problems refused to allow a male physician to examine her, thus delaying treatment and endangering her life.

(158) Arab man refused to allow male lab technicians into the room to draw blood from his wife.

(159) Culturally competent nurse was able to build a trusting relationship with the family of a Lebanese woman by engaging her son in conversation and asking how she could support them in a culturally appropriate manner.

(160) When a twelve-year-old Somalian girl was admitted to the hospital with high fever, clinicians discovered she was infibulated (female genital mutilation).

(161) Nurse from Sierra Leone talked about the year of festivities leading up to female circumcision and arranged marriage, and said if she were still living there, she would have her daughter circumcised.

(162) Two Nigerian nurses shared their very different experiences of being circumcised. For one, it was extremely traumatic; the other had no memory of it and no problems resulting from it.

(163) Doctors at American Air Force Hospital in Saudi Arabia discovered that the teenage Bedouin girl brought in with a gunshot wound to her pelvis was also pregnant. Doctors planned to fly her to London for a secret abortion in order to save her life because unmarried pregnant girls were stoned to death in order to restore family honor. However, an internist new to the country decided he couldn't live with his conscience and told her father, who then grabbed her and drove off. Two weeks later, she was dead. Honor had been restored.

Female Modesty

(164) Salvadoran receptionist at an imaging center took care to make sure patients getting mammograms were not exposed, reflecting her own concern for the importance of modesty.

(165) Vietnamese patient was uncomfortable during EKG until culturally sensitive nurse made sure she was completely covered with a blanket.

(166) Mexican woman refused to be dialyzed when her usual station (which was private) was unavailable because she did not want to be

exposed. The problem could have been resolved by putting a screen around her station.

(167) Problems with a "difficult" Afghani patient ended when culturally competent charge nurse made sure she was covered with an extra gown and assigned only female nurses.

(168) A Muslim woman's placed a washcloth on her sister's head to maintain her modesty, since she didn't have a headscarf with her. The culturally competent nurse then told the family to bring in a headscarf and made sure it was in place at all times.

(169) A German woman was amused by the modesty displayed by American women. The first time she visited an American gynecologist, she didn't know what to do with the drapes and gown she was handed.

Domestic Violence

(170) Iranian woman in traditional garb presented with multiple suspicious injuries. Her husband, who accompanied her, refused to allow her to answer questions, instead answering for her. When a male physician's assistant entered the room, he took his wife away because a man had seen his wife without her *chador*.

(171) A young Mexican male beat his fifteen-year-old wife (while she was holding their five-month-old son) so badly that she suffered head injuries and required sutures to her face and mouth.

(172) Mexican woman, beaten by husband, begged emergency department nurse to tell police it was an accident.

Chapter 8. Staff Relations

Nursing: The Role of the Nurse

(173) Vietnamese nurse was reluctant to do aspects of the job she never had to do in Vietnam—including bathing patients and cleaning bedpans—causing the other nurses to think she was "stuck-up."

(174) Foreign-born nurse had difficulty advocating for patient with authoritarian Pakistani physician because she shared his notion of the authority of the physician.

(175) When Anglo American nurse questioned an East Indian physician's orders regarding a patient, he became very angry and upset.

(176) When Anglo nurse refused to follow a Japanese physician's orders regarding patient medication because she thought it would harm the patient, he complained to her supervisor that she should have agreed to do it, and then not followed through.

(177) Iraqi physician was upset when an Anglo nurse questioned his order to discharge their patient.

(178) The working relationship of an authoritarian Asian physician and an Anglo nurse improved when she applied cultural competence skills. Rather than just asking him to sign orders for medication (which he probably perceived as showing a lack of respect), she began to explain the situation with the patient, tell him what she was considering and then asked him what he would like done.

(179) Thai nurse was hesitant to question Korean physician when she didn't understand his orders. Her concern with respect for authority and with self-esteem conflicted with her job as a patient advocate.

(180) Filipino nurse was responsible for the bad outcome of a patient because she did not use critical thinking skills.

Cultural Influences on Nursing

(181) Nigerian male nurse assistant would not take orders from a female supervisor.

(182) Filipina nurse did not get along with her coworkers. They had very different perceptions of each other's behavior. She thought they were taking advantage of her when they asked her for help; they thought she was snobbish and proud because she never asked them for help. What she saw as laziness, they saw as being a team player.

(183) Korean charge nurse in intensive coronary care unit had difficulty doing what the job required—counseling and reprimanding staff—because it conflicted with her cultural upbringing to be passive and avoid conflict.

(184) Older Filipina nurse criticized a younger Americanized Filipina nurse for calling doctors by their first name and letting them know when she disagreed with their orders.

(185) Filipina nurse with county health department was hurt by the constructive criticism of her Anglo supervisor when she served as interpreter for an elderly Filipina tuberculosis patient who had been violating a county health order to stay in her home.

(186) Filipina aide was insulted when her Anglo supervisor offered to help her out once she had finished her own work, because in her culture such an offer implies the recipient is incompetent. Later, rather than complain directly to her supervisor, she went to her coworkers, who then went to the supervisor. The supervisor was upset by what she saw as "going behind her back"; the nurse, however, was using the Asian third party approach designed to avoid conflict and show respect for authority.

(187) American nurse was having difficulties with a Vietnamese nurse she was preceptoring. The Vietnamese nurse avoided making eye contact and didn't ask

questions. The American nurse eventually realized that this was her way of show-
ing respect. When the preceptor changed her style, all went well.

Medicine: The Role of the Doctor

(188) Anglo patient was angry when a paternalistic Middle Eastern physician would not give her enough information about her condition. In
response, he resigned from her case.

Language and Communication Problems

(189) Vietnam veteran, disoriented due to anesthesia, thought he was
in prison in a foreign country when he awoke in the recovery room to
hear two nurses speaking in Tagalog.

(190) Eastern Orthodox Russian nurse was uncomfortable refusing
food from Filipino nurses during the 40-day period before Easter. Many
Filipino delicacies have meat, which, according to her religion, she
could not eat. They thought she was either discriminating against them
or anorexic. When she finally admitted why she refused their offers of
food, it opened the way to more open communication between them.

(191) Medical anthropologist (the author) unknowingly offended a
nurse at a conference by referring to having to "play nurse" to care for
her husband who had had knee surgery. It demonstrated how easily an
innocent remark can damage a relationship.

(192) Chinese nurse's tone of voice did not convey the seriousness of a
patient's condition because she had been raised to control her
emotions.

(193) Japanese nurse felt that Nigerian co-workers were yelling at their
patients and being rude and trying to overpower her, not realizing that
a loud tone of voice was the norm in their culture.

(194) Asian nurses, in order to maintain self-esteem, said they knew
how to do certain procedures when, in fact, they did not.

(195) Two young Filipina nurses helped an older Filipina nurse to
"cheat" on a CEU exam, probably out of respect for elders and to avoid
conflict. Anglo American nurse, valuing independence, refused to do
so, seeing it as a matter of integrity; the Filipina nurses, valuing *inter*dependence, did not see it that way.

(196) Anglo nurse had a hostile relationship with her Korean coworker
because of the latter's general formality and the fact that she never said
"please" or "thank you." In hierarchical Korean culture, the respect
was implied and understood.

(197) New Korean nurses hired on a unit were perceived as rude because they
did not say "please" or "thank you." When nurse taking cultural competence
course explained the reason to the other nurses, morale was greatly improved.

(198) American physician, visiting in Japan, was cautioned not to use the phrase "with your permission" when speaking to an audience of faculty members because it was inappropriate for someone of his stature to ask for permission and would diminish the audience's ability to respect anything else he said.

Religious Conflicts

(199) Nurse who was a Jehovah's Witness refused to hang blood when temporarily transferred to the intensive care unit.
(200) Filipino Catholic nurse was not comfortable circulating on a therapeutic abortion.
(201) Jewish nurse could not take a new position he had applied for because the unit director refused to give him Saturdays off to observe the Sabbath.

Chapter 9. Birth

Antepartum

(202) Pregnant Anglo American nurse was warned not to raise her arms above her head because it could cause her child to be born with the cord wrapped around his neck. She ignored the advice, and it happened. Even though she knew there was no medical connection, the next time she became pregnant she was careful not to lift her arms above her head.
(203) Roma (Gypsy) family was overly concerned about a young woman's bleeding after a miscarriage, and wanted her to remain in the hospital as long as possible. As long as she was bleeding, she was considered "polluted."
(204) African American woman believed her son's birthmark in the shape of a drumstick was the result of an unfulfilled craving for fried chicken she had during her pregnancy.

Labor and Delivery

(205) Filipina woman labored in silence.
(206) African American woman labored loudly.
(207) Cherokee woman labored silently.
(208) Husband of a "difficult" (loud) Iranian patient gave her a 3-karat diamond ring following the birth of their son to compensate for the "suffering" she had endured in giving birth.

(209) Orthodox Jewish husband was uncomfortable attending his wife during labor because birth is thought to render women "unclean" and it is thus forbidden for men to touch them.

(210) Arab husband was uncomfortable attending his wife during labor, since he believed it was a woman's place to help in birthing.

(211) Mexican husband was uncomfortable attending his wife during labor; doing so was seen as inappropriate in Mexico.

(212) Mexican father was upset when nurse insisted he join his mother-in-law and sister-in-law in the delivery room.

(213) Elderly Mexican woman had a tattoo on her upper thigh that, due to her modesty, neither her husband nor her children had ever seen.

(214) Hmong woman, pregnant with twins, would not consent to a caesarean section during a difficult delivery, perhaps because of fear that souls can leave the body during surgery. After the second twin died, the husband requested the placentas, explaining that they had to be separated in order to protect the live infant from death.

(215) Small hospital contacted the author because several Somali women refused to have caesarean sections for a second delivery, despite high risk for vaginal delivery after having a caesarean section the first time.

Postpartum

(216) When staff heard older Muslim Arab women talking about a "burial," they thought they wanted to kill the infant girl who had just been born. It turned out they wanted to bury the baby's placenta.

(217) Mexican woman did not want to breastfeed colostrum, thinking it was "bad" milk and not good for the baby.

(218) Nurse showed cultural sensitivity in respecting Chinese American woman's traditional practices (staying warm and resting) while promoting necessary medical care.

(219) Mexican immigrant would not drink ice water, so her culturally sensitive nurse replaced it with warm water, and asked her about other changes she would like to see in her treatment.

(220) Vietnamese woman appeared not to bond with her infant. It is likely she was trying to avoid attracting attention to the newborn in order to protect it from spirits who might want to "steal" the child.

(221) Nurses were upset when woman from India refused to hold her newborn twins except to feed them, a practice consistent with Indian tradition.

(222) Hospital personnel were extremely concerned when a Hindu nurse from India did not name her baby immediately after birth. She

was waiting the traditional seven days, during which time she would consult an astrologer and allow her husband's sisters the honor of choosing the name.

(223) Chinese woman from Vietnam believed her granddaughter grew up to be healthy, talented, and intelligent because her son and daughter-in-law took the precaution of giving her an "ugly" name. She believed her other son had suffered serious illnesses and died as a military prisoner because of the devils' jealousy over his "intelligent" name.

(224) Middle Eastern couple with two other daughters and no sons rejected their newborn baby girl; they had been hoping for a boy to carry on the family name and wealth.

(225) Middle Eastern husband refused to participate in any patient education in baby care techniques; he saw that as the job of women.

Chapter 10. End of Life

Dying

(226) Son of elderly Japanese patient asked medical and nursing staff not to let his mother know she had cancer. When they asked her if she wanted to know her diagnosis and why she was receiving medication (chemotherapy), she said no. She signed a durable power of attorney for her son to make all health care decisions.

(227) Filipino man living in the Philippines was not told that he had end-stage cancer because his wife chose not to tell him. After radiation therapy, the radiologist told him he was "cancer free," even though he wasn't. At the time, his daughter, a nurse living in the U.S. was upset that they didn't tell him the truth, but later was grateful that her father was able to live the last six months of his life to the fullest, unburdened by the loss of hope.

(228) Latino man whose his family was trying to "protect" him from knowing he had advanced pancreatic cancer, wanted to know the truth, so he asked the nurse. But he didn't want his family to know that he knew because he thought it would cause them to suffer if they did.

(229) Family of dying Latino man would not leave his bedside for fear that one of the staff might tell their father he was dying and thus cause him to lose the will to live and strength to fight the disease. To abide by their wishes, their request was documented and all staff informed. The patient was told he was critical, but that they were taking it one day at a time and hoping for the best. The family was pleased.

(230) One Filipino family told their loved one she was dying; another Filipino family chose to withhold the information. Afterward, each felt they had made the right decision.

(231) Physician who believed all patients should be told their diagnosis, even against the wishes of the family, had patients fail to show up for appointments and sometimes never return.

(232) Family of Mexican patient wanted hospice care for their dying mother until they learned she would have to sign informed consent for hospice and would thus learn that she was dying. They wanted to "protect" her from this knowledge.

(233) Culturally sensitive physician allowed a curandera *to perform a ritual healing with a Hispanic patient.*

(234) Iranian son refused to sign Do Not Resuscitate (DNR) order for his dying mother, perhaps believing that only Allah can decide when someone will die.

(235) African American patient refused to sign an advance directive or DNR because he felt it would be seen by God as giving up or losing faith. He died ten days later, after enduring a great deal of suffering.

(236) Vietnamese man's family refused to remove life support until astrologers deemed the time auspicious for the fate of his descendants.

Death

(237) Middle Eastern family did not want to turn off life support for boy who had suffered a brain aneurism and was pronounced brain dead because they did not see him as "dead" as long as his heart kept beating. The physicians gradually weaned him off vasopressors so his heart would stop beating "naturally."

(238) Sephardic man (author's brother) died while on life support in a small hospital where no physicians were immediately available to pronounce him and remove life support. Seeing his chest rise and fall with each (ventilator) breath made it difficult for the family to believe he was really dead.

(239) Sephardic family left the room of a dying family member every hour, believing it is too hard for the dying to let go of life in the presence of loved ones.

(240) Relatives of a Roma (Gypsy) king suffering from pneumonia insisted on keeping a lit candle by his bed, despite the presence of an oxygen tent, so at death his soul would be guided to heaven.

(241) Family of a Roma (Gypsy) king insisted on moving him outside just before he died in order to help free his soul.

(242) Culturally sensitive nurse assisted in preparing the body of a Buddhist patient after his death.

(243) Culturally sensitive nurse had a positive experience helping the family of an elderly male Vietnamese patient who died from a chronic illness.

(244) Family of Arab Muslim began loud wailing when he died, despite the fact that it was 2 A.M. and they were disturbing the other patients. Physician handled the situation with cultural competence by having his body moved to the chapel where they could continue mourning without disturbing the other patients.

Numbers and Death

(245) Japanese woman became upset when she saw she was being wheeled into operating room "4" for surgery because the number represents "death."

(246) Chinese member of board of directors of a hospital serving the Chinese community was upset when put in room 444 due to the association of the number with death.

Chapter 11. Mental Health

Mental Illness

(247) Japanese woman was put in a mental hospital by husband for wanting to go to college, and was not released because her culturally appropriate behaviors were seen as signs of psychosis—she did not make eye contact, had numerous somatic complaints with no medical basis, and didn't talk in therapy sessions.

(248) Japanese woman tried to kill herself because of the shame she felt over her daughter's arrest for drug trafficking, and her shame at failing at her suicide attempt. Culturally competent nurse created a bond with her and helped the psychiatric treatment team to help her.

(249) Mentally ill Puerto Rican woman's culturally appropriate behaviors—emotional expressiveness, dependency, and lack of eye contact—confused her diagnosis.

(250) Filipina nurse's visions and symptoms following the sudden death of her aunt and uncle were seen as signs of a nervous breakdown by an Anglo colleague but as normal by a Filipina colleague.

(251) Vietnamese woman visited student health services for a variety of physical complaints, and later attempted suicide. The medical student who examined her missed her depression because as is common in her culture, she somaticized her feelings.

(252) Korean doctor treated the attempted suicide of a young Korean woman as an "accidental" overdose, rather than follow procedure for a suicide attempt in order to avoid the stigma of mental illness. The Filipino admitting nurse did not question this obvious misdiagnosis due to respect for the physician.

Stress and Mental Health

(253) Mexican woman admitted with chest pains would not talk about the fact that her husband had recently left her, even though that was the likely source of her pain, because she was uncomfortable discussing personal problems outside the family.

(254) Mexican woman was hospitalized with depression because her husband feared she would harm their young child. Her husband believed she was suffering from susto *and needed treatment from a* curandero. *After the physicians reluctantly agreed to allow a curandero to treat her with prayer, massage, and herbal teas, she became less depressed and more responsive to the therapy prescribed by the psychiatrists.*

(255) Chinese college student felt suicidal over the conflict between the culture of her restrictive parents and that of her American friends, who were given much more freedom. The problem was exacerbated because she had been raised not to talk to outsiders about her problems, but since her family was the problem, she felt she had no one to talk to.

Chapter 12. Traditional Medicine

Traditional or "Folk" Remedies

(256) School nurse reported the parents of a Vietnamese girl for child abuse when she discovered red welts on the girl's neck. She didn't realize they were made by coining in an attempt to help her feel better.

(257) Vietnamese physician had his mother do coining on his chest after over-the-counter and prescription medications did not help his headaches, body aches, and flu symptoms. He claimed the coining was effective.

(258) Culturally competent nurse helped colleague confirm that marks on Asian patient's back were due to coining, rather than elder abuse.

(259) A nurse found round red marks all over the upper back of an Armenian man when doing a physical assessment for a myocardial infarction in the critical care unit. They were made by cupping.

(260) Culturally competent nurse interviewed parents, rather than assume suspicious marks on Cambodian child's body were due to child abuse. In fact, they were due to cupping.

(261) Anglo American woman went to acupuncturist who successfully used cupping to treat a cough that antibiotics had failed to cure.

(262) Japanese patient ignored doctor's instructions for treating his high fever by bundling up and refusing cold liquids and an ice blanket. The nurse eventually respected his wishes.

(263) Mexican woman refused a rectal temperature and bundled up in blankets despite her high fever and the efforts of the nurses to remove them.

(264) Mexican mother wrapped her feverish infant in blankets despite the nurses' instructions to cool him down.

(265) African American grandmother became very upset and hostile when she saw her grandson put naked into a cool mist tent to reduce his fever. She wanted to give him hot chamomile tea instead.

Medications

(266) Home health nurse discovered that a Mexican woman was applying her oral medication as a poultice to the incision site of her caesarean section since that was how she was used to using medication.

(267) Mexican woman was angry because she got pregnant using birth control pills; she had inserted them into her vagina.

(268) Mexican woman became pregnant while using contraceptive foam; she and her husband applied it to his penis.

(269) Elderly Vietnamese woman did not get the physician's prescription filled for her lung condition because she didn't understand how to fill a prescription. (See also case #118 involving the same patient.)

(270) Hispanic woman gave her infant a potentially dangerous traditional remedy for diarrhea her neighbor obtained from Guatemala.

(271) Nurse discovered that her Italian mother-in-law who was going in for colon cancer surgery was taking 18 different herbal supplements, some of which could cause bleeding and would have to be discontinued several days before surgery.

(272) Iranian man with gastrointestinal bleeding did not tell his physician he was taking two aspirins a day when the physician asked him what medications he was taking. Since they were over-the-counter, he didn't think of them or the vitamins he took as "medications." The nurse acting as interpreter learned the information when talking to him about his health.

"Folk" Diseases

(273) Medical student observing pediatric visit noticed that the Mexican infant's mother changed demeanor when she complimented the child (thus giving the child the evil eye). The mother relaxed when the student touched the child.

(274) Culturally competent nurse asked mother the meaning of a blue eye amulet worn by an infant at her clinic. It was thought to protect the child from the evil eye.

Traditional Healers

(275) Parents of Nigerian boy suffering an acute sickle cell crisis believed it was due to the spirit of their dead child "haunting" their son. The father consulted with a Nigerian medicine man over the phone while the medical team worked on the boy and the family, who was Christian, prayed for him.

(276) Cherokee woman refused to sign consent for surgery until she saw a medicine man. Her grandson drove to the reservation and brought back the medicine man, who conducted a healing ceremony. She then signed consent for the surgery. (277) Dying inmate began eating and taking medication again once his culturally competent nurse called in a medicine man to do a ceremony and arranged for him to do a sweat lodge.

Traditional Medical Systems

(278) Korean man admitted for depression refused to take his medications. The problem was he had been given water or juice to take his pills, and this violated hot/cold principles. When they gave him hot tea, he took his medication.

(279) Mexican woman ate nopales *to treat her diabetes. Her nurse learned that she ate fewer tortillas when she had* nopales *(a non-starchy, high-fiber vegetable), so rather than challenge her interpretation, he congratulated her and encouraged her to eat* nopales *and other non-starchy vegetables.*

(280) Mexican immigrant recovering from caesarean section was upset because staff would not allow her to give her infant *manzanilla* (chamomile tea) to treat his colic.

(281) Mexican man hospitalized with a stomach problem was upset because the nurse would not allow him to drink the *manzanilla* tea he believed would help.

(282) Mexican American teenage mother's infant would not stop crying. Her older sister, who had grown up in Mexico, successfully treated the infant for the Mexican folk disease, *empacho.*

(283) Angry Mexican mother accused home health nurse of giving her child the evil eye when she complimented her.

(284) Nurse spent time trying to convince Mexican patient that Bell's palsy could not have been caused by *susto.* She later realized this was the wrong approach and instead she should have conceded that the shock the patient had suffered (the *susto*) had weakened her immunity and made her more susceptible to the illness.

(285) Mexican patient felt belittled when physician told her there was no such thing as *susto* and it could not have caused her to become ill.

(286) Culturally competent nurse reassured parents of injured Mexican baby that he would not suffer from susto, but they could take the infant to see a curandero if that would make them feel better.

(287) African American woman refused an angiogram for acute chest pain, believing that she was being punished by God for a past sin, and He would cure her if her faith were strong enough. (An elaboration of case #5.) Culturally competent solution is suggested.

(288) Older African American woman presented with nausea and vomiting six years after diagnosis of high blood pressure. Thinking she had "high blood," she treated it with vinegar rather than prescribed medication. The vinegar caused the symptoms.

Chapter 13. Improving Adherence

Insufficient Instruction or Explanation

(289) Elderly patient (author's mother) was shown how to change a leg dressing by nurse who neglected to have the patient demonstrate her understanding. As a result, the patient had no idea how to do it.

Unclear Rationale

(290) Anglo American woman going in for uterine ultrasound followed the lab's instructions to drink several glasses of water before coming in, but because they didn't explain the reason, the water only replaced the fluids she had lost at the gym prior to coming in. If they had explained the reason, she would have gone to the gym *after* the ultrasound.

(291) African American man with congestive heart failure took his medication only when he was short of breath, rather than every day as prescribed. Physician should have explained why it had to be taken daily, even in the absence of symptoms.

Conflict with Cultural Beliefs or Practices

(292) Afghani Muslim man with stomach cancer refused chemotherapy because, unknown to the physician, the pump that would provide a continuous infusion—more convenient for most people—would cause him to be "unclean" and thus unable to pray. If he had been asked *why* he didn't want the pump, he could have explained and the physician could have offered an alternative to the pump.

(293) Latino man had problems doing intermittent cathertization because it didn't fit in with his lifestyle. He should have been offered the option of a leg bag.

Lack of Trust

(294) Vietnamese woman wasn't taking her diabetes medication because she believed that, like all Western medicine, it was "too hot" (yang). Culturally competent physician came up with a solution—take it with a yin (cold) tea.
(295) Elderly African American man was afraid to have surgery because he didn't trust the white hospital due to historical discrimination against African Americans, such as the Tuskegee Experiment.

Chapter 14. Making a Difference

Diet

(296) Nurse who interviewed Afghani Muslim patients learned that they usually order vegetarian meals to avoid food that has been contaminated by pork. She consulted with the director of food services and as a result, the hospital's poor vegetarian menu was greatly improved and a nutritionist is now on call to help family members provide a balanced menu should they want to bring in meals from home.

Respecting Cultural and Religious Beliefs and Practices

(297) Nurse proposed additional questions be added to the hospital's medical history questionnaire so the information could help them provide more culturally appropriate care.
(298) Nurse who discovered that many Filipino patients believed that covering their head could prevent heat loss leading to illness, contacted the volunteer services manager, who got volunteers to knit colorful caps for patients to wear if they choose.
(299) Nurse helped Catholic family by moving them to a larger room and purchasing small religious icons so they could pray for their family member; she suggested permanently turning a small quiet room near the emergency department into a makeshift chapel.
(300) Nurse got hospital to change policies to allow more visitors in the critical care cnit, including overnight visitors, and to allow family members to assist with nontechnical care. As a result, the hospital was able to reduce costs and increase patient satisfaction.

Bibliography

Ahmed, S. M., and J. P. Lemkau. (2000) Cultural issues in the primary care of South Asians. *Journal of Immigrant Health* 2 (2) (April): 89–96.

Ailinger, R., and M. Causey. (1995) Health concepts of older Hispanic immigrants. *Western Journal of Nursing Research* 17 (6): 605–13.

Al-Shahri, M, Z. (2002) Culturally sensitive caring for Saudi patients. *Journal of Transcultural Nursing* 13 (2) (April): 133–38.

Allan, B. (2009). Why Hispanics may be less comfortable with hospice. *Hispanic Marketing & Public Relations*, April 8. Accessed May 6, 2013, http://www.hispanicmpr.com/resources/articles/why-hispanics-may-be-less-comfortable-with-hospice/.

Alvord, L. A., and E. C. Van Pelt. (2000) *The Scalpel and the Silver Bear: The First Navajo Woman Surgeon Combines Western Medicine and Traditional Healing.* New York: Bantam Dell Doubleday.

American Cancer Society (2013) The Patient Self-Determination Act (PSDA). http://www.cancer.org/treatment/findingandpayingfortreatment/understandingfinancialandlegalmatters/advancedirectives/advance-directives-patient-self-determination-act.

American College of Cardiology Foundation. (2002) Racial/Ethnic Differences in Cardiac Care: The Weight of the Evidence. Henry Kaiser Foundation, Summary Report, September 29.

American Nurses Association. (1998) *Culturally Competent Assessment for Family Violence.* Washington, D.C.: American Nurses Association.

Anderson, R. (1996) *Magic, Science, and Health.* New York: Harcourt Brace.

Andrews, M. M., and J. S. Boyle. (2007) *Transcultural Concepts in Nursing Care.* 5th ed. Philadelphia: Lippincott Williams & Wilkins.

Arthur, D., H. K. Chan, et al. (1999) Therapeutic communication strategies used by Hong Kong mental health nurses with their Chinese clients. *Journal of Psychiatric and Mental Health Nursing* 6 (1) (February): 29–36.

Asakitikpi, A. E. (2008) Born to die: The Ogbanje phenomenon and its implication on childhood mortality in southern Nigeria. *Anthropologist* 10 (1): 59–63.

Athar, S. (1999) Information for health care providers when dealing with a Muslim patient. Islamic Medical Association of North America. www.islam-usa.com/e40.html.

Bacardi-Gascon, M. (2007) Lowering effect on postprandial glycemic response of nopales added to Mexican breakfasts. *Diabetes Care* 30 (5) (May): 1264–65. CCINAHL AN: 2009583074.

Baer, R. D., J. Garcia de Alba, et al. (1998) Mexican use of lead in the treatment of empacho: Community, clinic, and longitudinal patterns. *Social Science and Medicine* 47 (9) (November): 1263–66.

Barrett, B., K. Shadick, et al. (1998) Hmong/medicine interactions: Improving cross-cultural health care. *Family Medicine* 30 (3) (March): 179–84.

Barry, D. T., and M. G. Carlos. (2002) Cultural, psychological, and demographic correlates of willingness to use psychological services among East Asian immigrants. *Journal of Nervous and Mental Disease* 190 (1): 32–39.

Battaglia, B. (1996) Understanding Hispanic folk ailments and illnesses. *Cross Cultural Connection* 2 (2) (October–December): 1–2, 4.

———. (1997a) Cultural views on death and dying, part 1. *Cross Cultural Connection* 3 (1) (July–September): 1–2.

———. (1997b) Cultural views on death and dying, part 2. *Cross Cultural Connection* 3 (2) (October–December): 1–3.

———. (1998) Cultural views on death and dying, part 3. *Cross Cultural Connection* 3 (3) (January–March): 1–4.

Becerra, R. M., and A. P. Iglehart. (1995) Folk medicine use: Diverse populations in a metropolitan area. *Social Work in Health Care* 21 (4): 37–58.

Bechtel G. A., R. Davidhizar, and C. M. Tiller. (1998) Patterns of mental health care among Mexican Americans. *Journal of Psychosocial Nursing and Mental Health Services* 36 (11): 20–27.

Beck, S. E., and E. K. Goldberg. (1996) Jewish beliefs, values, and practices: Implications for culturally sensitive nursing care. *Advanced Practice Nursing Quarterly* 2 (2) (Fall): 15–22.

Bent, S. and R. Ko. (2004) Commonly used herbal medicines in the United States: A review. *American Journal of Medicine* 116 (7): 478–85.

Betancourt, J. R., and O. Ananeh-Firempong II. (2004) Not me! Doctors, decisions, and disparities in health. *Cardiovascular Review Report* 25 (3): 105–9.

Betancourt, J. R., J. E. Carrillo, and A. R. Green. (1999) Hypertension in multicultural and minority populations: Linking communication to compliance. *Current Hypertension Reports* 1: 482–88.

Betancourt, J. R., A. R. Green, and J. E. Carrillo. (2002) *Cultural Competence in Health Care: Emerging Frameworks and Practical Approaches.* New York: Commonwealth Fund.

Bhungalia, S., and C. Kemp. (2002) (Asian) Indian health beliefs and practices related to the end-of-life. *Journal of Hospice and Palliative Nursing* 4 (1) (January): 54–58.

Blackhall, L. (2013) Do patients need to know they are terminally ill? No. *BMJ* 346: 2560.

Blackhall, L. J., G. Frank, et al. (1999) Ethnicity and attitudes towards life sustaining technology. *Social Science and Medicine* 48 (12): 1779–89.

Blackhall, L. J., S. T. Murphy, G. Frank, V. Michel, and S. Azen. (1995) Ethnicity and attitudes toward patient autonomy. *JAMA* 274 (10): 820–25.

Bodenheimer, T., K. MacGregor, and C. Sharifi (2005) Helping patients manage their chronic conditions. California HealthCare Foundation, June.

Bodo, K., and N. Gibson. (1999) Childbirth customs in Vietnamese traditions. *Canadian Family Physician* 45 (March): 690–92, 695–97.

Bonura, D., M. Fender, M. Roesler, and D. F. Pacquiao. (2001) Culturally congruent end-of-life care for Jewish patients and their families. *Journal of Transcultural Nursing* 12 (3) (July): 211–20.

Braun, K. L., and R. Nichols. (1997) Death and dying in four Asian American cultures: A descriptive study. *Death Studies* 21 (4) (July/August): 327–59.

Braun, K. L., J. H. Pietsch, et al., eds. (1999) *Cultural Issues in End-of-Life Decision Making.* Thousand Oaks, Calif.: Sage.

Brink, S. (1988) Doctoring Gypsies. *Boston Magazine* 7: 80–86.

Bronner, Y. (1994) Cultural sensitivity and nutrition counseling. *Topics in Clinical Nutrition* 9 (2) (March): 13–19.

Brooks, G. (1995) *Nine Parts of Desire: The Hidden World of Islamic Women*. New York: Anchor Books.

Brown, P. L. (2009) A doctor for disease, a shaman for the soul. *New York Times*, September 20.

Browner, C. et al. (2003) Genetic counseling gone awry: Miscommunication between prenatal genetic service providers and Mexican-origin clients. *Social Science & Medicine* 56: 1933–46.

Bui, H. N., and M. Morash. (1999) Domestic violence in the Vietnamese immigrant community: An exploratory study. *Violence Against Women* 5 (7) (July): 769–95.

Bukaty, R. F. (2004) Revealing hospital gowns redesigned. *USA Today*, August 17.

Burrs, F. A. (1995) The African American experience: Breaking the barriers to hospices. *Hospice Journal* 10 (2): 15–18.

Burstyn, L. (1995) Female circumcision comes to America. *Atlantic Monthly* (October): 28–35.

Callister, L. C. (1995) Cultural meanings of childbirth. *Journal of Obstetric, Gynecologic, and Neonatal Nursing* 24 (3): 327–31.

Callister, L. C., K. Vehvilainen-Julkunen, and S. Lauri. (1996) Cultural perceptions of childbirth: A cross-cultural comparison of childbearing women. *Journal of Holistic Nursing* 14 (1): 66–78.

Campbell, J. C., and D. W. Campbell. (1996) Cultural competence in the care of abused women. *Journal of Nurse Midwifery* 41 (6) (November–December): 457–62.

Campinha-Bacote, J. (1992) Voodoo illness. *Perspectives in Psychiatric Care* 28 (1) (January–March): 11–17.

———. (1994) *The Process of Cultural Competence in Health Care: A Culturally Competent Model of Care*. 2nd ed. Wyoming, Ohio: Transcultural C.A.R.E. Associates.

———. (1997) *Readings and Resources in Transcultural Health Care and Mental Health*. Cincinnati: Transcultural C.A.R.E. Associates.

———. (1998) *The Process of Competence in the Delivery of Healthcare Services: A Culturally Competent Model of Care*. Cincinnati: Transcultural C.A.R.E. Associates.

———. (1999) A model and instrument for addressing cultural competence in health care. *Journal of Nursing Education* 38 (5): 203–7.

Carrese, J. A., and L. A. Rhodes. (2000) Bridging the cultural differences in medical practice: The case of discussing negative information with Navajo patients. *Journal of Internal Medicine* 15: 92–96.

Caswell, J. (2012a). Why not comply. Excerpted from *Stroke Connection Magazine*, May/June, 2004 for American Heart Association-Stroke Association, October.

———. (2012b) Why not comply part II. Excerpted from *Stroke Connection Magazine*, July/August 2004 for American Heart Association-Stroke Association, October.

Centers for Disease Control and Prevention. (1993) Lead poisoning associated with use of traditional ethnic remedies. *California: Morbidity and Mortality Weekly Report* 42: 521–54.

———. (1999) Guidelines for prevention of surgical site infection. http://www.cdc.gov/hicpac/SSI/004_SSI.html.

Cerrato, P. L. (1996) Customize diets with culture in mind. *Office Nurse* 9 (4) (April): 22–23, 26.

Chang, C. (2013) New mothers turn to an old Chinese diet. *Los Angeles Times*, January 14.

Chaudry, M. M. (1992) Islamic food laws: Philosophical basis and practical implications. *Food Technology* 46 (10) (October): 92.

Chen, Y. (2001) Chinese values, health and nursing. *Journal of Advanced Nursing* 36 (2) (October): 270–73.

Cheng, B. K. (1997) Cultural clash between providers of majority culture and patients of Chinese culture. *Journal of Long-Term Home Health Care* 16: 39–43.

Chrisman, N. (1991) Culture-sensitive nursing care. In M. Patrick, S. Woods, R. Craven, J. Rokosky, and P. Bruno, eds., *Medical-Surgical Nursing: Pathophysiological Concepts.* 2nd ed., 34–46. New York: Lippincott.

Chrisman, N. J., and P. A. Zimmer. (2000) Cultural competence in primary care. In P. V. Meredith and N. M. Horan, eds., *Adult Primary Care,* 65–75. Philadelphia: W.B. Saunders.

Collis, E., and K. E. Sleeman (2013) Do patients need to know they are terminally ill? Yes. *BMJ* 346: 2589.

Counihan, C., and S. Kaplan, eds. (1997) *Food and Culture.* New York: Routledge.

Cramer, J. A. (2004) A systematic review of adherence with medications for diabetes. *Diabetes Care* 27 (5): 1218–24.

Crawley, L., P. Marshall, and B. Koeing. (2002) Strategies for culturally effective end-of-life care. *Annals of Internal Medicine* 136 (9) (Supplement, May 7): 673–79.

Crawley, L., R. Payne, et al. (2000) Palliative and end-of-life care in the African American community. *Journal of the American Medical Association* (284): 2518–21.

Cross-Cultural Medicine. (1983) Special Issue. *WJM* 139 (6) (December).

Cross-Cultural Medicine—A Decade Later. (1992) Special Issue. *WJM* 157 (3) (September).

Crowe, K., L. Matheson, and A. Steed. (2000) Informed consent and truth-telling: Cultural directions for healthcare providers. *Journal of Nursing Administration* 30 (3) (March): 148–52.

Cuellar, I., and F. A. Paniagua, eds. (2000) *Handbook of Multicultural Mental Health.* San Diego: Academic Press.

Culhane-Pera, K. A., D. E. Vawter, et al., eds. (2003) *Healing by Heart: Clinical and Ethical Case Stories of Hmong Families and Western Providers.* Nashville, Tenn.: Vanderbilt University Press.

Culture in Medicine. (2001) Special Issue. *Academic Medicine* 76 (5) (May).

Danielson, B. L., A. J. LaPree, et al. (1998) Attitudes and beliefs concerning organ donation among Native Americans in the upper Midwest. *Nursing* 8 (3) (September): 153–56.

Dasgupta, S. D. (1998) Gender roles and cultural continuity in the Asian Indian immigrant community in the U.S. *Sex Roles: A Journal of Research* 38 (11): 953–75.

Davidhizar, R. and J. N. Giger. (2004) A review of the literature on care of clients in pain who are culturally diverse. *International Nursing Review* 51 (1): 47–55.

Davidson, M. N., and P. Devney. (1991) Attitudinal barriers to organ donation among Black Americans. *Transplantation Proceedings* 23: 2531–32.

Davis, R. E. (2000) Cultural health care or child abuse? The Southeast Asian practice of cao gio. *Journal of the American Academy of Nurse Practitioners* 12 (3) (March): 89–95.

Davis, R. E. (2001) The postpartum experience for Southeast Asian women in the United States. *MCN Maternal and Child Nursing* 26 (4) (July–August): 208–13.

DePacheco, M., and M. Hutti. (1998) Cultural beliefs and health care practices of childbearing Puerto Rican American women and Mexican American women: A review of the literature. *Mother Baby Journal* 3 (1) (January): 14–25.

Devi, S. (2012). U.S. guidelines for domestic violence screening spark debate. *The Lancet* 379 (9815): 506.

Dinh, A., C. Kemp, and L. Rasbridge. (2000) Culture and the end of life: Vietnamese health beliefs and practices related to the end of life. *Journal of Hospice and Palliative Nursing* 2 (3) (July–September): 111–17.

Dresser, N. (1996) *Multicultural Manners*. New York: Wiley.

Dupree, C. Y. (2000) The attitudes of Black Americans toward advance directives. *Journal of Transcultural Nursing* 11 (1) (January): 12–18.

Engebretson, J. (1994) Folk healing and biomedicine: Culture clash or complementary approach? *Journal of Holistic Nursing* 12 (3) (September): 240–50.

Erickson, C. D., and N. R. Al-Timimi. (2001) Providing mental health services to Arab Americans: Recommendations and considerations. *Cultural Diversity and Ethnic Minority Psychology* 7 (4) (November): 308–27.

Evanikoff del Puerto, L. and E. Sigal (2005), Russians. In J. G. Lipson and S. L. Dibble, eds., *Culture & Clinical Care*, 415–30. San Francisco: UCSF Nursing Press.

Fadiman, A. (1997) *The Spirit Catches You and You Fall Down: A Hmong Child, Her American Doctors, and the Collision of Two Cultures*. New York: Farrar, Straus, and Giroux.

Fernea, E. W., and R. A. Fernea. (1989) A look behind the veil. In E. Angeloni, ed., *Annual Editions: Anthropology 89/90*, 149–53. Guilford, CT: Dushkin.

Fetters, M. D. (1998) The family in medical decision making: Japanese perspectives. *Journal of Clinical Ethics* 9 (2): 132–46.

Fink, L. (2007) Culture, language, and equitable care: Clinician perspectives on caring for diverse patient populations. Accessed June 3, 2013, http://www.quantiamd.com/q-qcp/QuantiaMD_Culture_Language_Care_study.pdf.

Flaskerud, J. H. (2000) Ethnicity, culture, and neuropsychiatry. *Issues in Mental Health Nursing* 21 (1) (January–February): 5–29.

Flores, G. (2000) Culture and the patient-physician relationship: Achieving cultural competency in health care. *Journal of Pediatrics* 136 (1) (January): 14–23.

Flores, G., M. Abreu, I. Schwartz, and M. Hill. (2000) The importance of language and culture in pediatric care: Case studies from the Latino community. *Journal of Pediatrics* 137 (6): 842–48.

Gabler, M., S. E. Stern, et al. (1998) Latin American, Asian, and American cultural differences in perceptions of spousal abuse. *Psychological Reports* 83 (2) (October): 587–92.

Galanti, G. (2000a) An introduction to cultural differences. *WJM* 172 (5): 335–36.

———. (2000b) Commentary: American health care professionals should respect the traditions of other cultures. *WJM* 173 (5): 356.

———. (2000c) Iranian births. *WJM* 173 (1) (July): 67–68.

———. (2000d) Vietnamese family relationships. *WJM* 172 (6): 415–16.

———. (2000e) Filipino attitudes toward pain medication. *WJM* 173 (October): 278–79.

———. (2001a) Japanese Americans and self-care. *WJM* 174 (3): 208–9.

———. (2001b) The challenge of serving and working with diverse populations in American hospitals. *Diversity Factor* 9 (3): 21–26.

———. (2003) The Hispanic family and male-female relationships: An overview. *Journal of Transcultural Nursing* 14 (3): 180–85.

————. (2005) Culturally competent rehabilitation nursing. *Rehabilitation Nursing* 30 (4):123–126.

————. (2006a) *65 Tips for Foreign-Born Nurses Working in American Hospitals.* Oakland, Calif.: Support for Nurses.

————. (2006b) Applying cultural competence to perianesthesia nursing. *Journal of PeriAnesthesia Nursing* 21 (2): 97–102.

————. (2007) *Orienting Foreign-Born Nurses to Work Effectively in American Hospitals: A Training Manual for Health Educators.* Oakland, Calif.: Support for Nurses.

————. (2012) *Cultural Sensitivity: A Pocket Guide for Health Care Professionals,* 2nd ed. Oakbrook Terrace, Ill.: Joint Commission Resources.

Galanti, G., and A. Sheikh. (2009) How to provide culturally competent healthcare. *(E)Hospital* 11 (4): 22–24.

Gallagher, C. (1996) Religious attitudes regarding organ donation. *Journal of Transplant Coordination* 6 (4) (December): 186–90.

Gardenswartz, L., and A. Rowe (1998) *Managing Diversity in Health Care.* San Francisco: Jossey-Bass.

Gatrad, A. R. (1994) Muslim customs surrounding death, bereavement, post-mortem examinations, and organ transplants. *BMJ* 309 (August 20): 521–23.

Gaw, A. C. (2001) *Concise Guide to Cross-Cultural Psychiatry.* Washington, D.C.: American Psychiatric Publishing.

Gehi, A. K. et al. (2007) Self-reported medication adherence and cardiovascular events in patients with stable coronary heart disease. *Archives of Internal Medicine* 167 (16): 1798–1803.

Gelfand, D. E., H. Balcazar, et al. (2001) Mexicans and care for the terminally ill: Family, hospice and the church. *American Journal of Hospice and Palliative Care* 18 (6) (November–December): 391–96.

Getzel, G. S. (1995) Judaism and death: Practice implications. In J. K. Parry and A. S. Ryan, eds., *A Cross-Cultural Look at Death, Dying, and Religion*, 18–31. Chicago: Nelson-Hall.

Giger, J. N., and R. E. Davidhizar, eds. (2007) *Transcultural Nursing: Assessment and Intervention.* 5th ed. St. Louis: C.V. Mosby.

Gillman, J. (1999) Religious perspectives on organ donation. *Critical Care Nursing Quarterly* 2 (3) (November): 19–29.

Goode, T. D., M. C. Dunne, and S. M. Bronheim. (2006) *The Evidence Base for Cultural and Linguistic Competency in Health Care.* New York: Commonwealth Fund.

Gordon, S. M. (1994) Hispanic cultural health beliefs and folk remedies. *Journal of Holistic Nursing* 12 (3) (September): 307–22.

Graves D. L., R. C. Like, N. Kelly, and A. Hohensee. (2007) Legislation as intervention: An examination of cultural competence policy in health care. *Journal of Health Care Law and Policy* 10 (2).

Green, J. (1992a) Death with dignity: Christianity. *Nursing Times* 88 (3): 26–29.

————. (1992b) Death with dignity: Christian Science. *Nursing Times* 88 (4): 32–33.

————. (1992c) Death with dignity: Jehovah's Witnesses. *Nursing Times* 88 (5): 36–37.

————. (1992d) Death with dignity: The Afro-Caribbean community. *Nursing Times* 88 (8): 50–51.

Gross, J. (2007) Keeping patients' details private, even from kin. *New York Times,* July 3.

Haber, D. (1999) Minority access to hospice. *American Journal of Hospice and Palliative Care* 16 (1) (January–February): 386–89.

Haddad, L. G., and S. P. Hoeman. (2000) Home healthcare and the Arab-American client. *Home Healthcare Nurse* 18 (3) (March): 189–97.

Haffner, L. (1992) Translation is not enough: Interpreting in a medical setting. *WJM* 157 (3): 255–59.

Hafizi, H. (2005) Iranians. In J. G. Lipson and S. L. Dibble, eds., *Culture and Clinical Care*, 246–76. San Francisco: UCSF Nursing Press.

Hahn, R. A. (1995) *Sickness and Healing: An Anthropological Perspective.* New Haven, Conn.: Yale University Press.

Hall, E. T., and M. R. Hall. (1990) *Understanding Cultural Differences: Germans, French and Americans.* Yarmouth, Minn.: Intercultural Press.

Hammerschlag, C. A. (1988) *The Dancing Healers: A Doctor's Journey of Healing with Native Americans.* San Francisco: Harper and Row.

Hampton, R. L., and R. J. Gelles. (1994) Violence toward Black women in a nationally representative sample of Black families. *Journal of Comparative Family Studies* 25 (1) (Spring): 105–19.

Han, Y., R. D. Williams, et al. (1999) Breast self examination (BSE) among Korean American women: Knowledge, attitudes, and behaviors. *Journal of Cultural Diversity* 6 (4) (Winter): 115–23.

Hansen, K. K. (1998) Folk remedies and child abuse: A review with emphasis on *caída de mollera* and its relationship to shaken baby syndrome. *Child Abuse and Neglect* 22 (2) (February): 117–27.

Harris, M. (1974) *Cows, Pigs, Wars, and Witches: The Riddles of Culture.* New York: Vintage.

Hashwani, S. S. (2005) Pakistanis. in J. G. Lipson and S. L. Dibble, eds., *Culture and Clinical Care*, 360–74. San Francisco: UCSF Nursing Press.

Hasnain-Wynia, R., D. W. Baker, et al. (2007) Disparities in health care are driven by where minority patients seek care. *Archives of Internal Medicine* 167 (12): 1233–39.

Health Resources and Services Administration. (2001) *Cultural Competence Works: Using Cultural Competence to Improve the Quality of Care for Diverse Populations and Add Value to Managed Care Arrangements.* Merrifield, Va..: HRSA Information Center.

Healy, M. 2013. Physicians debate whether patients need to know they're dying. *Los Angeles Times*, April 25.

Helfgot, M. (2011). Hospitals take cultural sensitivity seriously. *Chicago Tribune*, July 27.

Helman, C. G. (2007) *Culture, Health and Illness: An Introduction for Health Professionals.* 5th ed. Boston: Butterworth-Heinemann.

Hern, J. H. E., B. A. Koenig, et al. (1998) The difference that culture can make in end-of-life decision making. *Cambridge Quarterly of Healthcare Ethics* 7 (1) (Winter): 27–40.

Higgins, B. (2000) Puerto Rican cultural beliefs: Influence on infant feeding practices in western New York. *Journal of Transcultural Nursing* 11 (1) (January): 19–30.

Ho, M., C. L. Bryson, and J. S. Rumsfelt (2009) Medication adherence: Its importance in cardiovascular outcomes. *Circulation* 119: 3028–35.

Holden W., J. Joseph, and L. Williamson. (2005) Use of herbal remedies and potential drug interactions in rheumatology outpatients. *Annals of the Rheumatic Diseases* 64: 790.

Horne, S. (1999) Domestic violence in Russia. *American Psychologist* 54 (1) (January): 55–61.

Hsieh, E. (2006) Conflicts in how interpreters manage their roles in provider—patient interactions. *Social Science & Medicine* 62:721–730.

Huff, R. M., and M. V. Kline. (1999) Tips for working with Hispanic populations. In R. M. Huff and M. V. Kline, eds., *Promoting Health in Multicultural Populations: A Handbook for Practitioners*, 189–97. Thousand Oaks, Calif.: Sage.

Hughes, C. C. (1998) The glossary of culture-bound syndromes in DSM-IV: A critique. *Transcultural Psychiatry* 35 (3) (September): 413–21.

Hung, P. (2001) Traditional Chinese customs and practices for the postnatal care of Chinese mothers. *Complementary Therapies in Nursing and Midwifery* 7 (4) (November): 202–6.

Hunt, L. M., N. H. Arar, and L. L. Akana. (2000) Herbs, prayer, and insulin: Use of medical and alternative treatments by a group of Mexican-American diabetes patients. *Journal of Family Practice* 49: 216–23.

Irish, D. P., K. F. Lundquist, and V. J. Nelsen, eds. (1993) *Ethnic Variations in Dying, Death, and Grief*. Washington, D.C.: Taylor and Francis.

Jehovah's Witnesses—Position Overview. *Penn Medicine*, accessed May 22, 2013. http://www.pennmedicine.org/health_info/bloodless/000206.html.

Jenkins, C. N. H., T. Le, et al. (1996) Health care access and preventive care among Vietnamese immigrants: Do traditional beliefs and practices pose barriers? *Social Science and Medicine* 43 (7) (October): 1049–56.

Johnson, S. K. (2002) Hmong health beliefs and experiences in the Western health care system. *Journal of Transcultural Nursing* 13 (2) (April): 126–32.

Johnson, S. K. and A.L. Hang. (2005) Hmong. In J. G. Lipson and S. L. Dibble, eds., *Culture and Clinical Care*, 250–63. San Francisco: UCSF Nursing Press.

Juarez, G., B. Ferrell, et al. (1998) Influence of culture on cancer pain management in Hispanic patients. *Cancer Practice* 6 (5) (September–October): 262–69.

Juckett, G. (2005) Cross-cultural medicine. *American Family Physician* 72 (11): 2267–74.

Kabat, G. (2012) *Natural does not mean safe*. Slate, November 26.

Kagawa-Singer, M. (1994) Diverse cultural beliefs and practices about death and dying in the elderly. *Gerontology and Geriatrics Education* 15 (1): 101–16.

Kagawa-Singer, M., and L. J. Blackhall. (2001) Negotiating cross-cultural issues at the end of life: "You've got to go where he lives." *JAMA* 286: 2993–3001.

Kagawa-Singer, M., I. M. Martinson, et al. (1998) Forum focus: A multicultural perspective on death and dying. *Oncology Nursing Forum* 25 (10) (November–December): 1751–63.

Kaiser Permanente National Diversity Council. (1999) *A Provider's Handbook on Culturally Competent Care: African American*. Oakland, Calif.: Kaiser Permanente National Diversity Council.

Kapp, M. B. (1993) Living and dying the Jewish way: Secular rights and religious duties. *Death Studies* 17: 267–76.

Kaptchuk, T. J. (1983) *The Web That Has No Weaver: Understanding Chinese Medicine*. New York: Congdon and Weed.

Katims, I. P. (1999) Buddhist ethics and implications for end-of-life issues. In L. Zhan, ed., *Asian Voices: Asian and Asian-American Health Educators Speak Out*, 106–16. Sudbury, Mass.: Jones and Bartlett.

Kaufert, J. M., and R. W. Putsch. (1997) Communication through interpreters in healthcare: Ethical dilemmas arising from differences in class, culture, language, and power. *Journal of Clinical Ethics* 8 (1) (Spring): 71–87.

Kelly, N. (2007) Telephone interpreting in health care settings: Some commonly asked questions. *ATA Chronicle* (June): 18–21.

Kemp, C. (1996) Islamic cultures: Health-care beliefs and practices. *American Journal of Health Behavior* 20 (3): 83–89.

———. (2001) Culture and the end of life: Hispanic cultures (focus on Mexican-Americans). *Journal of Hospice and Palliative Nursing* 3 (1) (January–March): 29–33.

Kennedy, J. G. (1967) Nubian Zar ceremonies as psychotherapy. *Human Organization* 26 (4): 185–94.

Keovilay, L., L. Rasbridge, et al. (2000) Cambodian and Laotian health beliefs and practices related to the end of life. *Journal of Hospice and Palliative Medicine* 2 (4): 143–51.

Kephart, W. M. (1989) The Gypsies. In E. Angeloni, ed., *Annual Editions: Anthropology 89/90*, 122–37. Guilford, Conn.: Dushkin.

Kim, B. S. K., P. H. Yang, et al. (2001) Cultural value similarities and differences among Asian American ethnic groups. *Cultural Diversity and Ethnic Minority Psychology* 7 (4) (November): 343–61.

Kleinman, A. (1980) *Patients and Healers in the Context of Culture*. Berkeley: University of California Press.

Kleinman, A., and P. Benson (2006) Anthropology in the clinic: The problem of cultural competency and how to fix it. *PLoS Medicine* 3 (10): e294.

Kleinman, A., L. Eisenberg, and B. Good. (1978) Culture, illness, and care: Clinical lessons from anthropologic and cross-cultural research. *Annals of Internal Medicine* 88: 251–58.

Klessig, J. (1992) The effect of values and culture on life-support decisions. *WJM* 157 (3): 316–22.

Kluckhohn, C. (1951). Values and value orientations in the theory of action. In T. Parsons and E. Shils, eds., *Toward a General Theory of Action*, 409–14. Cambridge, Mass.: Harvard University Press.

Kluckhohn, F. R. (1953) Dominant and variant value orientations. In P. Brink, ed., *Transcultural Nursing: A Book of Readings*, 63–81. Englewood Cliffs, N.J.: Prentice-Hall.

Koenig, B. (1995) Understanding cultural differences in caring for dying patients. *WJM* 163 (3): 244–49.

Korbin, J. E. (1995) Social networks and family violence in cross-cultural perspective. *Nebraska Symposium on Motivation* 42: 107–34.

Kramer, B. J. (1992) Health and aging of urban American Indians. *WJM* 157 (3): 281–85.

Kramer, J. (1996) American Indians, in J. G. Lipson, S. L. Dibble, and P. A. Minarik, eds., *Culture and Nursing Care: A Pocket Guide*, 11–22. San Francisco: UCSF Nursing Press.

Krane, J. E. (1996) Violence against women in intimate relations: Insights from cross-cultural analyses. *Transcultural Psychiatric Research Review* 33 (4): 435–65.

Kristof, N. D. (1991) Stark data on women: 100 million are missing. *New York Times*, November 5, Science section, C1, C12.

Kristy, S. (1998) Toward understanding Vietnamese attitudes, beliefs and practices regarding blood donation. *Social Sciences in Health: International Journal of Research and Practice* 4 (3) (August): 154–62.

Kuczewski, M., and P. J. McCruden (2001) Informed consent: Does it take a village? The problem of culture and truth telling. *Cambridge Quarterly of Healthcare Ethics* 10 (1) (Winter): 34–46.

Kulig, J.S. and S. Prak (2005) Cambodians (Khmer). In J. G. Lipson and S. L. Dibble, eds, *Culture & Clinical Care*, 63–84. San Francisco: UCSF Nursing Press.

Kung, W. W. (2001) Consideration of cultural factors in working with Chinese American families with a mentally ill patient. *Families in Society* 82 (1): 97–107.

Kuo, C., K. H. Kavanagh, et al. (1994) Chinese perspectives on culture and mental health. *Issues in Mental Health Nursing* 15 (6) (November–December): 551–67.

LaFraniere, S. (2007) Nouakchott journal: In Mauritania, seeking to end an overfed ideal. *NYTimes.com*, July 4 (in World section, Africa).

Lanier, S. A. (2000) *Foreign to Familiar.* Hagerstown, Md.: McDougal.

Lapine, A., R. Wang-Cheng, M. Goldstein, et al. (2001) When cultures clash: Physician, patient and family wishes in truth disclosure for dying patients. *Journal of Palliative Medicine* 4 (4): 475–80.

Lawrence, P., and C. Rosmus. (2001) Culturally sensitive care of the Muslim patient. *Journal of Transcultural Nursing* 12 (3): 228–33.

Lecca, P. J., I. Quervalu, J. V. Nunes, and H. F. Gonzales. (1998) *Cultural Competency in Health, Social, and Human Services: Directions for the Twenty-First Century.* New York: Garland.

Lee, S., J. Sobal, et al. (1999) Acculturation and dietary practices among Korean Americans. *Journal of the American Dietetic Association* 99 (9) (September): 1084–89.

Leininger, M., and M. R. McFarland. (2002) *Transcultural Nursing: Concepts, Theories, Research and Practice.* 3rd ed. New York: McGraw-Hill.

Levin, S. J., Like, R. C. and J. E. Gottlieb. (2000) ETHNIC: A framework for culturally competent clinical practice; Appendix: Useful clinical interviewing mnemonics. *Patient Care* 34 (9): 188–89.

Lightfoot-Klein, H. (1990) *Prisoners of Ritual: An Odyssey into Female Genital Circumcision in Africa.* Binghamton, N.Y.: Haworth Press.

Like, R. C. (1999) Culturally competent managed health care: A family physician's perspective. *Journal of Transcultural Nursing* 10 (4) (October): 288–89.

Lillie-Blanton, M., O. E. Rushing, and R. S. Boone. (2002) *Racial/Ethnic Differences in Cardiac Care: The Weight of the Evidence.* Menlo Park, Calif.: Henry J. Kaiser Family Foundation and American College of Cardiology Foundation.

Lin, K., and F. Cheung. (1999) Mental health issues for Asian Americans. *Psychiatric Services* 50 (6) (June): 774–80.

Lipson, J. G., and S. L. Dibble, eds. (2005) *Culture and Clinical Care.* San Francisco: UCSF Nursing Press.

Lipson, J. G., and A. I. Meleis. (1983) Issues in health care of Middle Eastern patients. *WJM* 139: 854–61.

Locks, S., and L. Boateng. (1996) Black/African Americans. In J. G. Lipson, S. L. Dibble, and P. A. Minarik, eds., *Culture and Nursing Care: A Pocket Guide*, 37–43. San Francisco: UCSF Nursing Press.

Longo, B. (1990) Traditional Southeast Asian medical techniques: What nurses should know. *Nurseweek* (February 5).

Loue, S., and M. Faust. (1999) Intimate partner violence among immigrants. In S. Loue, ed., *Handbook of Immigrant Health*, 521–44. New York: Plenum Press.

Loustanau, M., and E. J. Sobo. (1997) *The Cultural Context of Health, Illness, and Medicine.* Westport, Conn.: Bergin and Garvey.

Lu, H., While, A. E. and K. L. Barriball. (2008) Role perceptions and reported actual role content of hospital nurses in mainland China. *Journal of Clinical Nursing* 17 (8): 1011–22.

Manmohan, T., et al. (2012) Drug compliance and adherence to treatment. *Journal of Evolution of Medical and Dental Sciences* 1 (3): 142–59.

Martinelli, A. M. (1987) Pain and ethnicity. *AORN Journal* 46 (2): 273–81.

Mattson, S. (1995) Culturally sensitive perinatal care for Southeast Asians. *Journal of Obstetric, Gynecologic, and Neonatal Nursing* 24 (4) (May): 335–41.

Mattson, S., and E. Rodriguez. (1999) Battering in pregnant Latinas. *Issues in Mental Health Nursing* 20 (4) (July–August): 405–22.

McCullough-Zander K., ed. (2000) *Caring Across Cultures: The Provider's Guide to Cross-Cultural Health.* 2nd ed. Minneapolis: Center for Cross-Cultural Health.

McGoldrick, M., J. Giordano, and J. K. Pearce, eds. (2005) *Ethnicity and Family Therapy.* 3rd ed. New York: Guilford.

McKennis, A. T. (1999) Caring for the Islamic patient. *AORN Journal* 69 (6) (June): 1187–96, 1199–206.

Meleis, A. I. (2005) Arabs. In J. G. Lipson and S. L. Dibble, eds., *Culture and Clinical Care*, 42–57. San Francisco: UCSF Nursing Press.

Messer, E. (1981) Hot-cold classification: Theoretical and practical implications of a Mexican study. *Social Science and Medicine* 15: 133–45.

Mouton, C. (2000) Cultural and religious issues for African Americans. In K. Braun, J. H. Pietsch, and P. Blanchette, eds., *Cultural Issues in End-of-Life Decision Making*, 71–82. Thousand Oaks, Calif.: Sage.

Muecke, M. A. (1983a) Caring for Southeast Asian refugee patients in the USA. *American Journal of Public Health* 73, 4 (1983): 431–38.

———. (1983b) In search of healers: Southeast Asian refugees in the American health care system. *WJM* 129: 835–40.

Mukherjee, S. (2010) *The Emperor of All Maladies.* New York: Scribner.

Mull, D. S., P. F. Agran, et al. (1999) Household poisoning exposure among children of Mexican-born mothers: An ethnographic study. *WJM* 171 (1) (July): 16–19.

Mull, J. D., D. S. Mull, and N. Nguyen. (2001) Vietnamese diabetic patients and their physicians: What ethnography can teach us. *WJM* 175 (November): 307–11.

Mutha, S., C. Allen, and M. Welch. (2002) *Toward Culturally Competent Care: A Toolbox for Teaching Communication Strategies.* San Francisco: Regents of the University of California.

Nakamura, R. M. (1998) *Health in America: A Multicultural Perspective.* Boston: Allyn and Bacon.

Narruhn, R. A. (2008) Perinatal profile for patients from Somalia. *Ethnomed,* December 1. Accessed May 3, 2013, http://ethnomed.org/clinical/pedia trics/perinatal-profile-for-pat ients-from-so malia.

National Cancer Institute. (2008) Fact sheet on cancer health disparities. Accessed March 15, 2014, http://www.cancer.gov/cancertopics/factsheet/cancer-health-disparities.

———. (2013) Questions and answers about PC-SPES. Accessed June 18, 2013, http://www.cancer.gov/cancertopics/pdq/cam/pc-spes/Patient/Page2#Section_7.

National Conference of State Legislatures. (2013) Disparities in health. April. Accessed May 14, 2013, http://www.ncsl.org/issues-research/health/health -disparities-ove rview.aspx.

Neff, N. (n.d.) Folk medicine in Hispanics in the Southwestern United States. Accessed August 13, 2007, http://www.rice.edu/projects/HispanicHealth/Courses/mod7/mod7.htm l.

Nesse, R. M. and G. C. Williams (1994) *Why We Get Sick.* New York: Vintage.

Nobles, A. Y., and D. T. Sciarra. (2000) Cultural determinants in the treatment of Arab Americans: A primer for mainstream therapists. *American Journal of Orthopsychiatry* 70 (2) (April): 182–91.

Nzewi, E. (2001) Malevolent ogbanje: Recurrent reincarnation or sickle cell disease? *Social Science and Medicine* 52 (9): 1403–16.

Office of Minority Health. (2001) *National Standards for Culturally and Linguistically Appropriate Services in Health Care: Final Report.* Washington, D.C.: U.S. Department of Health and Human Services.

Ohnuki-Tierney, E. (1984) *Illness and Culture in Contemporary Japan.* New York: Cambridge University Press.

Olavarrieta, C. D., and J. Sotelo. (1996) Domestic violence in Mexico. *JAMA* 275 (24): 1937–41.

Orr, R. D. (1996) Treating patients from other cultures. *American Family Physician* 53 (6) (May): 2004–6.

Osterberg, L., and T. Blaschke. (2005) Adherence to medication. *New England Journal of Medicine* 353: 487–97.

Pacquiao, D. F., L. Archeval, et al. (2000) Hispanic client satisfaction with home health care: A study of cultural context of care. In M. L. Kelley and V. M. Fitzsimons, eds., *Understanding Cultural Diversity: Culture, Curriculum, and Community in Nursing,* 229–40. Sudbury, Mass.: Jones and Bartlett.

Palacios, J. L., R. Butterfly, and C. J. Strickland (2005) American Indians/Alaskan Natives. In J. G. Lipson and S. L. Dibble, eds., *Culture and Clinical Care,* 27–41. San Francisco: UCSF Nursing Press.

Pang, K. Y. (1998) Symptoms of depression in elderly Korean immigrants: Narration and the healing process. *Culture, Medicine, and Psychiatry* 22 (1) (March): 93–122.

Pang, M. C. (1999) Protective truthfulness: The Chinese way of safeguarding patients in informed treatment decisions. *Journal of Medical Ethics* 25 (3) (June): 247–53.

Payer, L. (1996) *Medicine and Culture: Varieties of Treatment in the United States, England, West Germany, and France.* New York: Holt.

Peir, F. L. 2011. In Queens, new mothers and old Asian custom. *New York Times,* June 3.

Perkins, H. S., C. M. Geppert, A. Gonzales, et al. (2002) Cross-cultural similarities and differences in attitudes about advance care planning. *Journal of Internal Medicine* 17 (1) (January): 48–57.

Pike, O. A. (1992) The Church of Jesus Christ of Latter-Day Saints: Dietary practices and health. *Food Technology* 46 (10) (October):118–21.

Pourat, N., J. Lubben, et al. (2000) Perceptions of health and use of ambulatory care: Differences between Korean and White elderly. *Journal of Aging and Health* 12 (1) (February): 112–34.

Price-Wise, G. (2008) Language, culture, and medical tragedy: The case of Willie Ramirez. Healthaffairs.org, November 19. Accessed May 17, 2013, http://healthaffairs.org/blog/2008/11/19/language-culture-and-med ical-tragedy-the-case-of-willie-ramirez/.

Puchalski, C. M. et al. Religion, spirituality, and end of life care. Accessed July 31, 2013, http://www.uptodate.com/contents/religion-spirituality-and-end-of-life-care.

Purnell, L. (1999) Panamanians' practices for health promotion and the meaning of respect afforded them by health care providers. *Journal of Transcultural Nursing* 10 (4) (October): 331–39.

Purnell, L., and B. Paulanka, eds. (2003) *Transcultural Health Care: A Culturally Competent Approach.* 2nd ed. Philadelphia: Davis.

Rajwani, R. J. (1996) South Asians. In J. G. Lipson, S. L. Dibble, and P. A. Minarik, eds., *Culture and Nursing Care: A Pocket Guide,* 264–79. San Francisco: UCSF Nursing Press.

Redfield, R. (1947) The folk society. *American Journal of Sociology* 52(4):293–308.

Reichman, D. E. and J. A. Greenberg. (2009) Reducing surgical site infections: A review. *Review of Obstetric Gynecology* 2 (4): 212–21.

Reizian, A., and A. I. Meleis. (1986) Arab-Americans' perceptions of and responses to pain. *Critical Care Nurse* 6 (6): 30–37.

Rhee, S. (1997) Domestic violence in the Korean immigrant family. *Journal of Sociology and Social Welfare* 24 (1) (March): 63–77.

Rivera-Andino, J., and L. Lopez. (2000) When culture complicates care. *RN* 63 (7) (July): 47–49.

Rodriguez, E. (1999) The heart of the matter: Worldview as a central concept in effective cross-cultural work. *Journal of the California Alliance for the Mentally Ill* 10 (1): 5–7.

Ross, H. M. (1998) Best practice: Jewish tradition in death and dying. *MedSurg Nursing* 7 (5) (October): 275–80.

Rotblatt, M. and I. Ziment. (2002) *Evidenced-Based Herbal Medicine.* Philadelphia: Hanley and Belfus.

Salimbene, S. (2000) *What Language Does Your Patient Hurt in?*™ *A Practical Guide to Culturally Competent Patient Care.* Amherst, Mass.: Diversity Resources.

Sarhill, N., S. LeGrand, R. Islambouli, et al. (2001) The terminally ill Muslim: Death and dying from the Muslim perspective. *American Journal of Hospice and Palliative Care* 18 (4) (July–August): 251–55.

SenGupta, I. (2010) Medical interpreting: A new era in professionalism. Seattle: Cross Cultural Health Care Program.

Shaw, E. (1985) Female circumcision. *American Journal of Nursing* 85 (6): 684–87.

Sheikh, A., and A. R. Gatrad, eds. (2000) *Caring for Muslim Patients.* Oxford: Radcliffe Medical Press.

Simpson, E., J. D. Mull, E. Longley, and J. East. (2000) Pica during pregnancy in low-income women born in Mexico. *WJM* 173: 20–24.

Smedley B. D., A. Y. Stith, and A. R. Nelson, eds. (2003). *Unequal Treatment: Confronting Racial and Ethnic Disparities in Health Care.* Washington, D.C.: National Academy Press.

Snow, L. F. (1977) Popular medicine in a Black neighborhood. In E. H. Spicer, ed., *Ethnic Medicine in the Southwest.* Tucson: University of Arizona Press.

———. (1983) Traditional health beliefs and practices among lower class Black Americans. *WJM* 139: 820–28.

———. (1993) *Walkin' over Medicine: Traditional Health Practices in African-American Life.* Boulder, Colo.: Westview.

Sobo, E. J. and M. O. Loustaunau (2010) *The Cultural Context of Health, Illness, and Medicine,* 2nd ed. Santa Barbara, CA: Praeger.

Sokol, M. C. et al. (2005) Impact of medication adherence on hospitalization risk and healthcare cost. *Medical Care* 43 (6): 521–30.

Spector, R. E. (2003) *Cultural Diversity in Health and Illness.* 6th ed. Upper Saddle River, N.J.: Prentice-Hall.

Starr, B. and R. Sacks. (2012) Improving outcomes for patients with chronic disease: The medication adherence project (MAP). A project of the Cardio-vascular Prevention & Control Program and the Fund for Public Health in

New York. Accessed March 19, 2013, http://www.nyc.gov/html/doh/down loads/pdf/cardio/cardio-map-tools -manual.pdf.

Stein, H. F. (1990) *American Medicine as Culture*. Boulder, Colo.: Westview.

Stolley, J. M., and J. Koenig. (1997) Religion/spirituality and health among elderly African Americans and Hispanics. *Journal of Psychosocial Nursing and Mental Health Services* 35 (11) (November): 32–38, 45–46.

Sue, S. (1998) In search of cultural competence in psychotherapy. *American Psychologist* 53: 440–48.

Sutherland, A. (1992) Gypsies and health care. *WJM* 157 (3): 276–80.

Takayama, J. I. (2001) Giving and receiving gifts: One perspective. *WJM* 175: 138–39.

Talamantes, M. A., W. R. Lawler, et al. (1995) Hispanic American elders: Caregiving norms surrounding dying and the use of hospice services. *Hospice Journal* 10 (2): 35–49.

Thiederman, S. (1991) *Bridging Cultural Barriers for Corporate Success*. Lexington, Mass.: Lexington Books.

Think Cultural Health General/CLAS Standards. Think Cultural Health, Office of Minority Health, U.S. Department of Health and Human Services. Accessed June 3, 2013, https://www.thinkculturalhealth.hhs.gov/Content/clas.asp.

Thomas, S. B., and S. C. Quinn. (1991) The Tuskegee syphilis study, 1932 to 1972: Implications for HIV education and AIDS risk education programs in the Black community. *American Journal of Public Health* 81 (11): 1498–505.

Torrecillas, L. (1997) Communication of the cancer diagnosis to Mexican patients: Attitudes of physicians and patients. *Annals of the New York Academy of Sciences* 809 (February): 188–96.

Torrey, E. F. (1986) *Witchdoctors and Psychiatrists: The Common Roots of Psychotherapy and Its Future*. New York: Harper and Row.

Trotter, R. T. (1997) *Curanderismo: Mexican American Folk Healing*. Athens: University of Georgia Press.

Tsai, J. H. (1999) Meaning of filial piety in the Chinese parent-child relationship: Implications for culturally competent health care. *Journal of Cultural Diversity* 6 (1): 26–34.

Turnbull, C. (1962) *The Forest People*. New York: Touchstone.

Vawter, D. E., and B. Babbitt. (1997) Hospice care for terminally ill Hmong patients: A good cultural fit? *Minnesota Medicine* 80 (11) (November): 42–44.

Vinciguerra, T. (2007). A bundle of joy isn't enough? *New York Times*, December 6.

Warda, M. R. (2000) Mexican Americans' perceptions of culturally competent care. *Western Journal of Nursing Research* 22 (2) (March): 203–24.

Waters, C. M. (2000) End-of-life care directives among African-Americans: Lessons learned: A need for community-centered discussion and education. *Journal of Community Health Nursing* 17 (1): 25–37.

Waters, C. M., and S. Locks (2005) African Americans. In J. G. Lipson and S. L. Dibble, eds., *Culture and Clinical Care*, 14–26. San Francisco: UCSF Nursing Press.

Weldon, M. M., M. S. Smolinski, et al. (2000) Mercury poisoning associated with a Mexican beauty cream. *WJM* 173 (1) (July): 15–18.

World Health Organization. (2003). Adherence to long-term therapies: Evidence for action. WHO, Essential Medicines and Health Products Information Portal.

Worlds Apart: Mohammad Kochi's Story (2005). Video by Fanlight Productions, accessed March 12, 2013, http://www.fanlight.com/catalog/films/912_wa.php.

Worsley, B. (n.d.) Noncompliance: A problem for patients and doctors. SCPIE Companies. Accessed March 12, 2013, http://www.scpcf.com/PDF/MLM-Noncompliance.pdf.

Wynia, M and J. Matiasek. (2006) Promising practices for patient-centered communication with vulnerable populations: Examples from eight hospitals. Commonwealth Fund 947, August.

Yeatman, G. W. (1980) *Cao gio* (coin rubbing): Vietnamese attitudes toward health care. *JAMA* 244: 2748–49.

Zachariah, R. (2005) East Indians. In J. G. Lipson and S .L. Dibble, eds., *Culture and Clinical Care*, 146–62. San Francisco: UCSF Nursing Press.

Zborowski, M. (1952) Cultural components in response to pain. *Journal of Social Issues* 8: 16–30.

Zevin, I. V., N. Altman, and L. V. Zevin. (1997) *A Russian Herbal: Traditional Remedies For Health and Healing*. Rochester, Vt.: Healing Arts Press.

Zimring, S. D. (2001) Multi-cultural issues in advance directives. *Journal of the American Medical Directors Association* 2 (5) (September–October): 241–45.

Zola, I. K. (1966) Culture and symptoms: An analysis of patients' presenting complaints. *American Sociological Review* 31: 615–30.

Zoucha, R. (1998) Understanding the significance of culture in emergency care and treatment. *Topics in Emergency Medicine* 20 (4) (December): 40–51.

Note: For further resources, including websites and films, see www.ggalanti.org.

WJM articles are available through PubMed at http://www.pubmedcentral.nih.gov/tocrender.fcgi?journal = 183&act ion = archive.

Index